Practical Clinical Microbiology and Infectious Diseases

Practical Clinical Microbiology and Infectious Diseases

A Hands-On Guide

Edited by
Firza Alexander Gronthoud, MD, DTM&H
Consultant Microbiologist
The Royal Marsden NHS Foundation Trust
United Kingdom

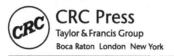

CRC Press
Taylor & Francis Group
Boca Raton London New York

CRC Press is an imprint of the
Taylor & Francis Group, an **informa** business

First edition published 2021
by CRC Press
6000 Broken Sound Parkway NW, Suite 300, Boca Raton, FL 33487-2742

and by CRC Press
2 Park Square, Milton Park, Abingdon, Oxon, OX14 4RN

Library of Congress Cataloging-in-Publication Data

Names: Gronthoud, Firza Alexander, editor.
Title: Practical clinical microbiology and infectious diseases : a hands-on guide / [edited by] Dr. Firza Alexander Gronthoud.
Description: First edition. | Boca Raton : CRC Press, 2020. | Includes bibliographical references and index. | Summary: "This book offers practical tips and essential guidance for the clinical microbiologist and healthcare professional to put theoretical knowledge into daily practice. This handbook is intended to support the healthcare professional from interpretation of laboratory results, to consultation and infection control"-- Provided by publisher.
Identifiers: LCCN 2020010640 (print) | LCCN 2020010641 (ebook) | ISBN 9781138721753 (hardback) | ISBN 9781138721715 (paperback) | ISBN 9781315194080 (ebook)
Subjects: MESH: Bacterial Infections | Mycoses | Virus Diseases | Microbiological Phenomena | Handbook
Classification: LCC RA644.B32 (print) | LCC RA644.B32 (ebook) | NLM WC 39 | DDC 614.5/7--dc23
LC record available at https://lccn.loc.gov/2020010640
LC ebook record available at https://lccn.loc.gov/2020010641

ISBN: 9781138721753 (hbk)
ISBN: 9781138721715 (pbk)
ISBN: 9781315194080 (ebk)

Typeset in Times LT Std
by Nova Techset Private Limited, Bengaluru & Chennai, India

Contents

SECTION I   Principles of Infection Management

SECTION II   Diagnosis of Infections

SECTION III   *Treatment of Infections*

SECTION IV Special Problems

SECTION V Difficult-to-Treat Organisms

SECTION VI Appendix

Preface

There are already many valuable medical textbooks available covering various aspects of clinical microbiology and infectious diseases. Although important fundamental concepts such as epidemiology, pathogenesis and clinical manifestations are being taught, reading these textbooks might not necessarily prepare the medical professional on how to deal with frequent issues that arise during the various stages of infection management, with common examples being interpreting and acting on laboratory results and adverse events related to antibiotic use such as drug toxicities and allergies, as well as preventing infections from difficult-to-treat organisms.

This book addresses this issue by drawing on the real-life clinical experiences of its authors, targeting those healthcare professionals working in the field of infection management, such as doctors training in clinical microbiology and infectious diseases or those who already have obtained their specialty degree or any medical professional interested in the management of infection.

The aim of this handbook is to concisely offer practical guidance on how to translate theoretical apply theory into clinical practice, as well as to provide guidance on how to deal with day-to-day scenarios and clinical problems encountered when managing infections.

Learning the tricks of the trade from experienced infection specialists supports the specialty trainee (and any medical professional interested in infection) to develop confidence and competence in dealing with common but sometimes challenging and complex clinical scenarios and ultimately improving patient safety and experience.

We hope that this handbook is a useful source and quick access reference.

Firza Alexander Gronthoud, MD, DTM&H

Acknowledgements

I dedicate this book to my parents and my sister. Everything I have achieved in life would not have been possible without their unconditional love, support and guidance. They have always been there for me during my entire personal and professional life. They taught me humbleness, discipline, manners, respect, compassion and kindness and so much more which has been instrumental in all my successes in life. I am truly blessed and eternal grateful to them.

I want to show my gratitude to the contributors of this book without whom this work could not have been completed: Dr. Anda Samson, Dr. Patrick Lillie, Dr. Caryn Rosmarin, Dr. Simon Tiberi, Dr. Marina Basarab, Dr. Julian Anthony Rycroft, Dr. Jennifer Tomlins and Dr. Devan Vaghela.

I want to express my special thanks to Dr. Riina Richardson and Professor Malcolm Richardson who have been mentors to me and provided invaluable guidance and counsel throughout my career in the UK and supported my transition from a newly qualified Dutch consultant to an NHS healthcare professional.

Finally, I would like to thank all my wonderful colleagues with whom I've had the honour and privilege of working with and who helped shape my career and contributed to my personal and professional growth: Dr. Lodewijk Spanjaard, Dr. Ruud van Ketel, Dr. Wies Langenberg, Dr. Caroline Visser, Dr. Caspar Hodiamont, Dr. Tom van Gool, Professor Menno de Jong, Professor Constance Schultsz, Professor Hans Zaaijer, Dr. Janke Schinkel, Dr. Katja Wolther, Dr. Wieke Freudenburg, Dr. Sacha de Graaf, Dr. Lia Kusumawati, Dr. Franciscus Ginting, Dr. Adhi Sugianli, Dr. Inke Nadia Lubis, Dr. Ayodhia Pitaloka Pasaribu, Dr. Ida Parwati Dr. Mari Cullen, Dr. Stephanie Thomas, Dr. Ibrahim Hassan, Dr. Sajad Mirza, Professor David Denning, Dr. Chris Kosmidis, Dr. Pippa Newton, Dr. Eavan Muldoon, Dr. Paschalis Vergidi, Dr. Caroline Moore, Dr. Sarah Glover, Dr. Graeme Jones, Dr. Tat S. Yam, Dr. Julian Sutton, Dr. Gillian Urwin, Dr. Sima Jalili, Dr. Tony Elston, Dr. Vasile Laza-Stanca, Dr. Dimitrios Mermerelis, Dr. Rella Workman, Dr. Anne Hall, Dr. Silke Schelenz, Dr. Darius Armstrong-James, Professor Michael Loebinger, Penny Agent, Dr. Unell Riley, Dr. Jackie Kenney, Dr. Angela George, Sue Alexander and Pat Cattini.

Editor

Firza Alexander Gronthoud, MD, DTM&H, obtained his primary medical degree in 2009 at Maastricht University (the Netherlands). He completed his specialty training in 2015 in medical microbiology and virology at the Amsterdam Medical Centre. During this period, he spent one year in Medan, Indonesia, as part of an international research collaboration between the Netherlands and Indonesia. In 2015, he moved to the United Kingdom to take up his first consultant post at Manchester University Hospital NHS Foundation Trust. In 2017, he completed the diploma course in tropical medicine and hygiene at the London School of Hygiene and Tropical Medicine. Dr. Gronthoud currently works as a consultant microbiologist at the Royal Marsden Hospital NHS Foundation Trust and is pursuing an MSc in clinical microbiology and infectious diseases at Edinburgh University (Scotland).

Contributors

Marina Basarab, MRCP, MFPH, FRCPath
Consultant in Infection
St. George's University Hospitals NHS
  Foundation Trust
London, United Kingdom

Patrick Lillie, MBChB, FRCP, DTM&H, PhD
Consultant in Infectious Diseases
Hull University Teaching Hospital
  NHS Trust
Kingston upon Hull, United Kingdom

Caryn Rosmarin, MBBCh, DTM&H, FRCPath
Consultant Microbiologist
Barts Health NHS Trust
London, United Kingdom

Julian Anthony Rycroft, PhD, MRCP, MB ChB(Hons), BSc(Hons)
Specialty Registrar in Infectious Diseases and
  General Internal Medicine
Royal London Hospital
Barts Health NHS Trust
London, United Kingdom

Annette Danielle (Anda) Samson, MD
Consultant in Internal Medicine and
  Infectious Diseases
Hull University Teaching Hospital NHS Trust
Kingston upon Hull, United Kingdom

Simon Tiberi, MD, FRCP
Infectious Diseases Consultant
Royal London Hospital
Barts Health NHS Trust
Honorary Clinical Reader
Blizard Institute
Queen Mary University of London
London, United Kingdom

Jennifer Tomlins MBBS, DTM&H, MRCP, MSc
Specialty Registrar
Infectious Diseases and Microbiology
Barts Health NHS Trust
London, United Kingdom

Devan Vaghela, MBBS, MRCP
Specialty Registrar
Barts Health NHS Trust
London, United Kingdom

Section I

Principles of Infection Management

1.1 Pillars of Infection Management

Firza Alexander Gronthoud

CLINICAL CONSIDERATIONS

Antibacterial agents (antibiotics) are used to treat bacterial infections, antiviral agents are used to treat viral infections, antiparasitic agents are used to treat infections caused by parasites and antifungal agents are used to treat infections caused by yeasts and moulds (commonly grouped as fungi). Together, these agents are also referred to as antimicrobials. There is widespread (mis)use of antimicrobials for both preventing and treating infections. An unintended consequence of antimicrobial treatment is the emergence of antimicrobial-resistant organisms as well as increased risk of drug toxicity, length of hospital stay, increased morbidity and mortality and increased costs. It is therefore worthwhile to consider the following.

VARYING DEGREES OF ANTIBIOTIC RESISTANCE

- *Multidrug resistant (MDR)*: Resistant to at least one antibiotic in three or more classes
- *Extensively drug resistant (XDR)*: Resistant to at least one antibiotic in all but two or fewer classes
- *Pan-drug resistant (PDR)*: Resistant to all antibiotics in all classes

FINDING THE BALANCE

High burden of infections (infection pressure) leads to increased use of antibiotics. Antibiotics exert pressure (antibiotic pressure) on the gut microbiota (commensal flora) which can lead to emergence and spread of antibiotic-resistant organisms to healthcare workers, patients and the environment. Gut commensal flora can resist colonization with drug-resistant organisms through secretion of antimicrobial products, competition for nutrients and help with maintenance of gut barrier integrity. This is called colonization resistance. High antibiotic pressure reduces colonization resistance and increases rates of patients colonized with drug-resistant organisms (colonization pressure). Increased colonization pressure further drives spread of MDR organisms (MDROs) and increased rates of infections caused by MDROs. This, in turn, leads to a vicious circle with increased use of broad-spectrum antibiotics, leading to increased antibiotic pressure on the gut, reduced colonization resistance and increased colonization pressure.

CLINICAL PEARL

Colonization resistance is also affected by drugs other than antimicrobials.

- Proton-pump inhibitors decrease intestinal pH, promoting colonization with MDRO and *Clostridioides difficile.*
- Metformine promotes the presence of butyrate-producing bacteria. Butyrate contributes to maintenance of gut barrier functions and has immunomodulatory and anti-inflammatory properties, thus contributing to colonization resistance.
- Antipsychotics have been shown to possess antibacterial effects.

GOALS OF INFECTION MANAGEMENT

- Diagnose and treat infections and prevent spread of infections to others.
- Reduce antibiotic pressure, colonization pressure, infection pressure and antibiotic resistance and keep the human microbiota healthy and maintaining its colonization resistance.

PILLARS OF INFECTION MANAGEMENT

The three pillars of infection management are diagnosis, treatment and prevention and control of infectious diseases and requires close collaboration among the microbiology laboratory staff, consultant microbiologist, consultant infectious diseases specialist, antimicrobial pharmacist and infection control nurses, supported by the executive board of the hospital.

CLINICAL APPROACH

To implement and execute the three pillars of infection management, it is essential to have diagnostic stewardship, antimicrobial stewardship and infection prevention and control initiatives in the hospital.

DIAGNOSTIC STEWARDSHIP

Accurate and fast microbiology results directly impact antimicrobial stewardship through early rationalization of antibiotics, shortening duration of treatment and facilitating intravenous to oral stepdown. It also allows for timely implementation of effective infection control precautions.

Key principles are taking the right samples at the right time, ensuring samples are collected according to hospital policies with optimized laboratory processes in place to ensure high-quality results with a short turnaround time and avoiding releasing meaningless results which can mislead clinicians and lead to inappropriate use of antimicrobials.

ANTIMICROBIAL STEWARDSHIP

Inappropriate antibiotic use may lead to increased adverse effects, secondary infections, drug interactions, additional costs, prolonged lengths of hospital stays and hospital readmissions.

The goal of antimicrobial stewardship is to ensure appropriate use of antimicrobial agents, improve patient outcome and reduce risk of both adverse drug events and emergence of antimicrobial resistance. Safety and effectiveness of antimicrobials including glycopeptides, aminoglycosides and certain azoles require therapeutic drug monitoring to ensure adequate blood levels.

INFECTION PREVENTION AND CONTROL

The absence of new, effective anti-Gram-negative antibiotics makes infection prevention and control the most important counter-measure against multidrug-resistant Gram-negative pathogens. Infection prevention and control can prevent additional infections and the spread of resistant pathogens and thereby reduce the need to use antibiotics.

These three pillars of infection management will be discussed in more details in Chapters 1.2–1.4.

Every patient is unique and may have individual infection risk factors influenced by personal lifestyle and underlying comorbidities. Effective implementation of the three pillars of infection management should be tailored to each individual by using a holistic but individualized approach.

This often involves a multidisciplinary team approach whereby individual infection risk factors are assessed and managed. Examples include smoking, alcohol use, diabetes, nutrition, wound care, intravascular and bladder catheter care and vaccination.

Finally, it is essential to maintain a healthy gut microbiota as there is a strong relationship between gut microbiota and the immune system, and an association with cancer and autoimmune disorders has been demonstrated.

BIBLIOGRAPHY

Barlam TF, Cosgrove SE, Abbo LM et al. Implementing an Antibiotic Stewardship Program: Guidelines by the Infectious Diseases Society of America and the Society for Healthcare Epidemiology of America. *Clin Infect Dis.* 2016 May 15;62(10):e51–e77.

Miller JM, Binnicker MJ, Campbell S et al. A Guide to Utilization of the Microbiology Laboratory for Diagnosis of Infectious Diseases: 2018 Update by the Infectious Diseases Society of America and the American Society for Microbiology. *Clin Infect Dis.* 2018 August 31;67(6):e1–e94.

Siegel JD, Rhinehart E, Jackson M et al. (Healthcare Infection Control Practices Advisory Committee). *Guideline for Isolation Precautions: Preventing Transmission of Infectious Agents in Healthcare Settings.* United States Centers for Disease Control and Prevention, 2007.

1.2 Diagnostic Stewardship

Firza Alexander Gronthoud

CLINICAL CONSIDERATIONS

More than half of all medical decisions are based on laboratory results. Approximately 25% have a negative impact on patient outcomes, raising the need to reduce laboratory error to as close to zero as possible. Fast, accurate microbiology results lead to quicker appropriate treatment decisions and timely implementation of infection control precautions.

Choosing the right test and collecting the right specimen using the correct method, reducing turnaround time and correctly interpreting results requires specialist knowledge, often not taught in medical school or higher medical training.

Similar to an antimicrobial stewardship programme to ensure correct use of antibiotics, there is a need for a diagnostic stewardship programme to prevent improper use of the clinical laboratory and optimize the quality of infection management. It is therefore worthwhile to consider the following.

NEGATIVE CONSEQUENCES OF IMPROPER USE OF THE MICROBIOLOGY LABORATORY

- Long transport time or inefficient laboratory processes can prolong long turnaround time of results, leading to unnecessary prolongation of broad-spectrum antimicrobials.
- Not distinguishing between colonization and infection can lead to inappropriate use of antimicrobials.
- Ordering the wrong test at the wrong time or collecting specimens incorrectly can yield false-negative or false-positive results.
- Failing to retrieve or ignoring a test result.

DISADVANTAGES OF NOT PERFORMING MICROBIOLOGY TESTS

- Prescribing antibiotics without knowing the cause of infection can lead to unnecessary use of broad-spectrum antibiotics or the use of antibiotics not active against the organism causing the infection.
- It can also lead to use of antibiotics when there is no infection at all.
- Increased risk of treatment failure or relapse of infection can lead to more antibiotic courses.

THE ROLE OF THE MICROBIOLOGY LABORATORY

- Report significant results and avoid risk of misinterpretation of nonsignificant results.
- Provide advice about best use of the laboratory and recommend antimicrobial treatment regimens through education and guidelines.
- Antimicrobial-resistance surveillance informs local antimicrobial guidelines and feeds into regional, national and international surveillance.
- Screening for multidrug-resistant organisms to aid timely implementation of infection control precautions.

ROLE OF CLINICIANS IN DIAGNOSTIC STEWARDSHIP

- To understand the advantages, disadvantages and clinical value of tests in different settings.
- To provide clinical information to ensure appropriate microbiological tests are performed on the sample.
- Accurate result interpretation to avoid inappropriate use of antimicrobials.

CLINICAL PEARL

The Dipstick

- Overuse of urine dipsticks in the diagnosis of urinary tract infections. Major cause of unnecessary antibiotic treatment.
- Asymptomatic bacteriuria is very common in the elderly and a positive dipstick test does not necessarily mean that the patient needs treatment.

IMPACT OF RAPID ACCURATE MICROBIOLOGY DIAGNOSIS

- Shortens duration of treatment
- Early de-escalation from broad-spectrum to narrow-spectrum agents
- IV to oral stepdown
- Rapid detection of alert organisms and multidrug-resistant organisms
- Reduces risk of toxic side effects
- Reduces risk of emergence of antimicrobial resistance
- Reduces total antimicrobial consumption and costs
- Improves patient outcomes and reduces length of hospital stay

TURNAROUND TIME

Long turnaround times lead to delays in diagnosis and unnecessary use of antimicrobials or use of ineffective antimicrobial treatments. Factors that can influence turnaround times of diagnosis include:

- Culture: Most tests for bacterial infection still rely on prolonged incubation to grow bacteria on culture media.
- Serological tests rely on the detection of antibodies to the infection, and these may not appear for at least 10–14 days after the onset of the infection.
- Transport time.

Diagnostic stewardship aims to improve all aspects of the laboratory diagnosis of infections. Diagnostic stewardship is an effective and important mechanism in the capacity-building and quality-improvement process in the healthcare system. It also helps to optimize resource utilization and to improve surveillance data. Stages in the diagnostic process that are covered within diagnostic stewardship are:

- Indication for test and specimen selection
- Provision of relevant clinical information
- Correct storage and transportation of specimens to the laboratory
- Booking in and processing specimens

- Selection of appropriate tests
- Reporting and interpretation of results
- Guiding patient management

CLINICAL APPROACH

Key interventions of diagnostic stewardship are as follows.

EDUCATION OF CLINICAL STAFF TO IMPROVE THE DIAGNOSTIC VALUE OF REQUESTED TESTS

Teaching sessions, development of guidelines and hospital wide campaigns can raise awareness of appropriate use of the microbiology laboratory and can upskill members of the staff. Some topics that could be covered in teaching sessions are:

- Ability of a test to differentiate between health and disease.
- Does the test result play a significant role in the management and/or outcome of the patient, i.e. to rule out infection or distinguish between bacterial and viral infection.
- Overview of the various microbiology tests (i.e. PCR, culture, serology) and their advantages and disadvantages.
- Basic understanding of the meaning of microbiology results and promoting correct interpretation of results.

Guidelines can offer guidance on appropriate collection and transport of specimens:

- Transport time should be less than two hours to prevent bacterial overgrowth.
- Most specimens should be stored between 2 and 8°C; exceptions include mycology samples, blood cultures and cerebrospinal fluid.
- Avoid blood culture contamination through aseptic techniques. Volume of blood is more important than timing (i.e. waiting until a patient spikes a fever).
- Urine: Send midstream urine. To avoid diagnosing a colonized catheter rather than infection, replace catheter first and then send new urine sample. Use boric acid containers.
- A positive dipstick or cloudy and offensive-smelling urine in the absence of urinary symptoms is not an indication for sending a urine culture or antimicrobial therapy.
- Wound swabs and sinus tracts often grow colonizing bacteria not involved in the infection. Irrigating the wound with saline, squeezing the edge of the wound until pus is discharged and sending pus for culture increases diagnostic yield.
- Avoid sending catheter urine or drain fluid which has been in the collecting bag for hours.
- If admitted more than 48 hours ago, then only test for *Clostridioides difficile* after other causes of diarrhoea have been excluded. (Appropriate testing for *C. difficile* is discussed in more detail in Chapter 5.9.)
- Stool cultures in afebrile outpatients with acute onset of watery diarrhoea is highly unlikely to yield positive results for a bacterial pathogen.
- Examination of stool for ova and parasites should be obtained only in patients with diarrhoea for more than 2 days plus an appropriate travel history or if there is a strong suspicion of *Giardia* or *Cryptosporidium* infection.
- Sterile fluids (pleural fluid, joint aspirate, peritoneal fluid): If a large volume can be obtained, it should be inoculated into blood culture bottles containing nutrient media. A small portion should also be sent to the laboratory in a sterile tube so that appropriate stains (e.g. Gram, acid-fast) can be prepared and direct culture can be performed.

- Therapeutic drug monitoring: Taking trough levels too early has a detrimental effect as clinicians may withhold the dose or reduce the dose, leading to treatment failure and worse patient outcome.
- Only send line tips if there is a suspicion of infection.
- Guidance on requesting serology: If the serum is taken too early, no antibodies will be detected, and serology test will be negative. Conversely, if the sample is taken too late, serology test may not be able to distinguish between past or active infection.
- With many arboviral infections, such as dengue, the period of viraemia may only be detectable in the first days of infection. After this period, it may be more useful to perform serology.

CLINICAL PEARL

It is common practice for clinicians to take a blood culture when a patient is febrile. Clinical signs of sepsis are a response to the release of endotoxins or exotoxins from the organisms, occurring as long as one hour after the organisms entered the blood. Thus, few to no organisms may be in the blood when the patient becomes febrile. For this reason, it is recommended that two to three blood samples should be collected at random times during a 24-hour period (Murray et al., 2013).

IMPROVING LABORATORY PROCESSES AND BETTER USE OF RESOURCES

- Complying with national and international guidance on laboratory test methods, i.e. UK Standard Methods for Investigation, United States ASM/IDSA guideline.
- Participating in laboratory accreditation requirements to assess compliance with the ISO15189 standard.
- For most bacterial culture requests, repeat testing should be rejected as it can lead to confusing results. Conversely, for some types of infections (viral, rickettsiosis, Lyme), repeat serologic testing is necessary to detect a rise in antibody titre which is seen in the acute infection.
- Adding comments to assist in interpreting results or advising on when to repeat the test.
- Improving turnaround time of results to guide earlier clinical decision-making:
  - Extending laboratory opening hours
  - Seven day per week working and reporting to meet deadlines of ward rounds or patient review
  - Substituting slow bacterial culture methods with rapid molecular techniques
- Introducing technological advances:
  - Lab automation to enable higher laboratory throughput of specimens at lower cost; they can also have positive benefit for stewardship activities. As well as improving laboratory turnaround times, automation can provide greater consistency of culture among samples and, in some cases, improve the yield of organisms from cultured samples.
  - Rapid bacterial identification with matrix assisted laser desorption ionization-time of flight mass spectrometry (MALDI-TOF MS); can be performed on both colonies or directly on clinical samples, i.e. blood cultures.
  - Rapid identification with MALDI-TOF without susceptibility testing but may not necessarily translate into empirical antimicrobial therapy changes.
  - Commercial or in-house molecular methods such as polymerase chain reaction (PCR) can not only detect the most common causes of respiratory tract, central nervous system, gastrointestinal and bloodstream infections but also detect antimicrobial-resistance genes.

- Presence of resistance genes may not necessarily correlate with *in vivo* susceptibility. For now, phenotypic susceptibility testing remains the gold standard.
- Molecular tests can also be used for rapid screening for multidrug-resistant organisms. Bacterial culture is slower but can provide extensive antimicrobial susceptibility testing.

RESTRICTIVE REPORTING OF ANTIMICROBIAL SUSCEPTIBILITY TESTING

- Reporting of susceptibility results should prevent inappropriate antimicrobial prescribing
- Influence clinician prescribing behaviour such as building experience and confidence that (combinations of) small spectrum antimicrobials are as effective as broad spectrum antimicrobials including carbapenems.

BETTER USE OF HOSPITAL IT

Building in rules in the electronic patient record to:

- Reject samples
- Advise on the best test
- Advise on when to repeat tests

AUDITS

Regular audits should be performed to evaluate the effect of each of the above interventions. Examples of metrics that can be used:

- Rate of specimen rejection
- Blood culture contamination rate
- Turnaround time of results
- Time from presentation of symptoms to diagnosis
- Rate of antimicrobial treatment modifications based on microbiology results
- Time to implementation of infection control precautions
- Duration of isolation
- Antimicrobial consumption

COMMUNICATION AND COLLABORATION WITH OTHER DISCIPLINES

- Optimal patient care depends on good communication between clinical staff at point-of-care, microbiology laboratories and surveillance staff.
- Standard operating procedures could stipulate how rapidly provisional results will be communicated, the on-call availability of laboratory staff and include provision for regular meetings to discuss results for individual care, to facilitate the development and adaptation of local treatment guidelines and to address performance and challenges.
- Joint ward rounds, with the presence of both clinicians and microbiologists, provide further opportunities for improving communication and patient management.
- Multidisciplinary team meetings facilitate and improve collaboration and build mutual understanding between clinical, laboratory and surveillance staff.

BIBLIOGRAPHY

Dik JW, Poelman R, Friedrich AW, Panday PN, Lo-Ten-Foe JR, van Assen S, van Gemert-Pijnen JE, Niesters HG, Hendrix R, Sinha B. An Integrated Stewardship Model: Antimicrobial, Infection Prevention and Diagnostic (AID). *Future Microbiol.* 2016;11(1):93–102.

Miller JM, Binnicker MJ, Campbell S et al. A Guide to Utilization of the Microbiology Laboratory for Diagnosis of Infectious Diseases: 2018 Update by the Infectious Diseases Society of America and the American Society for Microbiology. *Clin Infect Dis.* 2018 August 31;67(6):813–816.

Morency-Potvin P, Schwartz DN, Weinstein RA. Antimicrobial Stewardship: How the Microbiology Laboratory Can Right the Ship. *Clin Microbiol Rev.* 2016 December 14;30(1):381–407.

Murray P, Rosenthal K, Pfaller M. *Medical Microbiology.* 7th Edition, 2013.

Patel R, Fang FC. Diagnostic Stewardship: Opportunity for a Laboratory Infectious Diseases Partnership. *Clin Infect Dis.* 2018 August 16;67(5):799–801.

Roger PM, Montera E, Lesselingue D et al. collaborators. Risk Factors for Unnecessary Antibiotic Therapy: A Major Role for Clinical Management. *Clin Infect Dis.* 2019 Jul 18;69(3):466-472.

Sullivan KV. Advances in Diagnostic Testing that Impact Infection Prevention and Antimicrobial Stewardship Programs. *Curr Infect Dis Rep.* 2019 May 1;21(6):20.

Sullivan KV, Dien Bard J. New and Novel Rapid Diagnostics that are Impacting Infection Prevention and Antimicrobial Stewardship. *Curr Opin Infect Dis.* 2019 August;32(4):356–364.

1.3 Antimicrobial Stewardship

Firza Alexander Gronthoud

CLINICAL CONSIDERATIONS

Up to 50% of antimicrobial use in hospitals is inappropriate, leading to increased length of antimicrobial duration, increased length of stay, emergence of antimicrobial resistance and increased risk of drug toxicity. Antimicrobial stewardship is a multidisciplinary team effort and initiatives should be tailored to each healthcare institution owing to different practices, cultures and healthcare systems and processes in place. It is therefore worthwhile to consider the following:

THE GOAL OF ANTIMICROBIAL STEWARDSHIP

The primary goal of antimicrobial stewardship is to ensure that for each patient, the right antimicrobial is given at the right time using the right dose and route and reducing the risk of drug toxicity and emergence of antimicrobial resistance.

SECONDARY GOALS

- Improve patient outcome by improving infection cure rates and reducing mortality and morbidity
- Improve patient safety
  - Prevent colonization with multidrug-resistant organisms and infection with *Clostridioides difficile*
  - Reduce length of hospital stay and antimicrobial consumption
- Reduce healthcare costs

COMMON CAUSES OF INAPPROPRIATE USE OF ANTIBIOTICS

- Treating respiratory or gastrointestinal viral infections
- Treating asymptomatic bacteriuria in patients who are not pregnant or who are not undergoing urological procedures
- Not reviewing antimicrobial therapy when microbiology results are available
- Mismatch antimicrobial spectrum of activity and microorganisms (potentially) involved in the infection
- Not following local guidelines
- Intravenous route when oral can be used
- Incorrect duration and incorrect dose and frequency
- Not reviewing drug allergy status
- Not reviewing prescriptions for drug-drug interaction
- Prolonged use of surgical prophylaxis >24 hours
- In the ICU setting, failure to de-escalate or excessive duration of therapy

COLLATERAL DAMAGE OF ANTIBIOTICS

- Emergence and spread of antimicrobial resistance
- Reduced colonization resistance (See Chapter 1.1 'Pillars of Infection Management')
- Changes in metabolic capacity of microbiota causing overall health consequences

CLINICAL PEARL

Carriage of resistant bacteria in our microbiota can persist for many months, and the risk of prolonged carriage is increased by further antibiotic use.

DRIVERS OF (MIS)USE OF ANTIBIOTICS

- Lack of knowledge and education
- Lack of or inadequate diagnostics tests leads to uncertainty regarding presence of infection (see Chapter 1.2)
- Fear of a life-threatening infection
- Local culture and historical practice

CLINICAL CONSEQUENCES OF ANTIMICROBIAL RESISTANCE

- Longer time to resolution of symptoms
- Prolonged courses of antimicrobial therapy
- Increased use of broad-spectrum antibiotics
- Increased length of stay with risk of healthcare-acquired infections

UTILITY OF PK/PD TARGETS

- Suboptimal antimicrobial concentrations promote development of multidrug resistance. Improving outcomes from infection requires understanding of the interactions between the drug, host and infecting pathogen.
- Application of pharmacokinetic and pharmacodynamic drug targets can optimize antimicrobial killing and prevent emergence of antimicrobial resistance (see Chapter 3.8).

REDUCING RISK OF ADVERSE DRUG EVENTS

- Timely de-escalation to narrow-spectrum antimicrobials reduces risk of resistance or development of *C. difficile* infection.
- Renal dose adjustments will ensure patients are not over- or under-dosed, which may increase their risk for adverse effects, infection relapse or development of resistance.

POTENTIAL BARRIERS TO IMPLEMENTING ANTIMICROBIAL STEWARDSHIP INITIATIVES

- Executive teams with different priorities
- Opposition from prescribers
- Lack of trained staff (microbiology, infectious diseases, pharmacy and nurses)
- Outdated IT technology making it difficult to (1) monitor antimicrobial use and costs, and (2) obtain local antimicrobial susceptibility data
- Outdated guidelines

CLINICAL APPROACH

RATIONAL USE OF ANTIMICROBIALS

Antimicrobial stewardship is every prescriber's responsibility, and for each antimicrobial prescription, the following items need to be considered:

- Which organisms could be involved in this infection?
- Risk factors for drug-resistant bacteria (hospital admissions in past 3 months, previous antimicrobial courses)
- Take cultures before starting antimicrobials
- Tissue penetration
- Take into account renal and hepatic function
- In cases of positive microbiology cultures: distinguishing between infection or colonization can prevent unnessecary antibiotic prescriptions
- Limiting the use of broad-spectrum drugs when a narrower antimicrobial spectrum suffices
- Shortening duration of therapy when prolonged antibiotic courses do not provide benefit
- Avoiding drug-drug interactions
- Appropriate dose
- Therapeutic drug monitoring
- Intravenous or oral route
- Use empirical therapy first; narrow the spectrum later
- Use a proper dose first up; no point under-dosing patients
- Where possible, use monotherapy (it reduces cost and toxicity)
- If the microbiology suggests reduced susceptibility, think: Are the antibiotics working clinically? Is there direct bedside evidence that they are working? If the answer is yes, then you should continue them in spite of laboratory evidence. *In vitro* sensitivity does not predict *in vivo* effect. It might be good to liaise with the infection specialist to ensure the right dose is given.
- Limit 'prophylactic' use to appropriate situations
- Consider non-infective causes of inflammation (it's not always sepsis)

These are quite a few considerations and may seem daunting for the clinical team who are also dealing with other non-infectious problems. Fortunately, the antimicrobial stewardship team can provide support and guidance to clinicians through:

- Providing guidance on appropriate investigations and sampling, initiation of empiric therapy, streamlining to directed therapy
- Reviewing prescriptions for antimicrobial agents
- Providing advice on optimization of antimicrobial therapy, i.e. therapeutic drug monitoring and modifying doses in renal or hepatic impairment
- Reviewing drug interactions with existing medications
- Promoting IV to oral stepdown when appropriate
- Gathering data and feeding back to clinicians and executive board: point prevalence surveys, audit data, quality improvement data collection, primary care prescribing data
- Updating local guidelines, taking into account local resistance profiles
- Managing an outpatient parenteral antimicrobial therapy service
- Ensuring compliance with national quality standards or quality initiatives
- Providing education through a formal teaching session or ad hoc education on ward rounds (Education is an essential tool to influence prescribing behaviour and upskill members of staff to further enhance and increase acceptance of stewardship strategies.)

The antimicrobial stewardship team can choose from various approaches when performing the above activities:

- *Restrictive*: Formulary restrictions, pre-approval by a senior member of an antimicrobial stewardship team doctor (i.e. infection specialist or a specified expert on the ICU team) and automatic stop orders.

- *Collaborative or enhancement*: Education of prescribers, implementation of treatment guidelines, creating awareness of adverse drug events, use of PK/PD concepts and prospective audit and feedback to providers.
- *Structural*: Use of computerized antibiotic decision support systems, faster diagnostic methods for antimicrobial resistance, antibiotic consumption surveillance systems, ICU leadership commitment, staff involvement and daily collaboration between ICU staff, pharmacists, infection control units and microbiologists.

To organize these activities, an antimicrobial stewardship programme should consist of

- Antimicrobial committee
- Antimicrobial formulary
- Antimicrobial team executing the day-to-day antimicrobial stewardship activities with key members including consultant microbiologist, consultant infectious diseases, antimicrobial pharmacist and senior representatives from clinical teams

EXAMPLES OF METRICS TO ASSESS AND EVALUATE ANTIMICROBIAL STEWARDSHIP INITIATIVES

- *Outcome measures*: 30-day mortality, surgical site infection rates, length of hospital stay, hospital readmission rates, *C. difficile* rates, infection recurrences
- *Prescribing related measures*: Duration of therapy, percentages of prescriptions in line with hospital guidelines, IV to oral switch

SURVEILLANCE OF ANTIBIOTIC PRESCRIPTION

- Surveillance is a first and essential step to measure antimicrobial consumption.
- Document physicians' incentives to prescribe antibiotics and to identify areas of potential overuse or misuse which could then be a target for antimicrobial stewardship interventions.
- Surveillance metrics are derived from antibiotic prescription data (pharmacy-based), microbiology results (laboratory-based) or diagnostic codes (administration-based) or a combination thereof.
- Monitor adherence to hospital guidelines/formularies, time to de-escalation of antibiotics, rate of *C. difficile* infections and drug toxicities, antimicrobial consumption and antimicrobial resistance.

TACKLING ANTIMICROBIAL RESISTANCE IN THE HOSPITAL

- Raise awareness among staff and patients
- Improve sanitation and hygiene
- Prevent infections (and thus antibiotic use) by infection prevention and control strategies (including vaccinations)
- Surveillance
- Rapid diagnostics
- Rational use of antibiotics

ANTIMICROBIAL STEWARDSHIP PROGRAMMES SHOULD BE ADAPTED TO LOCAL INSTITUTIONS AND CULTURE

- Cultural background and habits for antibiotic prescription, MDRO prevalence, local organizational aspects and available resources.
- Identifying barriers and facilitators that impact the staff's compliance to guidelines in order to design and execute a structured plan for improvement is essential.

ANTIFUNGAL STEWARDSHIP

Although it follows the same general principles as antibiotic stewardship, there some key differences:

- Therapeutic drug monitoring plays a bigger role in antifungal stewardship owing to azoles being the most used class of antifungals.
- Azoles are cytochrome P450 enzyme inhibitors and monitoring for drug-drug interactions is essential.
- Fungal culture has low sensitivity and the use of biomarkers and radiology is an important part of antifungal stewardship.
- Antifungal stewardship interventions depend on the patient population and fungus involved:
  - Candidaemia
  - Neutropenic fever
  - Pre-emptive treatment versus prophylaxis

ANTIFUNGAL STEWARDSHIP FOR PATIENTS WITH CANDIDAEMIA

- Restrict or avoid antifungal prophylaxis; in particular fluconazole
- Differentiate infection from colonization and do not treat colonization
- Use non-culture-based diagnostics for early detection of invasive candidiasis (IC) (1,3-β-D-glucan, Mannan Antigen and Anti-Mannan Antibodies)
- Limit the use of empirical therapy based only on risk factors
- Promote early pre-emptive antifungal treatment based on risk factors, (heavy) colonization and biomarkers
- Have adequate source control within 48 h (catheter removal, appropriate drainage, surgical control)
- Use an adequate dose; low dose is associated with resistance
- De-escalate whenever possible (if possible, within 5 days) from echinocandins to azoles
- Antifungal therapy (usually echinocandin or fluconazole) should be discontinued if there is a negative 1,3-β-D-glucan in serum combined with negative blood cultures and/or negative drain cultures.
- *Candida* scoring systems or a colonization index may be used to either withhold treatment for IC or to prompt the use of 1,3-β-D-glucan to enhance its positive predictive value.

ANTIFUNGAL STEWARDSHIP IN PATIENTS WITH PROFOUND NEUTROPAENIA

Patients with profound neutropaenia (i.e. intensive chemotherapy for acute myeloid leukaemia or allogeneic haematopoietic stem cell recipients) are at risk of invasive mould infections, predominantly caused by *Aspergillus* spp. Close monitoring of clinical and radiological findings, complemented by detection of fungal biomarkers in serum and bronchoalveolar lavage, might substantially reduce the inappropriate use of empirical mould active therapy.

Effective management of invasive fungal infections (IFIs) depends on early individualized therapy that optimizes efficacy and safety (See Chapter 3.2 'Basic principles of antifungal treatment'). Considering the negative consequences of IFI, for some high-risk patients, the potential benefits of prophylactic therapy may outweigh the risks. When using a prophylactic, empiric or pre-emptive therapeutic approach, clinicians must take into account the local epidemiology, spectrum of activity, pharmacokinetic and pharmacodynamic parameters and safety profile of different antifungal agents, together with unique host-related factors that may affect antifungal efficacy or safety.

THE USE OF BIOMARKERS

The use of biomarkers plays a big role in antifungal stewardship owing to the low sensitivity of standard culture techniques.

BIBLIOGRAPHY

Barlam TF, Cosgrove SE, Abbo LM et al. Implementing an Antibiotic Stewardship Program: Guidelines by the Infectious Diseases Society of America and the Society for Healthcare Epidemiology of America. *Clin Infect Dis.* 2016 May 15;62(10):e51–e77.

Dellit TH, Owens RC, McGowan JE Jr et al. Infectious Diseases Society of America; Society for Healthcare Epidemiology of America. Infectious Diseases Society of America and the Society for Healthcare Epidemiology of America Guidelines for Developing an Institutional Program to Enhance Antimicrobial Stewardship. *Clin Infect Dis.* 2007 January 15;44(2):159–177. Epub 2006 December 13.

Nathwani D, Sneddon J. Practical Guide to Antimicrobial Stewardship in Hospitals. *BiomérieuxR. Disponível em*: http://bsac.org.uk/wpcontent/uploads/2013/07/Stewardship-Booklet-Practical-Guide-to-Antimicrobial-Stewardship-in-Hospitals.pdf. 2015.

National Institute for Health and Care Excellence. Antimicrobial Stewardship: Systems and Processes for Effective Antimicrobial Medicine Use (NG15). 2015 August.

Ruhnke M. Antifungal stewardship in invasive *Candida* infections. *Clin Microbiol Infect.* 2014 June;20(Suppl 6):11–18.

1.4 Infection Prevention and Control

Firza Alexander Gronthoud

CLINICAL CONSIDERATIONS

The goal of infection control in a hospital setting is to prevent transmission of infectious agents which are difficult to treat or have the potential to cause severe illness. The type of isolation precautions is mainly determined by the mode of transmission and the severity of illness. Prevention and control of infections is an integral part of routine clinical care and should not be regarded as an additional set of practices and care. It is therefore worthwhile to consider the following.

INFECTIOUS AGENT

An infectious agent is any bacterium, virus, fungus, parasite or prion causing disease. The type of precautions used to prevent transmission to others depends on the agent's treatability, mode of transmission and severity of illness.

CLINICAL PEARL

All body fluids are potentially infectious (except sweat): blood and blood-tinged fluids including open wounds, stools, urine, vomit, respiratory secretions, saliva, semen, vaginal secretions, breast milk and sterile fluids including blood, pericardial fluid, pleural fluid and synovial fluid.

COLONIZATION VERSUS INFECTION

Colonization is when an infectious agent is present without causing symptomatic disease. Infection is when the infectious agent is present and causes symptomatic disease. Colonization does not require treatment with antimicrobials but does require infection control precautions.

HOSPITAL SOURCES OF TRANSMISSION

- Infectious agents transmitted during healthcare come primarily from human sources, including patients, healthcare workers and visitors. Source individuals may be actively ill or may be temporary or chronic carriers of an infectious agent without symptoms.
- Infectious agents may arise from endogenous flora of patients (e.g. bacteria residing in the respiratory or gastrointestinal tract) or from environmental sources such as air, water, medications or medical equipment and devices that have become contaminated.

MODES OF TRANSMISSION

- *Direct transmission*: Infectious agent transferred directly from one person to another person.
- *Indirect transmission*: Infectious agent transferred through a contaminated intermediate object (fomite) or person.

- *Large droplets (>5 microns)*: When a person coughs, sneezes or talks, and during certain procedures, large respiratory droplets are expelled which can enter other people through the nose, conjunctivae or oropharynx. Transmission via large droplets requires close contact as the droplets do not remain suspended in the air and generally only travel short distances (<2 metres). Droplets can also be transmitted by hands.
- *Airborne*: Small respiratory droplets, also called aerosols, which can travel over long distances and can remain suspended in the air for a prolonged time. Transmission similar to large droplets.
- Contaminated food, water, medications, devices or equipment.

DROPLETS VERSUS AEROSOLS

Small aerosols are inhaled deep into the lung and cause infection in the alveolar tissues of the lower respiratory tract, whereas large droplets are trapped in the upper airways. Droplets travel over 1–2 metres and do not stay suspended in the air. Infection via aerosols may therefore lead to more severe disease and require more strict infection control precautions.

CLINICAL PEARL

Certain procedures, particularly those that induce coughing, can promote airborne transmission. These include diagnostic sputum induction, bronchoscopy, airway suctioning, endotracheal intubation, positive pressure ventilation via face mask and high-frequency oscillatory ventilation.

CLINICAL PEARL

The modes of transmission vary by type of organism. In some cases, the same organism may be transmitted by more than one route (e.g. influenza and respiratory syncytial virus [RSV] can be transmitted by contact and droplet routes).

RISK OF INFECTION

Factors important to consider when risk assessing the need for specific infection control precautions or administration of post-exposure prophylaxis following infection exposure include:

- Age
- Immune status
- Comorbidities, i.e. diabetes mellitus, malignancy
- Virulence of infectious agent

CLINICAL APPROACH

RISK ASSESSMENT

For any given procedure, clinical situation or new admission/transfer, a risk assessment needs to be undertaken which involves going through the five pillars of infection prevention and control to ensure that besides clinical care, also appropriate infection control measures are in place.

- *Pillar 1*: Prevention of transmission
- *Pillar 2*: Source control

- *Pillar 3*: Environmental decontamination
- *Pillar 4*: Antimicrobial stewardship
- *Pillar 5*: Diagnostic stewardship

PILLAR 1: PREVENTION OF TRANSMISSION

The use of standard precautions is the primary strategy for preventing transmission of healthcare-associated infections. Transmission-based precautions are used in addition to standard precautions, where the suspected or confirmed presence of infectious agents represents an increased risk of transmission and/or severe illness.

Standard Precautions

The minimum standard of infection control precautions are to be used for all patients. Standard precautions are used by healthcare workers to prevent or reduce the likelihood of transmission of infectious agents from one person or place to another, and to render and maintain objects and areas as free as possible from infectious agents. Standard precautions include:

- Hand hygiene is the best evidence from the literature compared to other interventions in reducing transmission of infectious agents
- Use of personal protective equipment (PPE) during procedures that may result in exposure to bodily fluids
- Appropriate handling and disposal of sharps to protect healthcare workers against bloodborne diseases
- Appropriate handling of waste and linens
- Appropriate reprocessing of reusable equipment and instruments, including appropriate use of disinfectants
- Cleaning and spills management
- Hygiene and cough etiquette
- Implementation of intravascular and catheter care bundles

CLINICAL PEARL

The five WHO moments of hand hygiene:

- Before touching a patient
- Before clean/aseptic procedures
- After body fluid exposure/risk
- After touching a patient
- After touching patient surroundings

The process of hand washing using the correct technique takes 40–60 seconds. There can be as many as five opportunities per patient contact to wash the hands using the correct technique and duration. As a result, there is an overall low compliance with healthcare workers. Education is key in promoting good hand hygiene to prevent hospital-acquired infections.

Transmission-Based Precautions

Transmission-based precautions should be tailored to the particular infectious agent involved and its mode of transmission (see Chapter 6.5). For infectious agents that have multiple routes of transmission, more than one transmission-based precaution category is applied. Transmission-based precautions should be used until the patient is not actively excreting the infectious agent anymore. This is usually when signs and symptoms of the infection have resolved. In immunocompromised individuals, the period of excretion may be prolonged until long after the patient has become asymptomatic.

Transmission-based precautions include continued implementation of standard precautions and, in addition:

- Intensified use of PPE (including gloves, apron or gowns, surgical masks or respirators [FFP2, FFP3 or N95] and protective eyewear) according to likelihood of exposure to bodily fluids and probable type and route of transmission
- Patient-dedicated equipment
- Allocation of single rooms or cohorting of patients when required
- Appropriate air-handling requirements
- Enhanced cleaning and disinfecting of the patient environment
- Restricted transfer of patients within and between facilities

The three categories of transmission-based precautions are:

- *Contact precautions*: When there is known or suspected risk of direct or indirect contact transmission of infectious agents that are not effectively contained by standard precautions alone.
- *Droplet precautions*: For patients known or suspected to be infected with agents transmitted over short distances by large respiratory droplets. Because of the short travel distance, special air handling and ventilation are not required.
- *Airborne precautions*: For patients known or suspected to be infected with agents transmitted person to person by the airborne route.

Hand hygiene must be performed before putting on PPE and after removing PPE. Don PPE before patient contact and generally before entering the patient room and remove before leaving patient area. Respirators should be taken off outside the patient room, once the door is closed. To ensure effective protectiveness of respirators, healthcare workers are required to face-fit testing.

Pillar 2: Source Control

The goal of source control is to further reduce the risk of transmission to patients and healthcare workers and to prevent environmental contamination. This includes:

- All beds should be spaced apart 1–2 metres
- Single-room isolation for high risk of transmission: droplet, airborne, infective diarrhoea or highly virulent organisms, i.e. carbapenemase-producing organisms (CPOs) and methicillin-resistant *Staphylococcus aureus* (MRSA)

Prioritization of Single Rooms
- Airborne > droplet > contact; *C. difficile* > CPO > MRSA > extended spectrum beta-lactamase (ESBL)-producing bacteria > vancomycin-resistant *Enterococcus* (VRE)
- Patients who are infected with the same pathogen may be cohorted in the same room or bay
- In the absence of diarrhoea, patients colonized with extended spectrum beta-lactamase (ESBL) producing bacteria and VRE can be nursed in an open bay using contact precautions

Types of Single Rooms
- *Positive pressure*: Protective isolation to keep organisms out of the room; to be used for severely immunocompromised individuals such as bone marrow transplant recipients

- *Negative pressure*: To prevent airborne transmission; 6–12 air cycles per hour; air exhausted directly to the outside or HEPA filtration on exhaust
- *Normal pressure*: Carbapenemase producing organisms, infectious diarrhoea, MRSA

Transportation of Colonized/Infected Patients

- Patients who are under respiratory precautions (droplet and airborne) and who need to be transported should wear a surgical mask
- Patients should follow respiratory hygiene and cough etiquette
- Skin lesions should be covered

Pillar 3: Environmental Decontamination

Preventing transmission of infectious agents from the environment to patients and healthcare workers:

- Frequently touched surfaces should be cleaned daily with detergent solution, as well as when visibly soiled and after every known contamination.
- For specific organisms, enhanced cleaning with chlorine, H_2O_2 fogging and ultraviolet light is indicated.

Pillar 4: Antimicrobial Stewardship

- Appropriate use of antibiotics ensures the best treatment outcome and minimizes risk of toxicity, emergence of resistance and aims to preserve the gut flora, which can act as a reservoir for multidrug-resistant organisms.
- Healthcare worker vaccination against influenza and hepatitis B, and in some countries, tuberculosis.
- Post-exposure prophylaxis, vaccines or immunoglobulins are indicated in pregnant women, neonates and immunocompromised individuals following exposure with influenza, measles and varicella zoster.
- Immunosuppressed individuals may require extra vaccinations, i.e. asplenia patients, bone marrow transplant recipients, individuals with severe liver or renal disease.
- MRSA decolonization treatment suppresses the bacterial load and reduces transmission. It is not 100% effective in eradicating MRSA and recolonization does occur.
- Monitoring of antimicrobial consumption is also part of antimicrobial stewardship.

Pillar 5: Diagnostic Stewardship

Rapid and accurate diagnosis of infections enables timely instigation of infection control precautions, as well as early de-isolation of patients. Besides rapid diagnosis, rapid and effective monitoring of infection rates (passive screening) and rates of patients colonized with drug-resistant organisms (active screening) can help to efficiently allocate resources and identify areas that are at high risk, as well as assess effectiveness of local infection control programmes.

- Screening can act as a tool to monitor the quality of infection control practices.
- Screening can also identify patients who need to be isolated in a single room.
- During outbreaks, screening for carriers helps identify those who need isolation as well as monitor the effectiveness of the implemented actions to stop the outbreak.
- Screening may also be indicated in hospitals where drug-resistant organisms are endemic or when a patient is transferred from a setting of high endemicity of specific organisms.
- Screening also has downsides: Depending on the laboratory method used, it can have a long turnaround time, increased costs, block patient flow and lead to increased use of single

rooms and PPE, especially when patients are prematurely isolated pending the result. Each facility needs to determine whether screening for specific organisms is cost-effective and which laboratory method to use (culture versus PCR).

PRIORITIZING NEEDS

In the case of infection control nurse capacity issues, it may be beneficial to initially focus efforts on wards with high antibiotic pressure, infection pressure and colonization pressure as patients on these wards are at particular risk of developing severe, difficult-to-treat infections. These wards are also important infection reservoirs with risk of transmission to other units.

CLINICAL PEARL

Educating and empowering patients and visitors ensures that patients are actively involved in decision-making about care, and able to participate in reducing the risk of transmission of infectious agents.

BIBLIOGRAPHY

Loveday HP, Wilson JA, Pratt RJ, Golsorkhi M, Tingle A, Bak A, Browne J, Prieto J, Wilcox M, UK Department of Health. epic3 National Evidence-Based Guidelines for Preventing Healthcare-Associated Infections in NHS Hospitals. *J Hosp Infect.* 2014 January;86(Suppl 1):S1–70.

Sehulster LM, and Chinn RYW. *Guidelines for Environmental Infection Control in Health-care Facilities.* Recommendations of the CDC and the Healthcare Infection Control Practices Advisory Committee (HICPAC). Chicago IL: American Society for Healthcare Engineering/American Hospital Association, 2003.

Siegel JD, Rhinehart E, Jackson M et al. (Healthcare Infection Control Practices Advisory Committee). *Guideline for Isolation Precautions: Preventing Transmission of Infectious Agents in Healthcare Settings.* United States Centers for Disease Control and Prevention, 2007.

Section II

Diagnosis of Infections

2.1 Commensal Flora

Firza Alexander Gronthoud

CLINICAL CONSIDERATIONS

The human body is colonized with many organisms, collectively called the microbiota (or commensal flora). Most bacterial infections are endogenous, meaning they are caused by our own commensal flora. Under normal conditions, our commensal flora doesn't cause disease, but disease can occur when organisms from our commensal flora invade body sites where they don't belong.

Composition of the commensal flora depends on a person's location (community versus hospital setting) and a variety of medical factors, including use of antimicrobials, age, diet, hormonal state, health and personal hygiene.

Knowledge of the human commensal flora and under what circumstances it causes disease helps inform empirical antimicrobial therapy. Conversely, detection of bacteria in clinical samples may help determine the source of infection. It is therefore worthwhile to consider the following:

PROTECTIVE ROLE OF COMMENSAL FLORA

The human commensal flora is involved in food metabolism, provides essential growth factors, protects against infections with highly virulent bacteria and stimulates the immune system. A major negative consequence of antibiotics is disruption of the commensal flora, enabling colonization and overgrowth by the pathogen by reducing the colonization resistance (see Chapter 1.1).

COMMENSAL FLORA AS PATHOGENS

Exposure to bacteria can lead to (1) transient colonization, (2) permanent colonization or (3) clinical disease. Some organisms are strict pathogens—*Mycobacterium tuberculosis, Neisseria gonorrhoeae, Francisella tularensis, Plasmodium* spp. and rabies virus—while others only cause disease when the immune system is compromised or when anatomical barriers are broken—*Actinomyces* spp. or opportunistic pathogens such as *Pseudomonas aeruginosa* and *Acinetobacter baumannii*.

EYE

The surface of the eye is colonized with coagulase-negative staphylococci and *Haemophilus* spp., *Neisseria* spp., *Moraxella* spp., *Streptococcus* pneumoniae and viridans streptococci.

OROPHARYNGEAL FLORA

The commensal flora in the oropharynx consists mainly of anaerobes and streptococci. Coliforms can be transient colonizers, mainly in hospitalized patients. The most common anaerobes are *Actinomyces, Bacteroides, Prevotella, Fusobacterium, Corynebacterium, Veillonella, Rothia* and *Capnocytophaga*. Other members of the commensal flora are streptococci, *Gemella* and *Granulicatella, Neisseria* spp. and *Haemophilus* spp. Infections with oropharyngeal flora are seen in periodontal diseases, endocarditis and aspiration pneumonia. Oropharyngeal flora associated with endocarditis are viridans streptococci, *Haemophilus* spp. and members belonging to the HACEK group. Periodontal infections, perioral abscesses, sinusitis and mastoiditis may involve predominantly *P. melaninogenica, Fusobacterium* spp. and *Peptostreptococcus* spp. Aspiration of saliva may result in necrotizing pneumonia, lung abscess and empyema. *Streptococcus mutans* plays a particularly important role in dental plaques and caries. *Eikenella corrodens* is an important pathogen in human bites.

CLINICAL PEARL

The HACEK group constitutes a group of fastidious Gram-negative bacteria that are associated with infective endocarditis. Members are *Haemophilus aphrophilus* (renamed as *Aggregatibacter aphrophilus* and *Aggregatibacter paraphrophilus*), *Actinobacillus actinomycetemcomitans* (renamed as *Aggregatibacter actinomycetemcomitans*), *Cardiobacterium hominis, Eikenella corrodens* and *Kingella kingae*. With modern blood culture systems, prolonged incubation is no longer necessary and they generally can be detected within five days.

NOSE

The flora of the nose consists of corynebacteria, coagulase negative staphylococci (*Staphylococcus epidermidis S. haemolyticus and S. warneri*) and streptococci. Around one-third of the population carry *Staphylococcus aureus* in the nose.

LOWER RESPIRATORY TRACT

Streptococci, staphylococci, *Corynebacterium* spp., *Moraxella* spp., *Neisseria* spp. (including *Neisseria meningitidis*) and *Haemophilus* spp. can be found in the respiratory tract. The lower in the respiratory tract, the lower the bioburden. Common causes of upper and lower respiratory tract infections are *S. pneumoniae* and *H. influenzae*. Atypical pneumonia is caused by bacteria which don't have a cell wall and are not considered to be true members of the commensal flora: *Mycoplasma pneumoniae, Legionella pneumophila* and *Chlamydia pneumophila* (see Chapter 4.4 for diagnosis and treatment of atypical pneumonia). *Candida* spp. and *Aspergillus niger* can also be found in the ear canal and are common causes of otomycosis.

The larynx, trachea, bronchioles and lower airways are considered to be sterile, although transient colonization with secretions of the upper respiratory tract may occur after aspiration.

GASTROINTESTINAL TRACT

The commensal flora in the oesophagus contains a mixture of oropharyngeal flora and commensal flora inhabiting the stomach by swallowing or from the stomach by reflux.

The low pH and rapid peristalsis in the stomach suppress persistent colonization by many bacteria; only *Helicobacter pylori* persist in this environment. The most prevalent bacteria in the stomach are *Prevotella* spp., streptococci, *Veillonella* spp. and *Rothia* spp. Acidic pH and bile in the small intestine prevent bacterial colonization. Bacteria found in the lower parts of the small intestine are lactobacilli, enterococci, Gram-positive aerobes and facultative anaerobes with *Streptococcus* being the dominant genus.

The colon has the highest bacterial density and variety, approximately 10^{11} bacteria/mL, of which the most prevalent bacteria are the group of *Bacteroides* spp. Other prevalent microbes are streptococci, enterococci, *Clostridium*, lactobacilli, *Enterobacterales*, *Bifidobacteria* and *Corynebacteria*.

Infections with gastrointestinal flora are seen in gut perforation or anastomotic leakage, cholangitis and cholecystitis; most commonly, *Escherichia coli, Klebsiella* spp., viridans streptococci and *Bacteroides fragilis*. Streptococci of the milleri group are associated with abscess formation. Persistent fever despite antibiotic treatment should prompt for abdominal imaging to exclude liver abscesses or intra-abdominal collections.

In patients with prolonged antibiotic therapy and inadequate source control, antibiotic-resistant organisms such as *Enterococus*, *Pseudomonas aeruginosa* and *Candida* spp. become involved in the infection.

Bacterial translocation to the bloodstream can occur in patients with mucositis caused by chemotherapy.

The most common bacteria seen are viridans streptococci, enterococci and *E. coli*. Finally, diet has a marked influence on the relative composition of the intestinal microbiota.

VAGINAL FLORA

The composition of the vaginal microbiota varies with age, pH and hormonal levels. It is further influenced by menstrual cycle and during pregnancy. Sexual and hygienic practices may also play a role. A healthy vaginal microbiota consists mostly of *Lactobacilli* spp. Bacterial vaginosis is a common cause of vaginal discharge caused by vaginal inflammation and is a result of overgrowth of anaerobic microorganisms such as *Gardnerella vaginalis* and *Prevotella*, *Peptostreptococcus* and *Bacteroides* spp. Group B streptococci are present in up to 40% of women and can cause severe neonatal sepsis and meningitis. Many women are asymptomatic carriers of *Ureaplasma urealyticum* in the cervix or vagina. However, it can be sexually transmitted and cause urethritis in men and genital tract infections in women.

SKIN

In the first few days or weeks of life, the skin of newborns becomes colonized with coagulase-negative staphylococci, with *S. epidermidis*, *S. warneri* and *S. haemolyticus* as the most prevalent species. Other skin flora are *Propionibacterium acnes*, *Staphylococcus aureus*, beta-haemolytic streptococci, α-haemolytic streptococci (viridans streptococci), *Corynebacterium* spp., enterococci and anaerobes. Yeasts are often present in skin folds.

Because of constant exposure to the environment, the skin is prone to transient colonization. For instance, *Enterobacterales*, which are predominantly gastrointestinal colonizers, can also been found on the extremities.

Cellulitis and erysipelas are caused by *S. aureus* and *Streptococcus pyogenes*, also called group A *Streptococcus* (GAS). Necrotizing fasciitis is a life-threatening, rapidly spreading, often polymicrobial infection involving GAS, *Clostridium perfringens*, *Bacteroides* spp. and coliforms. Major pathogens associated with diabetic ulcer infections are *S. aureus*, β-haemolytic streptococci, *Pseudomonas aeruginosa* and also anaerobes and coliforms.

URINARY TRACT

With new molecular techniques, it has now been found that the urinary tract has its own commensal flora. The most common cause of urinary tract infections are *Escherichia coli* and *Klebsiella pneumoniae*. In patients with an indwelling catheter, *Pseudomonas aeruginosa* and enterococci are more frequently seen.

HOSPITAL FLORA

During hospitalization, the respiratory tract, gastrointestinal tract and skin can become colonized with multidrug-resistant bacteria including *Enterobacterales*, methicillin-resistant *Staphylococcus aureus*, *Pseudomonas aeruginosa*, *Acinetobacter baumannii* and vancomycin-resistant enterococci. Depending on local epidemiology, empirical therapy for hospital acquired infections should be targeted against these organisms.

CLINICAL PEARL

Most pathogenic bacteria that are part of our commensal flora are associated with a wide spectrum of clinical diseases. Bacteria that infect us through vectors typically cause specific diseases. Examples are *Borrelia burgdorferi*, which causes Lyme disease, and *Rickettsia* spp.

CLINICAL APPROACH

Clinical symptoms and radiology findings can help determine the site of infection. Knowledge of the commensal flora can then inform choice of empirical antibiotics.

Conversely, detection of bacteria in clinical specimens can help determine the source of infection and guide medical imaging and source control.

Medical conditions, drugs and medical procedures are risk factors for bacterial infections. In combination with the clinical picture, often an assumption can be made as to which organisms may be involved.

POOR DENTAL HYGIENE

Poor dental hygiene is a risk factor for periodontitis involving bacteria such as *Porphyromonas gingivalis*, *Tannerella forsythia* and *Treponema denticola*. *Aggregatibacter actinomycetemcomitans* has been linked to highly aggressive periodontitis. Transient bacterial translocation from oropharynx into the bloodstream is common. Poor dental hygiene and dental procedures are known contributors. Although often asymptomatic, in the presence of an abnormal heart valve, such bacteraemia can cause endocarditis. Common causes of endocarditis are viridans streptococci and bacteria from the HACEK group, all of which are part of the oropharyngeal commensal flora.

UNDERLYING MEDICAL CONDITIONS

Patients with Barrett's oesophagus and oesophageal carcinoma have a shift towards Gram-negative anaerobes in oesophageal flora. Colorectal cancer is associated with infections with *Streptococcus bovis*, causing bloodstream infection and endocarditis. *Clostridium septicum* can cause bloodstream infection or gas gangrene in patients with colorectal cancer, haematological malignancy, immunosuppression or diabetes mellitus.

Gallstones can lead to biliary stasis, bacterial overgrowth causing cholangitis and cholecystitis and bacterial translocation. Bacteria involved are predominantly *Enterobacterales*. Nasolacrimal duct obstruction can cause infection of the lacrimal sac, also called dacryocystitis. The main pathogens are *S. pneumoniae* and *S. aureus*.

DRUGS

Treatment of gastroesophageal reflux and peptic ulcer disease with antacids, H2-receptor antagonists and proton-pump inhibitors decreases acidity of the stomach and allows pathogens like *Salmonella* spp. to survive and cause gastrointestinal infections. Especially, treatment with proton-pump inhibitors is a well-known risk factor for *Clostridioides difficile*.

Antimicrobial drugs directly alter gut microbiota, decreasing its colonization resistance and facilitating colonization with drug-resistant bacteria and infection with *C. difficile*.

WOUNDS AND BREAKS IN THE SKIN AND MUCOSA

The bacterial flora on the skin protects individuals against colonization by pathogens. Conversely, skin flora can become pathogenic if the organisms penetrate the skin (e.g. when there is a wound). Cellulitis and erysipelas are predominantly caused by *S. aureus* and *Streptococcus pyogenes*. *Staphylococcus epidermidis* is a common skin colonizer and not associated with wound infections. However, this species may cause bloodstream infections in the presence of indwelling devices. Patients who receive chemotherapy for treatment of their underlying malignancy are at risk for mucositis, which increases the risk of bacterial translocation with gut flora. Patients with graft-versus-host disease affecting the skin or gut are at risk for infection.

VIRAL INFECTIONS

A complication of viral respiratory infections is bacterial superinfections with *Streptococcus pneumoniae* and *Staphylococcus aureus*. Group A streptococcal soft tissue infections can complicate varicella zoster infection.

MEDICAL DEVICES

Coagulase-negative staphylococci form biofilms on intravascular catheters and are the leading cause of intravascular catheter-associated bloodstream infections. Other major pathogens are *S. aureus*, enterococci, Gram-negative rods and *Candida* spp. Bladder catheters are a risk factor for catheter-associated urinary tract infections, predominantly caused by *E. coli*, *K. pneumoniae*, *P. aeruginosa* and enterococci.

PROSTHETIC DEVICES

The most common cause of prosthetic joint infections are coagulase-negative staphylococci and *Propionibacterium acnes* introduced during or after surgery. They adhere to foreign bodies and form biofilms, making these infections difficult to treat. Prosthetic joint infections can also arise from haematogenous spread with predominantly *S. aureus*.

INFECTIONS IN THE IMMUNOCOMPROMISED HOST

Pseudomonas aeruginosa and *Acinetobacter baumannii* are low-virulent, environmental bacteria that can colonize and cause infections in immunocompromised hosts. They are also called opportunistic agents, and because of multiple antibiotic-resistance mechanisms, they are difficult to treat. Profound neutropaenia is a significant risk factor for fungal infections with *Aspergillus* spp. and *Candida* spp.

BIBLIOGRAPHY

Bennett JE, Dolin R, Blaser MJ. *Mandell, Douglas, and Bennett's Principles and Practice of Infectious Diseases*. Philadelphia, PA: Elsevier/Saunders, 2015.
Versalovic J, Carroll KC, Funke G, Jorgensen JH, Landry ML, Warnock DW. *Manual of Clinical Microbiology*, 10th ed. American Society of Microbiology, 2011.

2.2 Diagnosing Bacterial Infections

Firza Alexander Gronthoud

CLINICAL CONSIDERATIONS

Bacterial infections are most often caused by our own commensal flora (endogenous infection). Commensal flora can cause infection when organisms gain entrance to body sites outside their natural habitat. Diagnosis of bacterial infections depends on taking an appropriate specimen from the suspected site of infection for microbiological investigations. To determine which body site and which bacteria are involved, it is worthwhile to consider the following.

SYNDROMIC APPROACH

Clinical symptoms and radiological findings can give clues to which organ system may be involved (see Appendix 6.1).

PATIENT-RELATED FACTORS

If the site of infection is not clear from the initial diagnostic work-up, it may be helpful to consider patient-specific risk factors to guide microbiological work-up and choosing which empirical antimicrobials to use:

- *Skin defects* including skin abrasions, eczema and wounds can become colonized with potential pathogens which may either harmlessly colonize the skin defect or, via contiguous spread, cause deep wound infections, soft tissue infections, bone infections and bloodstream infections. Commensal flora involved: *Staphylococcus aureus*, coagulase-negative staphylococci, beta-haemolytic streptococci (including groups A, C and G) or environmental flora including *Pseudomonas aeruginosa*, *Serratia marcescens* and *Acinetobacter baumannii*.
- *Mucositis* due to chemotherapy and radiotherapy increases risk of bacterial translocation into the bloodstream. Commensal flora involved are oropharyngeal and gastrointestinal flora, including streptococci, enterococci and anaerobes.
- *Reduced gastric acidity* due to use of proton-pump inhibitors or H2 blockers increases gastric pH and allows for survival of ingested bacteria such as *Salmonella* and *Clostridium difficile*.
- *Gut defects*: Gut contents may leak into the peritoneum after an anastomotic leak or gut perforation. Commensal flora involved are *Enterobacterales*, anaerobes, and streptococci. Early pathogenic role of enterococci is controversial.
- *Preceding viral infections* may facilitate a bacterial superinfection. Most common examples are influenza followed by *Streptococcus pneumoniae* pneumonia or chickenpox followed by group A *Streptococcus* soft tissue infection.
- *Dehydration* is linked to increased risk of urinary tract infection (UTI). Main pathogens involved are *Escherichia coli* and *Klebsiella pneumoniae*. Especially, elderly patients may present with confusion, acute kidney injury and hypotension.

- *Immunodeficiency*
  - *Asplenia*: Decreased ability of macrophages to filter the blood from capsulated bacteria including *S. pneumoniae, Haemophilus influenzae, N. meningitidis.*
  - *Neutropenia*: Neutrophils of less than 500 μmol/L significantly increase risk of bacterial infections from Gram-negative rods—members of the *Enterobacterales*, non-fermenters including *P. aeruginosa*—and Gram-positive cocci—streptococci, enterococci.
  - *Chronic granulomatous disease*: Due to a lack of NADPH oxidase, phagocytes are unable to kill foreign invaders and neutrophil activity is not regulated. Increased risk of infections due to catalase-positive bacteria and bacteria resistant to nonoxidative killing: *S. aureus, S. marcescens, E. coli, K. pneumoniae, Nocardia* spp. and *Burkholderia cepacian* complex.
  - *HIV*: Increased risk of non-typhoidal *Salmonella* bloodstream infections.
  - *Genetic or acquired deficiencies*: Patients with genetic or acquired deficiencies in early complement components are primarily susceptible to invasive bacterial disease.
- *Underlying pulmonary disease*: Asthma, COPD and bronchiectasis are important risk factors for pneumonia. Common pathogens include *S. pneumoniae, H. influenzae, S. aureus* and non-fermenters including *P. aeruginosa, Stenotrophomonas maltophilia, B. cepacian* complex and *Achromobacter xylosoxidans*.
- *Intravascular catheter and bladder catheter* results in increased risk of bloodstream infection or UTI. The most common pathogens causing intravascular catheter-associated bloodstream infections include coagulase-negative staphylococci, enterococci and *S. aureus*. Most common pathogens associated with catheter-associated UTIs are *E. coli, K. pneumoniae*, enterococci and *P. aeruginosa*.
- *Prosthetic joints or prosthetic valves*: Bacteria infect devices during implantation or after surgery via hematogenous spread or contiguous spread from an overlying wound or injury. Infection during implantation is caused by skin flora such as *S. aureus*, coagulase-negative staphylococci or *Propionibacterium* spp. Antibacterial treatment in late infections should cover *Staphylococcus aureus*, streptococci, *Enterobacterales* and *P. aeruginosa*.
- *Post-operative infections*: Anastomotic leak or perforation with developing intra-abdominal collection, surgical site infection, pneumonia or UTI.

ANIMAL EXPOSURE

Some bacteria have an animal reservoir and can cause infections through direct or indirect exposure to animals:

- Pneumonitis/hepatitis/pericarditis/endocarditis and contact with sheep, cattle or goats: Q fever caused by *Coxiella burnetii*
- Respiratory symptoms and contact with horses: *Rhodococcus equi*
- Wound infection with sepsis or haemorrhagic pneumonia and history of contact with sheep: Suspicion of anthrax caused by *Bacillus anthracis*
- Wound infection and/or sepsis and history of recent dog or cat bite: *Pasteurella multocida, Capnocytophaga canimorsus* and *Staphylococcus intermedius*
- Undifferentiated chronic fever with night sweats and weight loss or signs of arthritis/spondylitis and contact with sheep and goats or consuming unpasteurized dairy products, i.e. milk: *Brucella melitensis* or *Brucella abortus*
- Gastroenteritis, septic profile or meningoencephalitis and consuming unpasteurized dairy products: *Listeria monocytogenes*
- Endocarditis and previous contact with sheep and goats: *C. burnetii* and *Brucella* spp.
- Freshwater exposure, i.e. rafting, waterfalls or local canals and rivers: Leptospirosis

Arthropod-borne infections are infections transmitted through vectors carrying the pathogen and transmitting them to humans through bites.

- *Rickettsial disease*: Fever, lymphadenopathy, rash, splenomegaly; eschar usually seen.
  - Rocky Mountain spotted fever (*Rickettsia rickettsia*); tick-borne (*Ixodes* spp.)
  - African typhus (*R. conorii, R. africae*); tick-borne (*Ixodes* spp.)
  - Epidemic typhus (*R. prowazeckii*); louse-borne (*Pediculus humanus*)
  - Endemic murine typhus (*R. typhi*); rat flea-borne (*Xenopsylla cheopis*)
  - Scrub typhus (*Orientia tsutsugamushi*); chigger-borne (larval form of trombiculid mite)
- *Lyme disease*: Caused by *Borrelia burgdorferi*; tick-borne (*Ixodes* spp.)
  - Erythema migrans (stage 1 after days–1 month)
  - Arthritis/myocarditis/arrhythmia/Bell's palsy/fatigue (stage 2 after weeks–months)
  - Encephalitis/meningitis (stage 3 after months–years)

FOOD-BORNE INFECTIONS

Improper handling and cooking of food can increase risk of food-borne infections. After an initial incubation period (see Chapter 6.5), symptoms such as fever, diarrhoea and vomiting, and in severe cases, bloody diarrhoea, sepsis and neurological complications, may occur:

- Gastroenteritis and seafood: *Plesiomonas shigelloides, Aeromonas* spp.
- Gastroenteritis and rice: *Bacillus cereus, Staphylococcus aureus* and *Clostridium perfringens*
- Gastroenteritis and undercooked meat or chicken: *Salmonella* spp., *Campylobacter* spp.
- Bloody diarrhoea and vegetables: Enterohaemorrhagic *E. coli* (EHEC) O105:H7 and *E. coli* O104
- Gastroenteritis, sepsis +/− meningoencephalitis and unpasteurized milk: *Listeria monocytogenes*
- Undifferentiated fever and unpasteurized milk: *Brucella*

SEXUALLY TRANSMITTED DISEASES

- Genital ulcer with or without local lymphadenopathy: *Treponema pallidum* (syphilis or lues), *Haemophilus ducreyi*
- Genital discharge: *Chlamydia trachomatis* and *Neisseria gonorrhoea, Mycoplasma genitalium*

CLINICAL APPROACH

Chapter 2.8 outlines how to collect samples and how to interpret microbiology results.
   General rules to ensure optimal sample quality, microbiology results and antibiotic therapy:

- *Timing of cultures*: Samples taken after administration of antibiotic may lead to false-negative results, which can increase the cost, length of stay for the patient and unnecessary prolongation or broad-spectrum antibiotics.
- Common specimens for sepsis of unknown source are two sets of blood cultures, a urine culture and a sputum sample.
- *Choosing the right specimen*: Avoid sending a urine sample in a patient with a respiratory tract infection as it may lead to unnecessary treatment of asymptomatic bacteriuria.
- Samples should be collected aseptically.
- Transport time should be less than 2 hours. Otherwise samples should be stored between 2°C and 8°C, except blood cultures and cerebrospinal fluid (CSF), which should ideally be stored at 37°C in an incubator. Blood cultures may alternatively be stored at room temperature.

BIBLIOGRAPHY

Bennett JE, Dolin R, Blaser MJ. *Mandell, Douglas, and Bennett's Principles and Practice of Infectious Diseases*. Philadelphia, PA: Elsevier/Saunders, 2015.

Jorgensen JH et al. *Manual of Clinical Microbiology*, 11th ed. American Society of Microbiology, 2015.

Miller JM et al. A guide to utilization of the microbiology laboratory for diagnosis of infectious diseases: 2018 update by the Infectious Diseases Society of America and the American Society for Microbiology. *Clin Infect Dis*. 31 August 2018;67(6):e1–e94.

2.3 Diagnosing Viral Infections

Firza Alexander Gronthoud

CLINICAL CONSIDERATIONS

Diagnosis of bacterial infections depends on isolating microbes from a specimen collected from the site of infection. Viruses, on the other hand, may disseminate from one site to another during the course of infection. The indication for virology testing, specimen type, the choice between serology or PCR and timing of specimen collection is intrinsically linked to the clinical syndrome and the stage of infection. It is therefore worthwhile to consider the following.

INCUBATION PERIOD AND WINDOW PHASE

The period between inoculation and clinical symptoms is called the incubation period. The window phase is the time between infection and development of antibodies (immunity). It is useful to be familiar with the incubation period and window phase of common viral infections because:

- They determine when to request either serology or PCR as it takes the human body time to develop antibodies and the virus may only have a limited period of viraemia.
- The type of exposure and occurrence of symptoms may help to determine if a virus could be involved.

TRANSMISSION

Viruses can be transmitted through various routes of exposure. Combining this with clinical symptoms and laboratory findings can narrow down the potential viruses involved.

- Fecal-oral route, i.e. enterovirus, hepatitis A
- Inhalation of aerosols and droplets, i.e. measles, varicella zoster
- Arthropod-borne, i.e. dengue virus, Zika virus and West Nile virus
- Sexually transmitted, i.e. hepatitis B and HIV
- Blood-borne, i.e. HIV, hepatitis B and C

SHEDDING

Depending on the stage of infection, viruses can be directly found in bodily fluids such as blood, urine, respiratory secretions, stool and CSF by using molecular tests aimed at detecting viral DNA or RNA. Viruses can be transmitted to the environment and people via shedding in urine, stool and respiratory secretions. Viral shedding can occur before symptoms develop until even after the infection has been resolved and the individual is asymptomatic. Immunocompromised individuals can shed the virus for a longer time than immunocompetent individuals. Viruses which cause latent infections can intermittently reactivate during life and be shed in bodily fluids. This may or may not cause any symptoms. Knowledge of shedding and transmission of viruses helps determine the type and duration of infection control precautions to use.

BEHAVIOUR OF VIRUSES (CELL TROPISM)

Viruses are intracellular organisms and can be transmitted via various routes. Once inside the human body, they can replicate at the site of inoculation and have the ability to disseminate throughout the human body and reach various organs, causing organ-specific symptoms. Viruses have a preference to infect specific cells and tissues (cell tropism), and the clinical picture may thus give a clue which viruses may be involved.

LATENT INFECTIONS

Some viruses such as herpesviruses, adenovirus and polyoma viruses are not cleared by the human body. After an initial infection, they remain latent present in specific cells. After a dormant period, they can reactivate and cause both symptomatic and asymptomatic infection. The serologic status of patients may help decide whether some herpes viruses are latent present to decide whether prophylactic antiviral treatment should be started when a period of immunocompromise is expected.

METHODS TO DETECT VIRAL INFECTIONS

The main tools to directly detect the virus are using molecular tests such as polymerase chain reaction (PCR) and Loop Mediated Isothermal Amplification (LAMP). If the period of viraemia or viral shedding stage has passed, it may then be useful to investigate whether virus specific antibodies or antigens can be detected in serum. The first type of antibodies produced is IgM and usually disappears after weeks to months. IgG can be formed simultaneously but, more often, are produced in later stages and detectable for life, which may confer lifelong protection. Because some antibodies are produced early in the infection and can persist for life or fall below the detectable limit again, it may be necessary to repeat the serological test after several weeks to see if there are any changes in antibody titre.

CLINICAL PEARL

Rapid diagnosis of viral infections can:

- Prevent unnecessary diagnostic procedures
- Facilitate early discontinuation of antibiotic therapy
- Minimize risk of antibiotic resistance
- Facilitate rapid implementation of infection control precautions

RECURRENT INFECTIONS

It may take some time before the immune system offers adequate protection against viral infections. This is why children may experience recurrent infections with some viruses, whilst in adults, these viral infections are rare, i.e. rotavirus. For some viruses, the immune system may only provide temporary protection, i.e. respiratory viruses. Viruses can have many serotypes and protection against one virus may not guarantee protection against a different serotype, i.e. dengue virus.

EMPIRICAL ANTIVIRAL TREATMENT

Empirical treatment of bacterial infections consists of empirical antibiotic therapy with the highest likelihood of treating the infection before any pathogens are identified, whereas empirical treatment of viral infections is more challenging because:

- Antiviral agents have specific antiviral activity, are potentially toxic and are therefore only started upon strong clinical suspicion (i.e. in the case of herpes simplex) or a positive result.

- Different viruses may cause the same clinical syndrome but require different antiviral agents.
- There are no effective antiviral drugs for many viral infections including arboviruses, parainfluenza, polyoma viruses, parvovirus and measles.

CLINICAL APPROACH

MONONUCLEOSIS

- *Main viral causes*: Cytomegalovirus (CMV) and Epstein–Barr virus (EBV)
- *Route of infection*: Close contact with individuals shedding the virus in bodily fluids
- *Specimen type*: Serum
- *Test requests*: CMV IgM, CMV IgG, EBV VCA IgM, EBV VCA IgG, EBV EBNA
- *Specific for EBV*: Presence of atypical lymphocytes and presence of heterophile antibodies using Paul Brunel test
- *Caveat*: Cross-reaction may occur between CMV and EBV antibodies; antibodies against both viruses should be tested simultaneously and, if necessary, a convalescent serum sample in 3–4 weeks

CLINICAL PEARL

Throughout life, latent viruses can reactivate and cause asymptomatic shedding. These individuals are sources of transmission. Examples: Oropharyngeal shedding with CMV, EBV and herpes simplex virus (HSV); urinary shedding of BK virus and genital shedding of HSV.

RESPIRATORY INFECTIONS

- *Main viral causes*: Rhinovirus, enterovirus, adenovirus, coronavirus, respiratory syncytial virus (RSV), human metapneumovirus, influenza and parainfluenza.
- *Route of infection*: Respiratory transmission through aerosols and droplets.
- *Specimen type*: Upper and lower respiratory infection; nasopharyngeal swab (preferred) or an oropharyngeal swab in combination with a nose swab. A flexible swab should be used for nasopharyngeal sampling. Lower respiratory infection, a sputum sample or bronchoalveolar lavage may have a higher diagnostic yield but is more difficult to obtain.
- *Test request*: PCR for respiratory viruses. Most laboratories nowadays have a multiplex PCR which can detect common viral causes of respiratory tract infections.
- *Caveat*: Detection of the virus does not necessarily mean it is the cause of infection, as even after clinical infection, there may be a period of shedding. No official thresholds exist to differentiate between viral shedding post-infection and active infection. This is because PCR cannot differentiate between a viable infectious virus and residual viral nucleic acid.
- During seasonal periods, rapid point-of-care tests for influenza A and RSV may be useful. However, they have limited sensitivity, and especially in the beginning of the season when prevalence is still low, the negative predictive value is low and cannot be used to de-isolate a patient or hold off or even stop antiviral treatment.
- Some coronaviruses are linked to geographical areas and require a specific PCR assay: Middle East respiratory syndrome–coronavirus (MERS-CoV) and SARS.

GASTROENTERITIS

- *Main viral causes*: Rotavirus, enterovirus, adenovirus, norovirus, sapovirus and astrovirus
- *Route of infection*: Oral fecal transmission

- *Specimen type*: Stool
- *Test request*: Depending on local laboratory arsenals, rapid point-of-care tests for rotavirus, adenovirus and norovirus; molecular laboratories may have a multiplex PCR assay detecting the most common viral causes of gastroenteritis
- *Caveats*:
  - In immunocompromised patients with colitis, CMV, Epstein–Barr virus and HSV should also be considered. Colon biopsy, EDTA blood and stool should be collected for PCR. For CMV, the best specimen is a gut biopsy for the presence of nuclear inclusion bodies. A PCR-positive tissue sample does not discriminate between latent infection and active infection.
  - Rotavirus is the most important cause of gastroenteritis in young children. Because large amounts of rotavirus are shed in the stool during acute infection, an antigen detection test performed on a stool specimen is a cheap, rapid and sensitive test. Immunity against rotavirus takes years to develop, and that's why rotavirus is mainly seen in children. Severity of symptoms declines with repeated infections.

- Specimen collection date and relevant clinical data including antiviral chemotherapy should be documented on the request form.
- Viral swabs should be transported in viral transport medium. Pending transport, these swabs should be stored in a fridge between 2 and 8°C.
- Serum (or plasma) should be stored at –20°C unless nucleic acid detection is required such as for hepatitis C virus (HCV) or human immunodeficiency virus (HIV) viral load, in which case –70°C is recommended.
- Antenatal sera from pregnant women should be stored for at least one year.

MUCOCUTANEOUS LESIONS

- *Main viral causes*: HSV, varicella zoster virus (VZV), enterovirus
- *Specimen type*: For HSV or VZV samples, obtained by scraping the base of a lesion with a scalpel blade or rubbing it vigorously with a polyester or rayon swab and transport it in a sterile container with virus transport medium. In immunocompromised individuals, also EDTA blood
- *Test request*: For all specimen types, PCR
- *Caveats*:
  - Vesicular or ulcerative lesions are mostly caused by HSV or VZV and occasionally by enteroviruses.
  - Specific coxsackie viruses cause hand, foot and mouth disease.
  - Counterintuitively, the method of choice for detecting enteroviruses is a throat swab and stool sample for PCR.
- Other common viral infections of the skin or mucous membranes are caused by sexually transmitted viruses: human papilloma virus and molluscum contagiosum. Molluscum contagiosum is mainly a clinical diagnosis. Infection with HPV can be established with PCR on cervical smears.

HEPATITIS

Meningitis

- *Main viral causes of acute infection*: Enteroviruses, HSV type 2 (HSV-2) and VZV
- *Route of infection*: Reactivation or following primary infection
- *Specimen type*: CSF

- *Test request*: PCR
- *Caveats*:
  - HSV meningitis, usually caused by HSV-2, is a common cause of aseptic meningitis. This illness occurs with or without concomitant genital lesions and can have recurrent episodes.
  - Varicella zoster meningitis can occur as a complication of either chickenpox or herpes zoster and can occur with or without cutaneous lesions. Varicella zoster can be detected in CSF from patients with herpes zoster without any CNS involvement.

Encephalitis

- *Main viral causes*: HSV-1 is the most common cause
- *Route of infection*: Reactivation
- *Specimen type*: CSF
- *Test request*: PCR
- *Caveats*:
  - HSV-1 encephalitis typically shows haemorrhagic lesions in the temporal lobe and, untreated, is associated with high morbidity and mortality. If strong suspicion of HSV encephalitis and initial PCR on CSF was negative, repeat PCR after a few days.
  - *Opportunistic infections in immunocompromised individuals*: Besides HSV, VZV and enterovirus, the PCR panel should include other neurotropic viruses including CMV, EBV and adenovirus. Epstein–Barr virus causes primary CNS lymphoma in patients with AIDS. It rarely presents with neurological manifestations including encephalitis, aseptic meningitis, transverse myelitis, acute cerebellar ataxia and acute demyelinating encephalomyelitis. Reactivation of John Cunningham virus in HIV and transplant recipients leads to progressive multifocal leukoencephalopathy (PML). A negative PCR may not rule out PML as the sensitivity is around 70%.

CLINICAL PEARL

Arboviruses are transmitted through arthropods and cause endemic CNS infections: St Louis and West Nile viruses in the United States, tick-borne encephalitis in central and eastern Europe and Russia and Japanese encephalitis in Asia, western Pacific countries, and northern Australia. Diagnosis relies on detecting IgM antibodies in serum and CSF. The sensitivity of these tests approaches 100% by the tenth day of illness. Molecular testing is only useful in the first few days of infection because of the transient and low viral load in blood and CSF.

VIRAL RASHES IN PREGNANT WOMEN

- *Main viral causes*: Measles, parvovirus, VZV, rubella
- *Route of transmission*: Droplet
- *Specimen type*: Serology on clotted blood, PCR on respiratory samples, EDTA blood and urine

CONGENITAL INFECTIONS

- *Main viral causes*: CMV, HSV, parvovirus
- *Route of transmission*: Intra-uterine
- *Specimen type*: CMV: mother, EDTA blood; fetus, urine for CMV PCR in first week of life. HSV: mother, if genital vesicle, swab; neonate, oropharyngeal swab for PCR. Parvovirus: mother, EDTA blood; fetus, amniotic fluid for PCR
- *Test request*: PCR on fetal samples; mother, PCR on blood and vesicle. Also parvovirus IgM and IgG, CMV IgM and IgG

SCREENING

Serology can be used to determine the immune status. Depending on the nature of screening (prenatal or pre-transplant or before starting biologicals), the following tests may be requested:

- CMV IgG, EBV VCA IgG, EBV EBNA IgG, HSV IgG, VZV IgG, measles IgG, rubella IgG, parvovirus B19 IgG, hepatitis A IgG, HbsAg. Although not a virus, toxoplasma IgG and syphilis are often included.

BIBLIOGRAPHY

Bennett JE, Dolin R, Blaser MJ, Mandell, GL, Douglas, RG. *Mandell, Douglas, and Bennett's Principles and Practice of Infectious Diseases*, Philadelphia, PA: Elsevier/Saunders, 2015.
Fields BN, Knipe DM, Howley PM. *Fields Virology*. Philadelphia [u.a.]: Wolters Kluwer|Lippincott Williams & Wilkins, 2013.

2.4 Diagnosing Invasive Fungal Infections

Firza Alexander Gronthoud

CLINICAL CONSIDERATIONS

Invasive fungal infections (IFI) are caused by yeasts and moulds, each with their own population at risk and clinical manifestations. Candidaemia and intra-abdominal candidiasis are the leading causes of fungal infections in critically ill patients; profound neutropaenia is a major risk factor for invasive pulmonary mould infections, predominantly caused by *Aspergillus* spp. *Cryptococcus* spp. are a major cause of meningitis in patients with HIV. *Pneumocystis jirovecii* is an opportunistic pathogen in patients with HIV and other immunocompromised individuals. The choice of diagnostic tests depends on the population at risk and diagnosis is often delayed, leading to high morbidity and mortality. It is therefore worthwhile to consider the following.

POPULATION AT RISK FOR MOULD INFECTION

- Most mould infections are caused by *Aspergillus* spp.
- Diabetes mellitus: Rhino-orbital-cerebral infection caused by *Aspergillus* spp. and Mucorales
- Critically ill patients with influenza, on high-dose steroids for severe COPD or patients with Child-Pugh C hepatic cirrhosis or immune paralysis post-sepsis are at high risk for pulmonary aspergillosis
- Profound neutropaenia, most often seen in patients with haematological malignancies, i.e. allogeneic HSCT recipient or patients receiving induction chemotherapy for AML and ALL treatment. Predominantly caused by *Aspergillus* spp., less often Mucorales, *Fusarium* spp. and *Scedosporium* spp.
- Solid organ transplant recipients: Pulmonary infection caused by *Aspergillus* spp. and Mucorales
- Individuals on high-dose corticosteroid treatment (16–25 mg of prednisolone per day or ≥ 4 mg dexamethasone daily for ≥ 4 weeks)

RISK FACTORS FOR INVASIVE CANDIDOSIS

- Long-term or repeated treatment with broad-spectrum antibacterial agents promotes *Candida* colonization.
- Chemo- or radiotherapy causes mucositis, facilitating *Candida* translocation into the bloodstream.
- Intravascular catheter (dialysis, total parenteral nutrition) is a risk factor for candidaemia.
- Intra-abdominal surgery: *Candida* translocation into the blood stream or intra-abdominal candidosis.
- Immunocompromise further facilitates invasive disease.
- Critically ill patients often have one or more of the above risk factors and are at particular risk for invasive candidosis (IC).

POPULATION AT RISK FOR *CRYPTOCOCCUS* SPP.

- *Cryptococcus* spp. are mainly associated with meningitis, rarely pneumonia
- HIV: CD4 counts <150 cells/μL, with a median CD4 count of 50 cells/μL
- Solid organ transplant recipients

POPULATION AT RISK FOR *PNEUMOCYSTIS JIROVECII*

- Individuals infected with HIV and CD4 cell count <200 cells/μL who are not on *Pneumocystis jirovecii* pneumonia (PJP) prophylaxis
- Haematological or solid organ malignancies receiving chemotherapy or undergoing transplant and not on PJP prophylaxis
- High-dose corticosteroid therapy

DISEASE PRESENTATIONS AND MOST COMMON FUNGI ISOLATED

- Brain abscess: *Aspergillus* spp., *Candida* spp., less commonly *Scedosporium* spp., Mucorales
- Meningitis: *Cryptococcus, Candida* spp.
- Sinusitis: *Aspergillus* spp., *Fusarium* spp., less commonly *Scedosporium* spp., Mucorales
- Ocular infection: *Candida* spp., *Aspergillus* spp. and *Fusarium* spp.
- Pulmonary infection: *Aspergillus* spp., *Pneumocystis jirovecii*, Mucorales, *Cryptococcus* spp.
- Intra-abdominal: *Candida* spp.
- Bone and joint: *Candida* spp.
- Fungaemia: *Candida* spp., *Fusarium* spp., *Histoplasma capsulatum, Scedosporium* spp., *Aspergillus terreus*
- Skin and soft tissue: *Fusarium* spp., *Scedosporium* spp., Mucorales

DIAGNOSTIC METHODS

- *Microscopy*
  - Can rapidly give an identification at genus level, i.e. *Candida* spp., *Aspergillus* spp. or Mucorales.
  - Presence of fungus in tissue is diagnostic for proven fungal infection.
  - Visualization of fungi by direct microscopy helps to confirm that the organism is in the sample rather than contamination.
  - Common stains used are lactophenol cotton blue stain and fluorescent dyes.
- *Culture*
  - Provides species identification and antifungal susceptibility testing.
  - Sensitivity of blood cultures for invasive candidosis is ~50%.
  - Blood cultures are rarely positive in mould infections, except disseminated infections with *Fusarium* spp.
  - For pulmonary infections, a bronchoalveolar lavage (BAL) or >3 sputum samples for microscopy and culture should be obtained. Overall sensitivity is ~50%.
  - Growth of *Aspergillus* spp. from respiratory samples represents infection, colonization or laboratory contamination and needs to be correlated with the clinical picture.
- *Serology*
  - Cryptococcal antigen in CSF or serum by rapid latex agglutination tests or lateral flow assay is highly sensitivity, >90%.
  - Galactomannan is a cell wall component of *Aspergillus* spp. and can be detected in serum and BAL. Sensitivity in serum from patients with haematological disease who are not on antimould prophylaxis is ~80% and drops to 20% if on antifungal

prophylaxis. Sensitivity is lowest in non-neutropaenic individuals, patients on intensive care or solid organ transplant recipients.

- 1,3-β-D-glucan (BDG) is a cell wall component of many fungi including *Aspergillus* spp., *Candida* spp. and *P. jirovecii*, but not *Cryptococcus* or Mucorales.
- BDG has an excellent negative predictive value for ruling out *P. jirovecii* and *Candida* spp. in all populations and ruling out invasive aspergillosis in neutropaenic patients with haematological malignancies.
- False-positive results with BDG can be seen with surgical gauzes containing glucan, dialysis with cellulose membrane, thrombocyte infusion with leukocyte-removing filters, human blood products, amoxicillin-clavulanate, piperacillin-tazobactam (old formulations) and Gram-negative bacteraemia.
- *Aspergillus* IgE is as part of diagnostic work-up for allergic bronchopulmonary aspergillosis and *Aspergillus* IgG is used for chronic pulmonary aspergillosis. A galactomannan is more useful in neutropaenic patients, whilst an Aspergillus IgG should be used in nonneutropaenic patients.
- *PCR*: Commercial and in-house PCRs have been developed for *Candida* spp., *Aspergillus* spp., Mucorales, *Cryptococcus* spp. and *P. jirovecii* with generally high sensitivities and can be used on various samples.
- *Pneumocystis jirovecii* PCR is more sensitive than microscopy and has high sensitivity on BAL and sputum. A PJP PCR should always be used in combination with a BDG on blood. A weak positive PCR and a negative BDG may indicate colonization rather than infection. A quantitative PCR may differentiate between colonization and infection, but no official cut-off values exist.

FACTORS AFFECTING ACCURACY OF FUNGAL TESTS

- Antifungal agents reduce sensitivity of antifungal tests.
- Blood culture, BAL and sputum sensitivity depend on fungal burden, and high volumes should be used, i.e. 40–50 mL blood for candidaemia.
- *Pneumocystis jirovecii* PCR sensitivity is highest within the first week of therapy.

CLINICAL PEARL

- Galactomannan, BDG, and *Aspergillus* PCR have a high negative predictive value to rule out invasive aspergillosis in patients with profound neutropaenia. Positive predictive value is higher if disease prevalence is higher.
- BDG has excellent negative predictive value for ruling out *Pneumocystis jirovecii*, especially if the lactate dehydrogenase (LDH) is < 350 U/mL.

CLINICAL PEARL

Tissue samples should be sent to:

- Microbiology laboratory for microscopy and culture (and PCR if available) AND
- Histopathology for H&E on histopathology slides, Grocott silver stain or periodic acid-Schiff (PAS) for fungi, Ziehl–Neelsen stain for mycobacteria and Gram stain for bacteria and fungi

IMAGING

- Chest radiographs may be normal in neutropenic patients with invasive pulmonary aspergillosis and preferred method is high-resolution CT.
- Common CT finding of *P. jirovecii* is bilateral ground-glass with peripheral sparing.
- The halo sign is an early feature of invasive aspergillosis, but may also be caused by other fungi and bacteria.
- The inversed halo sign is more common with mucormycosis than aspergillosis.
- Nodules larger than 1 cm are suggestive of invasive fungal disease; in mucormycosis >10 nodules can be seen.
- Areas of consolidation on CT provide locations for targeted BAL.
- Early bone destruction can be subtle with fungal sinusitis, and a repeat imaging should be performed.
- Fungal cerebral abscesses appear as enhancing ring lesions on neuroimaging.
- Cerebral aspergillosis and mucormycosis might also appear as cerebral infarction with haemorrhage.

CLINICAL APPROACH

SUSPICION OF INVASIVE FUNGAL INFECTION (IFI)

The following questions can help determine the presence of an IFI:

- Is the patient persistently febrile despite ≥36 hours of antibiotic treatment?
- Does the patient belong to a population at risk for IFI?
- Is the patient on any antifungal prophylaxis?
  - Fluconazole reduces likelihood of invasive candidiasis
  - Voriconazole or posaconazole reduces likelihood of invasive candidiasis and aspergillosis if prophylactic levels have been attained
  - Trimethoprim/sulfamethoxazole significantly reduces the risk of *Pneumocystis jirovecii* pneumonia. Alternatively pentamidine inhalation, dapsone or atovaquone can be used, but there is less evidence regarding their effectiveness

NEUTROPAENIC PATIENT WITH PERSISTENT FEVER *OR* NEW PULMONARY SYMPTOMS/NEW INFILTRATES ON CHEST X-RAY

- High-resolution CT.
- Blood culture from any intravascular device and peripheral set.
- Depending on CT finding and underlying risk factors: Bronchoscopy for PCR: cytomegalovirus, *Pneumocystis jirovecii*, respiratory viruses AND microscopy + culture: bacteria, fungi and mycobacteria (Ziehl–Neelsen stain).
- Galactomannan preferably on BAL, alternatively on serum.
- Serum BDG with LDH if no respiratory sample for *Pneumocystis jirovecii* available.
- If travel to endemic region: histoplasma antigen in urine or serum for *Coccidioides* antibody.
- Review with CT finding, microbiology results and biomarkers.
- If CT chest is compatible with fungal infection, pending results from microbiological investigations and biomarkers: start antifungal therapy with caspofungin or liposomal amphotericin B.
- If CT chest is negative and patient was on prophylactic antifungal therapy with prophylactic levels, continue antifungal prophylaxis but look for other sources of infection and review with microbiology results.

NEUTROPAENIC SEPSIS WITH SKIN LESIONS

- Cutaneous lesions with papules: *Candida* spp., *Aspergillus* spp., *P. marneffei*, *Cryptococcus* spp., histoplasmosis
- Necrotizing skin lesion(s)s: *Fusarium* spp., *Aspergillus* spp.; less often, Mucorales
- In <10%, candidaemia can be accompanied by erythematous small papules and macules
- Blood cultures from any intravascular device and peripheral set
- Biopsy of skin lesions for microscopy and culture for bacteria, fungi and mycobacteria and for histopathology
- Serum1,3-β-D-glucan or galactomannan if aspergillosis is suspected. If the patient is nonneutropaenic, an Aspergillus IgG instead of a galactomannan should be requested
- If travel to endemic region: histoplasma antigen in urine

ICU PATIENTS WITH PERSISTENT SEPSIS

- Most likely fungi involved: *Candida* spp. or *Aspergillus* spp.
- Most common presentations are candidaemia and intra-abdominal candidiasis; less often, invasive pulmonary aspergillosis
- Blood cultures from any intravascular line + peripheral blood culture set
- Drain fluids or aspiration from any pus collection for microscopy and culture OR BAL if aspergillosis is suspected
- Chest X-ray and consider high-resolution CT
- CT abdomen with contrast if abdomen a possible source
- Serum1,3-β-D-glucan or galactomannan if aspergillosis is suspected. If the patient is nonneutropaenic, an Aspergillus IgG instead of a galactomannan should be requested
- Consider dilated fundoscopy and echocardiogram
- If travel to endemic region, histoplasma antigen in urine

CLINICAL PEARL

Persistently positive tests despite on appropriate antifungal therapy might suggest resistance, low antifungal concentrations or a source control issue, i.e. inadequate drainage or presence of intravascular device, foreign bodies or aspergilloma requiring surgical resection.

SUSPECTED MENINGITIS OR ENCEPHALITIS IN IMMUNOCOMPROMISED PATIENTS

- CT or MRI brain
- Blood cultures from any intravascular device and peripheral set
- Lumbar puncture (LP) for opening pressure (elevated in cryptococcosis) and CSF for cryptococcal rapid antigen or lateral flow test or India ink stain or cryptococcal PCR AND microscopy + culture for bacteria, fungi, mycobacteria AND PCR for cytomegalovirus, Epstein–Barr virus, herpes simplex, varicella zoster, enterovirus, parechovirus, JC virus (HIV and HSCT recipients), HHV6 (HSCT recipients) and Toxoplasma (in HSCT recipients with a positive toxoplasma IgG)
- HIV serology
- In HIV-infected patients with CD4 count <100 cells/mL and travel to Southeast Asia, also consider *Talaromyces marneffei* (formerly known as *Penicillium marneffei*)

Fungal Sinusitis

- *Aspergillus* is the most common pathogen in immunocompromised people, also *Fusarium* spp., *Scedosporium* spp. and Mucorales
- Typical physical findings include sinus tenderness, ophthalmoplegia and proptosis
- Oropharyngeal necrotic black eschar-like lesions can be seen and should raise particular concern for mucormycosis
- CT scans or MRI show evidence of soft tissue masses and bony destruction.
- A biopsy or aspirated material should be obtained

BIBLIOGRAPHY

Brown GD, Denning DW, Gow NA, Levitz SM, Netea MG, White TC. Hidden killers: Human fungal infections. *Sci Transl Med*. 19 December 2012;4(165):165rv13.

Colombo AL, de Almeida Júnior JN, Slavin MA, Chen SC, Sorrell TC. Candida and invasive mould diseases in non-neutropenic critically ill patients and patients with haematological cancer. *Lancet Infect Dis*. November 2017;17(11):e344–e356.

Kosmidis C, Denning DW. The clinical spectrum of pulmonary aspergillosis. *Thorax*. March 2015;70(3):270–277.

Schelenz S, Barnes RA, Barton RC, Cleverley JR, Lucas SB, Kibbler CC, Denning DW; British Society for Medical Mycology. British Society for Medical Mycology best practice recommendations for the diagnosis of serious fungal diseases. *Lancet Infect Dis*. April 2015;15(4):461–474.

2.5 Diagnosing Parasitic Infections

Firza Alexander Gronthoud

CLINICAL CONSIDERATIONS

A parasite is an organism that needs a host to replicate and spread, causing harm to the host in the process. The most common reason to test for parasites are diarrhoea with or without a travel history, febrile illness after visiting known endemic areas or unexplained eosinophilia. Parasites can cause various clinical syndromes and occur in certain geographical areas or have a global distribution. Although for intestinal parasites, stool microscopy or PCR is the gold standard, diagnosis of blood- and tissue-dwelling parasites remains more challenging, with specific tests to be requested on appropriate specimens. It is therefore worthwhile to consider the following.

CLASSIFICATION OF PARASITES

Parasites can be classified as protozoa, helminths (worms) and ectoparasites. Protozoa are unicellular organisms and can be broadly divided into intestinal and luminal protozoa such as *Giardia lamblia*, *Cryptosporidium* spp. and blood- and tissue-dwelling protozoa such as malaria, *Leishmania*, *Trypanosoma cruzi* (Chagas) and *Trypanosoma brucei* (African sleeping sickness). Helminths are multicellular organisms and are associated with intestinal infections or tissue infections. They can be divided into nematodes (*Ascaris* spp., *Strongyloides stercoralis* and hook worm), trematodes or flukes (*Schistosoma* spp., *Fasciola hepatica*, *Paragonimus westermani*) and cestodes (*Taenia* spp. and *Hymenolepis nana*). Ectoparasites are also multicellular organisms that infest the skin and feed on it. Examples of ectoparasites are scabies, myiasis, tungiasis, fleas and lice.

LIFE CYCLE

All parasites have a life cycle whereby different stages may be spent in one or more hosts. Knowledge of the different life cycles may help decide which therapy and interventions to prevent transmission are likely to be effective.

DIARRHOEA

- *Giardia lamblia* is the most common cause. Classical symptoms are a chronic non-bloody, foul smelling, and greasy diarrhoea with weight loss.
- *Entamoeba histolytica* causes dysentery.
- *Cystoisospora belli* (formerly known as *Isospora belli*, *Cyclospora cayetanensis* and *Cryptosporidium* cause self-limiting watery diarrhoea in immunocompetent individuals which can last several weeks. Immunocompromised individuals are at risk of developing severe and prolonged infection with malabsorption and weight loss.
- *Enterocytozoon bieneusi* causes a persistent watery diarrhoea in patients with AIDS and bone marrow transplant recipients.
- *Necator americanus* and *Ancylostoma duodenale* (hookworm) may present with diarrhoea and anaemia.
- *Trichuris trichiura* (whipworm) infections present with rectal prolapse.

Weight Loss + Intestinal Symptoms (i.e. Steatorrhoea, Borborygmus, Flatulence, Abdominal Pain)

- *Giardia lamblia*
- Nematodes (*Strongyloides* and capillariasis)
- Schistosomiasis

Eosinophilia

Eosinophilia is typically seen in helminth infections and common in infections caused by filariasis, *Trichinella*, strongyloidiasis, hookworm, schistosomiasis and *Ascaris*. A more pronounced eosinophilia is seen in infections with helminths residing in tissues compared to intestinal helminths. A greater degree of eosinophilia is seen with nematodes compared to cestodes. As an exception, eosinophilia can be seen in infection with *Cystoisospora belli*. Tropical (pulmonary) eosinophilia causes a chronic bronchitis or asthma with marked eosinophilia and is caused by a hypersensitivity reaction to *Wuchereria bancrofti* microfilariae.

Anaemia

Anaemia is commonly seen in malaria, hookworm, visceral leishmaniasis and schistosomiasis. Hookworm causes intestinal bleeding, resulting in anaemia. Malaria parasites replicate in red blood cells and the degree of anaemia is correlated to the parasitic load. Anaemia in visceral leishmaniasis is a result of invasion of the reticuloendothelial system and bone marrow and is accompanied by pancytopaenia. Anaemia in schistosomiasis is a consequence of malnutrition.

Dermatitis

- *Leishmania* can cause skin macules, papules, nodules or mucosal lesions.
- When *Schistosoma* cercariae penetrates the skin, it causes a localized pruritus rash known as swimmer's itch.
- Penetration of the skin by *Strongyloides* or hookworm can cause a localized reaction which can be more severe in hookworm with formation of papules or vesicles.
- *Onchocerca volvulus* causes itchy skin rashes and nodules under the skin.
- Myiasis is a skin infection caused by fly larvae invading the skin and feeding on the soft tissue, causing papules, nodules, and subcutaneous swellings with or without pain.
- *Tunga penetrans* (chigoe flea or jigger) produces local pruritus as it partly buries itself in the skin and lays eggs, causing swelling and local skin irritation, which may be complicated by bacterial superinfection.
- Itchy migrating macular and papular eruptions with or without serpiginous tunnels is seen in infections caused by *Strongyloides stercoralis* and cutaneous larva migrans (CML), and human hookworm infections as the worms penetrate the skin. *Strongyloides* larvae migrate at a higher speed compared to CML.
- *Enterobius vermicularis* (pinworm) causes severe perianal itching.
- Scabies is caused by the mite *Sarcoptes scabiei*, whereby it burrows in web spaces, wrists, waistline, and genitals, causing itchy erythematous papules.

Myositis

Circumorbital oedema, eosinophilia and a history of consumption of insufficiently cooked pork is diagnostic of trichinella. Myositis is caused by larval migration into the muscle. Myositis is also seen in infections caused by *Sarcocystis species*.

FEBRILE ILLNESS

- Malaria
- Visceral leishmaniasis (fever, pancytopaenia, hepatosplenomegaly; also think histoplasmosis)
- Katayama syndrome
- Amoebic liver abscess
- *Trypanosoma cruzi*
- African trypanosomiasis
- Filariasis (fever occurs in early infection or recurrent attacks of lymphangitis and lymphadenitis)
- *Toxocara* species

FEVER + LYMPHADENOPATHY

- *Toxoplasma gondii*
- Filariasis
- Chagas disease
- African trypanosomiasis

FEVER + HEPATOMEGALY + ABDOMINAL PAIN + JAUNDICE

- *Fasciola* species
- *Echinococcus* species
- Amoebic liver abscess
- *Schistosoma* species
- Malaria

PULMONARY SYNDROMES

Symptoms of cough, dyspnoea and wheezing with eosinophilia occurs due to infection with the filarial parasite *Wuchereria bancrofti*, but can also be seen with migration into the lung of larvae of the *Ascaris* spp., hookworm, or *Strongyloides stercoralis*.

Invasion of the pulmonary parenchyma with formation of cavitary lesions can occur with parasites that can invade the lung directly, such as paragonimiasis and echinococcosis.

OCULAR SYNDROMES

Acute ocular presentations of parasitic infections are mostly limited to visual loss caused by *Toxoplasma gondii*. The parasite mostly infects newborns, infants and immunocompromised individuals and causes chorioretinitis leading to vision loss. Adult Loa loa worms can also migrate to the eye.

Onchocerca volvulus may lead to blindness due to an inflammatory response and high parasite burden. This is also known as river blindness and is seen almost exclusively in areas endemic for this parasite. *Acanthamoeba* can cause keratitis through infected contact lenses.

NEUROLOGIC SYNDROMES

Parasitic infections can present as meningitis. *Angiostrongylus cantonensis* and *Gnathostoma* cause disease by direct invasion of the meninges and cause eosinophilic meningitis. Meningitis due to *Strongyloides stercoralis* infection occurs almost exclusively in exposed patients treated with steroids or with concurrent HTLV-1 infection.

Severe malaria caused by *Plasmodium falciparum* can be complicated by encephalitis. Neurocysticercosis a common cause of seizures in endemic areas. Neuroimaging shows a ring-enhanced lesion.

Schistosomal infections can cause tropical spastic paraplegia. Primary amoebic meningoencephalitis occurs when *Naegleria fowleri* gains entrance to the brain through the nose after exposure to contaminated water.

TRAVEL AND EXPOSURE

The list of suspected parasites can be further narrowed down by taking a detailed travel history and asking for typical exposure:

- Mosquito bite in South America, Africa and Asia: Malaria
- Risk factors, i.e. certain food or animal contact
- Freshwater, i.e. Lake Malawi: Schistosomiasis
- Insect bites: *Trypanosoma cruzi*, *Leishmania* species, malaria, filariasis, African trypanosomiasis
- Soil: *Strongyloides stercoralis* or hookworm
- Food, i.e. pork: *Taenia solium*; carnivores: *Toxoplasma gondii*
- Animal, i.e. dogs: *Echinococcus* species, *Toxocara* species; cats: *Toxoplasma gondii*

CLINICAL PEARL

The five most-neglected parasitic infections are Chagas disease, toxocariasis, cysticercosis, toxoplasmosis and trichomoniasis and are public health priorities.

CLINICAL APPROACH

- Is this clinical syndrome compatible with a parasitic infection?
- Has there been a travel history and were there any exposures?
- Does the incubation period fit?

Once it has been determined which parasites could be involved, the next step is to obtain the correct specimen and request specific tests.

INTESTINAL PARASITES

- Stool
- Visualization of trophozoites and eggs: Protozoa
- Visualization of eggs: Nematodes, trematodes and cestodes
- Trophozoites: Stool not older than 30–50 minutes (hot stool) or in a fixative
- Microscopy: Wet prep or on fecal concentrate (increased sensitivity)
- Molecular: Gastrointestinal panel: *Giardia lamblia*, *Cryptosporidium*, *E. histolytica*

BLOOD- AND TISSUE-DWELLING PARASITES

- The microscopic examination of thick and thin peripheral blood smears stained with Giemsa or other appropriate stains is used for detection and identification of *Plasmodium*, *Babesia* and *Trypanosoma* species and of the filarial nematodes species (i.e. *Brugia*, *Mansonella* and *Wuchereria*).

- Sensitivity of these methods may be enhanced by concentration procedures (e.g. buffy coat test, centrifugation and filtration).
- Microscopic examination and/or culture of ulcer, bone marrow, tissue aspirate and biopsy samples are useful for the diagnosis of African trypanosomiasis, onchocerciasis, trichinosis and leishmaniasis.

SEROLOGY

- Serology can be used to screen for presence of parasites or used as an additional diagnostic test.
- Cross-reaction occurs between helminths.
- Serologic assays exist for:
  - Malaria
  - *Leishmaniasis*
  - Amoebic liver abscess
  - Schistosomiasis
  - *Fasciolasis*
  - Tissue cysticercosis
  - Filariasis

BIBLIOGRAPHY

Gillespie S and Pearson RD. *Principles and Practice of Clinical Parasitology.* John Wiley & Sons, 2001.
John DT and Petri WA. Jr. *Markell and Voge's Medical Parasitology.* W. B. Saunders, 2006.

2.6 Laboratory Detection of β-Lactam Resistance in *Enterobacterales*

Firza Alexander Gronthoud

CLINICAL CONSIDERATIONS

Routine antimicrobial susceptibility testing may be unreliable in detecting antimicrobial resistance mechanisms. This can lead to treatment failure, increased mortality and emergence and spread of multidrug resistance. Hospital-acquired infections are most commonly caused by Gram-negative rods. β-lactam agents are the mainstay of treatment of Gram-negative infections. However, multidrug resistance is increasingly occurring worldwide. Knowledge of the clinically most important β-lactam resistance mechanisms and extra tests to detect them enhances and guides antimicrobial stewardship and infection prevention and control. It is therefore worthwhile to consider the following.

β-LACTAM RESISTANCE

- Production of β-lactamase enzymes which destroy (hydrolyse) β-lactam agents is the most important mechanism of resistance in *Enterobacterales* against β-lactam antibiotics.
- There are many different β-lactamase enzymes, each with different activities against β-lactam antibiotics. The two main families of β-lactamase enzymes are the TEM and SHV.
- β-lactamases can be classified into four classes (A, B, C and D) based on their amino acid sequences (Ambler classification).
- β-lactamases can also be characterized by their spectrum of activity, the degree to which their activity is inhibited by β-lactamase inhibitors (BLIs), such as clavulanic acid and tazobactam, and the location and expression of the enzyme (Bush–Jacoby–Medeiros classification)
- Some *Enterobacterales* naturally produce a β-lactamase, others have acquired one through plasmids (mobile genetic elements).

β-LACTAMASE INHIBITORS (BLIs)

- β-lactamase inhibitors have been developed to protect the β-lactam antibiotic from hydrolysis.
- β-lactamase inhibitors used in clinical practice are clavulanic acid, sulbactam, tazobactam and the newer avibactam, relebactam and vaborbactam.
- β-lactamase inhibitors vary in the degree to which they inhibit β-lactamase enzymes.

KLEBSIELLA OXYTOCA

- *Klebsiella oxytoca* is resistant to amoxicillin because it naturally produces a β-lactamase called K1.
- Around 10%–20% of *K. oxytoca* isolates hyperproduce K1 and are resistant to aztreonam, cefuroxime, ceftriaxone and cefpodoxime, have variable resistance to cefotaxime but remain susceptible to ceftazidime.

- K1 hyperproducers are resistant to β-lactam-β-lactamase inhibitor combinations (amoxicillin/clavulanic acid, ampicillin/sulbactam and piperacillin/tazobactam).

INHIBITOR-RESISTANT TEM (IRT)

- With the widespread use of BLIs, a group of β-lactam-inhibitor-resistant mutant TEM β-lactamases have emerged.
- IRTs are spread on plasmids and enable *Enterobacterales* to become resistant to ampicillin/sulbactam and amoxicillin/clavulanic acid.
- IRT-producing isolates remain susceptible to second- and third-generation cephalosporins and carbapenems.
- There is no clinical data on the activity of piperacillin/tazobactam against IRT.

COMPLEX MUTANT TEM (CMT) β-LACTAMASES

- CMT β-lactamases are TEM β-lactamases and contain IRT and extended-spectrum β-lactamase (ESBL)-like mutations conferring resistance to ampicillin/sulbactam and amoxicillin/clavulanic acid and third-generation cephalosporins.
- CMT β-lactamases have mainly been documented in *Escherichia coli*.

EXTENDED-SPECTRUM β-LACTAMASE (ESBL)

- ESBLs are the commonest cause of resistance to third-generation cephalosporins in *Klebsiella* spp. and *E. coli*.
- ESBLs are variants of SHV and TEM β-lactamase enzymes which hydrolyze aztreonam, penicillins, and second- and third-generation cephalosporins, i.e. cefuroxime, cefotaxime, ceftazidime and ceftriaxone.
- ESBLs are inhibited by clavulanic acid and tazobactam.
- A third group of ESBL enzymes, CTX-M, has emerged and has become the dominant ESBL type and is mostly seen in *E. coli*.
- A specific CTX-M enzyme, CTX-M-15, is commonly associated with OXA-1 which is not inhibited by clavulanic acid.
- SHV- and TEM-type ESBLs are generally much more active against ceftazidime than cefotaxime or ceftriaxone, whereas for CTX-M-type ESBLs, the opposite applies.
- EUCAST and CLSI MIC breakpoints for cephalosporins and aztreonam have been reduced in the past years to identify ESBLs.
- It is important to realize that EBSLs can still appear cephalosporin sensitive with routine susceptibility tests and clinical failures with cephalosporins have been documented for high-inoculum ESBL infections.

AMPC-TYPE CEPHALOSPORINASES IN SPACE-M ORGANISMS (*SERRATIA* SPP., *PROVIDENCIA* SPP., *PSEUDOMONAS AERUGINOSA*, *C. FREUNDII*, *ENTEROBACTER* SPP. AND *M. MORGANII*)

- AmpC-type enzymes are β-lactamases that destroy penicillins and first-, second- and third-generation cephalosporins.
- The group of SPACE-M naturally produce low-level chromosomal-encoded AmpC enzymes and are *in vitro* resistant to amoxicillin, amoxicillin/clavulanic acid, cefoxitin and appear susceptible to aztreonam, piperacillin/tazobactam and third-generation cephalosporins.
- AmpC-type enzymes are not inhibited by clavulanic acid, sulbactam and tazobactam.
- If SPACE-M organisms are exposed to β-lactams that induce their chromosomal AmpC gene, depending on the level of induction, mutations will occur in the AmpC gene, leading to de-repression of the chromosomal AmpC gene, leading to hyperproduction of AmpC.

- De-repressed AmpC mutants are also resistant to aztreonam, cefuroxime, third-generation cephalosporins and piperacillin/tazobactam (de-repressed mutants).
- First-generation cephalosporins, ampicillin and amoxycillin are labile, strong inducers of AmpC.
- Cefuroxime, third-generation cephalosporins, piperacillin/tazobactam and aztreonam, although also labile, are weak AmpC inducers.
- However, treatment with these antibiotics may select for de-repressed mutants with subsequent therapy failure and risk of transmission of these mutants. This risk can be as high as 20% for *Enterobacter* spp.
- *E. coli* and *Shigella* spp. constitutively produce AmpC at a clinically nonsignificant low level. These AmpC genes are non-inducible.
- AmpC genes may also be transmissible via plasmids, particularly in *E. coli*, *K. pneumoniae*, *Salmonella enterica* and *Proteus mirabilis*.
- The most prevalent and most widely disseminated are the CMY-2-like enzymes.
- The acquired AmpCs are expressed constitutively, conferring resistance similar to that in the de-repressed or hyperproducing mutants of natural AmpC producers.
- Cefepime is a fourth-generation cephalosporin and more stable than third-generation cephalosporins to AmpC activity and is a treatment alternative for certain infections caused by inducible AmpC producers.
- Laboratory reports should warn clinicians against the use of third-generation cephalosporins in infections caused by these and other AmpC-inducible species, except when the infection is in the urinary tract, where very high cephalosporin concentrations can be attained.

CARBAPENEMASE

- Carbapenemases are β-lactamases that hydrolyze penicillins, in most cases cephalosporins, and to various degrees, carbapenems and monobactams (the latter are not hydrolyzed by metallo-β-lactamases).
- The three most common groups of carbapenemases are KPC (class A), metallo-β-lactamases including VIM, IMP and NDM (class B), and OXA-48 (group D).
- The majority of the carbapenemase-producing *Enterobacterales* (CPE) isolates also produce CTX-M type ESBLs.
- Carbapenemase-producing strains also often have resistance mechanisms to different classes of antibiotics.
- Carbapenem resistance can also be caused by ESBL or AmpC production in combination with decreased permeability due to porin loss (especially ertapenem is prone to this).
- OXA-48 carbapenemases typically have the lowest minimum inhibitory concentrations (MICs) to carbapenems and are the hardest to identify, followed by MBLs and lastly KPCs, which have the highest MICs.

CLINICAL PEARL

Limitations of phenotypic antimicrobial susceptibility testing:

- Bacteria can have several resistance mechanisms.
- Resistance mechanisms can be difficult to detect phenotypically because they are expressed at low basal levels.
- Inducible resistance mechanisms may not be apparent until after antibiotic treatment is started.
- Some laboratory AST measurement methods are less accurate than others, i.e. disk diffusion versus microbroth dilution.

CLINICAL APPROACH

- In *Enterobacterales*, resistance to β-lactam/β-lactamase inhibitors and/or second/third generation cephalosporins should raise the suspicion of various possible β-lactamases.

DETECTING K1 HYPERPRODUCTION IN *KLEBSIELLA OXYTOCA*

K1 hyperproduction should be suspected if *K. oxytoca* has high-level resistance to piperacillin/tazobactam, cefuroxime and aztreonam—but only borderline resistance or susceptibility to cefotaxime and full susceptibility to ceftazidime.

K1 hyperproducers may give weak positive clavulanic acid synergy tests with cefotaxime or cefepime (not ceftazidime) and as such may be confused with ESBL producers. The differences between K1 hyperproducers and ESBLs producer are:

- K1 hyperproducers have high-level resistance to piperacillin/tazobactam, whereas ESBL is inhibited by tazobactam.
- Although a K1 hyperproducer may give a weak positive clavulanic acid synergy test result, in an ESBL producer, the clavulanate will markedly increase the zone of inhibition by more than 5 mm.

DIFFERENTIATING K1 HYPERPRODUCTION FROM ESBL IN *KLEBSIELLA OXYTOCA*

- A ceftazidime MIC of > 2 µg/mL is indicative of ESBL production.
- In an ESBL producer, the ceftriaxone and cefotaxime MICs are equally elevated, whilst in a K1 hyperproducer, the ceftriaxone MIC is ≥8-fold higher than the cefotaxime MIC.

DETECTION OF INHIBITOR-RESISTANT TEM (IRT)

- IRT production should be suspected if the isolate is resistant to β-lactam inhibitors but sensitive to cephalosporins.
- Standard *in vitro* susceptibility tests are not sufficiently reliable for identification of IRTs, and discrepancies have been observed when comparing disk-diffusion and MIC results.
- There is no international standard for the amount of clavulanic acid that should be combined with amoxicillin for detection of IRT, and low-level IRT production can be missed when using a 2:1 disk ratio amoxicillin/clavulanic acid.
- Until an official standard is published for detection of IRT, expert opinion is to use an amoxicillin/clavulanic acid disk with a fixed concentration of 2 µg/mL clavulanic acid.

DETECTION OF COMPLEX MUTANT TEM β-LACTAMASES (CMT)

- CMT should be suspected in *E. coli* resistant to third-generation cephalosporins and β-lactam inhibitors.
- There is no phenotypic test for detecting CMT, and ultimately, detection of CMT relies on the use of molecular methods.
- Ruling out the following phenotypes may suggest the presence of CMT in *E. coli*:
  - *ESBL production*: ESBLs are inhibited by tazobactam and clavulanic acid whilst CMT are unaffected.
  - *De-repressed AmpC*: This is primarily seen in the SPACE-M group. Rarely, *E. coli* may acquire a plasmid-mediated AmpC gene.
  - *Combined ESBL and AmpC profile*: CMT is mostly seen in *E. coli*, whereas inducible AmpC occurs in the SPACE-M group. Detectable co-production of both ESBL and AmpC is most likely to occur in the SPACE-M group.

DETECTING ESBL PRODUCERS FROM CLINICAL SAMPLES

ESBL production should be suspected in isolates resistant to ceftazidime, cefotaxime or cefpodoxime and should be confirmed with the ESBL confirmatory test.

STANDARD ESBL CONFIRMATORY TEST

- Compares the degree of inhibition of growth of the isolate by a third-generation cephalosporin in the presence or absence of clavulanic acid.
- The preferred method is using cefotaxime and ceftazidime or cefpodoxime with and without clavulanic acid (combination disk method).
- ESBL test is positive when the zone diameter of the cephalosporin is expanded by the clavulanic acid by more than 5 mm.
- For CTX-M types, the zone size difference is seen with cefotaxime, whilst for TEM and SHV ESB types, the difference is seen with ceftazidime.
- Note:
    - If the isolate is an AmpC producer or K1 hyperproducer, no or little zone size difference is seen with clavulanic acid as neither AmpC nor K1 are inhibited by clavulanic acid.
    - On the other hand, see the section 'Detection of ESBLs in Organisms with Inducible AmpC or De-Repressed AmpC'.

ALTERNATIVE ESBL CONFIRMATORY TESTS

- Double disk method in which amoxicillin/clavulanic acid disk is placed near a third-generation cephalosporin. ESBL test is positive if there is a 'keyhole' in the direction of amoxicillin/clavulanic acid. Disadvantage: Requires optimal distance between the disks.
- Use of a combined MIC strip containing cefotaxime or ceftazidime with and without clavulanic acid. ESBL test is positive if clavulanic acid causes a ≥8-fold reduction in the MIC or if a phantom zone or deformed ellipse is present. Disadvantage: Difficulties in interpretation of phantom zones or sporadic mutants inside the inhibition zone. Furthermore, this test is less accurate for *K. oxytoca* hyperproducing K1 or ESBL.
- Automated systems either infer ESBL production based on the MIC profile, cross-referencing it with a database containing MIC profiles of ESBL producers, or detect ESBL using a third-generation cephalosporin with or without clavulanic acid. The Vitek2 (bioMerieux) system yields a more indeterminate result compared to the Phoenix (Becton Dickinson). Automated systems may fail to detect resistance to piperacillin/tazobactam, as described for isolates coproducing CTX-M-15 and OXA-1.

DIFFERENTIATION BETWEEN ESBL AND DE-REPRESSED AMPC

De-repressed AmpC produces high level AmpC and, similarly to ESB, will be resistant to third-generation cephalosporins.

Piperacillin/tazobactam can differentiate between ESBL and a de-repressed AmpC. Isolates that produce ESBL only will be susceptible, whereas isolates with a de-repressed AmpC only will be resistant. However, in a strain which has both de-repressed AmpC and ESBL, the piperacillin/tazobactam will be attacked by AmpC enzymes and ESBL production will be masked.

DETECTION OF ESBLs IN ORGANISMS WITH INDUCIBLE AMPC OR DE-REPRESSED AMPC

ESBLs are more difficult to detect in the SPACE-M group because clavulanic acid used in the ESBL confirmatory test will induce the AmpC enzymes to attack the indicator cephalosporin, masking any ESBL activity.

ESBL production in the SPACE-M group should be suspected if there is resistance to third generation cephalosporins and cefepime.

- Use either a cefepime/clavulanic acid combination disk or combined MIC strip.
- Cefepime is more stable than third-generation cephalosporins to AmpC activity, meaning that although clavulanic acid will induce AmpC production, cefepime and its antibacterial effect will remain intact.
- Similar to the ESBL confirmatory test, a >8-fold MIC reduction or >5 mm zone expansion with clavulanic acid indicates a positive ESBL result.

DETECTING ESBL IN PSEUDOMONAS AERUGINOSA

- ESBL detection in *P. aeruginosa* is challenging owing to the presence of multiple resistance mechanisms: inducible AmpC enzyme, greater degree of impermeability than *Enterobacterales* and efflux-mediated resistance (see Chapter 5.4).
- ESBL production in *P. aeruginosa* will show high-level ceftazidime resistance (MIC > 64 mg/L and growth up to the edge of a ceftazidime 30 μg disk), whereas hyperproduction of AmpC and/or impermeability/efflux function gives lower-level resistance.
- The ESBL confirmatory test cannot be used for *P. aeruginosa* because most of the ESBL types in *P. aeruginosa* are OXA variants, which are not inhibited by clavulanic acid.

DETECTION OF DE-REPRESSED AmpC IN SPACE-M GROUP

De-repressed AmpC mutants can be recognized by resistance to cefoxitin and third-generation cephalosporins and susceptibility to cefepime.

DETECTION OF ACQUIRED AmpC IN ENTEROBACTERALES OTHER THAN SPACE-M

Acquired AmpC should be suspected if the cefoxitin MIC >8 mg/L (zone size <19 mm) and the organism is resistant to a third-generation cephalosporins.
   Note:

- This strategy will detect plasmid-mediated CMY-1 but not the ACC-1 AmpC enzyme, which does not hydrolyze cefoxitin.
- Cefoxitin resistance may also be due to porin deficiency.

CARBAPENEMASE ENZYMES

Carbapenem MICs for CPE may still be below the clinical breakpoint and appear susceptible *in vitro*. However, the carbapenem MIC will still be higher in CPE compared to wild-type *Enterobacterales*. The epidemiological cut-off value (ECOFF) can then be used as a screening method for potential carbapenemase producers. If the MIC is greater than the ECOFF, carbapenemase production should be suspected.

   Tests that can be used are combination disk test methods, colorimetric assays based on hydrolysis of carbapenems and other methods detecting carbapenem hydrolysis. The various tests are described below.

COMBINATION DISK TESTING

- Disks containing meropenem with and without an inhibitor.
- The inhibitors used are:
  - Boronic acid to inhibit class A KPC.

- EDTA to inhibit class B metallo-β-lactamase.
- Cloxacillin to inhibit class C AmpC β-lactamases. This test is used to differentiate between AmpC hyperproduction plus porin loss and carbapenemase-production.
- In addition, a disk containing temocillin or E-test strip is placed as well. High-level temocillin (MIC >128 mg/L, or zone diameter <11 mm) is used as a marker for OXA-48 production.
- If the isolate produces carbapenemase, then in the presence of a corresponding inhibitor, an increase in zone size is visible.
- This test has sensitivity and specificity issues caused by the following:
  - Additional mechanisms of resistance are often present (i.e. ESBL or AmpC).
  - Low-level carbapenem resistance may be missed.
  - EDTA may also exert other effects on the bacterial cell, i.e. permeabilization causing a false-positive result.

CARBANP TEST

This is a rapid (<2 h) test for detection of carbapenem hydrolysis, which causes a drop in pH with a subsequent change in colour from red to yellow with phenol red solution. Disadvantages: Subjective colour reading and less sensitive for detecting OXA-48.

METALLO-B-LACTAMASE TEST (MBL TEST)

- Combined MIC strip containing imipenem with and without EDTA.
- An eight-fold MIC reduction in the presence of EDTA indicates metallo-ß-lactamase production.

MODIFIED HODGE TEST

- Phenotypic test for detection of CPE.
- Modified Hodge test does not distinguish between carbapenemase types, is less sensitive for MBL detection and is time-consuming.

Commercial PCR kits are emerging which can rapidly detect the most common carbapenemase enzymes with high sensitivity, including KPC, OXA-48, NDM-1 and VIM. Disadvantages are costs, detection of limited panel of carbapenemase enzymes and emerging enzymes remain undetected.

BIBLIOGRAPHY

Cantón R, Morosini MI, de la Maza OM, de la Pedrosa EG. IRT and CMT β-lactamases and inhibitor resistance. *Clin Microbiol Infect*. January 2008;14(Suppl 1):53–62.

Livermore DM and Brown DF. Detection of beta-lactamase-mediated resistance. *J. Antimicrob Chemother*. 2001;48(Suppl 1):59–64.

EUCAST guidelines for detection of resistance mechanisms and specific resistances of clinical and/or epidemiological importance Version 2.01 July 2017

Thomson KS. Extended-Spectrum-β-Lactamase, AmpC, and Carbapenemase Issues. *J Clin Microbiol*. April 2010;48(4):1019–1025.

UK Standards for Microbiology Investigations Laboratory Detection and Reporting of Bacteria with Extended Spectrum β-Lactamases. www.gov.uk/government/collections/standards-for-micro biology-investigations-smi

2.7 Understanding the Antibiogram

Firza Alexander Gronthoud

CLINICAL CONSIDERATIONS

Microbiology laboratories determine antimicrobial susceptibility through tests whereby organisms are cultured in the presence of antimicrobial agents (phenotypic tests). Based on the minimum concentration of an antibiotic needed to inhibit growth (also called MIC; measured by microbroth dilution or MIC gradient strips) or based on the zone of inhibition (when using disk diffusion), the result is reported as sensitive, resistant or intermediate sensitive. Intermediate sensitive means that treatment may still be effective if a higher dose is used and if the infection is in a body compartment where the antibiotic has a good tissue penetration, i.e. β-lactams in the urinary tract.

In the past years, molecular tests have emerged which can detect specific antimicrobial-resistance genes or can sequence the genome, enabling detection of all known resistance genes as well as new genes. Care must be taken when interpreting these findings because the presence of resistance genes does not necessarily confer in vivo resistance.

An antibiogram is a list of antimicrobial sensitivity results based on phenotypic tests and is the main tool used to select an antimicrobial drug.

The downside of an antibiogram is that it may mask underlying resistance mechanisms, giving false sensitive results. This is because some resistance mechanisms are only triggered under certain conditions not easily simulated in the lab. This is especially the case with inducible β-lactamase enzymes or the presence of biofilms at the site of infection.

Interpretative reading refers to predicting antimicrobial resistance mechanisms based on a sensitivity report and unmasking hidden antimicrobial resistance mechanisms, leading to both correction of false sensitive/resistant results and extrapolating which other antimicrobials can be used without the need for further testing. It is therefore worthwhile to consider the following.

INTRINSIC RESISTANCE IN GRAM-NEGATIVE ORGANISMS

- SPACE-M organisms (*Serratia marcescens*, *Pseudomonas aeruginosa*, *Acinetobacter baumannii*, *Citrobacter freundii*, *Enterobacter cloacae* complex and *Morganella morganii*) are intrinsically resistant to amoxicillin, amoxicillin/clavulanic acid and second-generation cephalosporins because these agents are strong inducers of the AmpC gene, leading to resistance. Third-generation cephalosporins are weak inducers *in vitro*, and results may initially appear as sensitive; however, *in vivo* resistance will occur eventually.
- *Proteus* spp., *Morganella morganii*, *Serratia* spp., *Providencia* spp. and *Burkholderia* spp. are intrinsically resistant to colistin.
- *Proteus* spp., *Morganella morganii* and *Pseudomonas* spp. are resistant to all tetracyclines and tigecycline.
- *Serratia marcescens*, on the other hand, is intrinsically resistant to tetracycline and doxycycline but not to minocycline or tigecycline.
- *Pseudomonas aeruginosa* may appear *in vitro* to be sensitive to trimethoprim/ sulfamethoxazole and chloramphenicol, but these agents should probably be avoided in clinical practice, although clinical success has been seen in cystic fibrosis.

- *Proteus* spp., *Morganella morganii* and *Providencia* spp. are resistant to nitrofurantoin and tigecycline.
- Most Gram-negative organisms are intrinsically resistant to amoxicillin; exceptions are wild-type *E. coli* and *Proteus mirabilis.*
- *Stenotrophomonas maltophilia* is intrinsically resistant to carbapenems.
- *Burkholderia* spp. and *S. maltophilia* are intrinsically resistant to aminoglycosides.

INTRINSIC RESISTANCE IN GRAM-POSITIVE ORGANISMS

- Gram-positive bacteria are intrinsically resistant to aztreonam and temocillin.
- Although ceftazidime may have *in vitro* activity to penicillin-sensitive Gram-positive bacteria, this agent should probably be regarded as resistant.
- Although streptococci and enterococci are intrinsically resistant to aminoglycosides, these antibiotics display synergism with β-lactam agents. This phenomenon can be exploited when treating endocarditis.
- *Listeria monocytogenes* is resistant to cephalosporins.
- Intrinsic vancomycin resistance is seen in most *Lactobacillus* spp., *Leuconostoc* and *Pediococcus* spp., *Enterococcus casseliflavus* and *Enterococcus gallinarum.*

INTRINSIC RESISTANCE IN ANAEROBES

- All anaerobes are resistant to aminoglycosides.
- *Propionibacterium acnes* is resistant to metronidazole.

RESISTANCE MECHANISMS WHICH SHOULD RAISE ATTENTION

- Methicillin-resistant *Staphylococcus aureus.*
- Vancomycin resistance in staphylococci is very rare and most likely represents an erroneous result. On the other hand, coagulase-negative staphylococci can be teicoplanin resistant but vancomycin sensitive, most notably observed in *S. haemolyticus.*
- Vancomycin-resistant enterococci (*E. faecium* and *E. faecalis*).
- *Enterococcus faecium* is sensitive to amoxicillin (90% are amoxicillin resistant).
- Extended Spectrum β-lactamase (ESBL) and carbapenemase-producing organisms (CPOs).
- Colistin resistance in most Gram-negative organisms (*Serratia* spp., *Proteus* spp., *Morganella morganii* and *Burkholderia* spp. are intrinsically resistant).
- Metronidazole and carbapenem resistance in *Bacteroides* spp.
- Third-generation cephalosporin resistance in *Haemophilus influenzae*, *Neisseria* spp. and *Moraxella catarrhalis.*
- Linezolid and daptomycin resistance in Gram-positive organisms.

Detection of these organisms requires the use of confirmation tests to ensure that the result is correct as it has major clinical and infection control implications.

EXTRAPOLATING SUSCEPTIBILITY RESULTS

- All Gram-positive and Gram-negative organisms sensitive to amoxicillin are also sensitive to piperacillin.
- Organisms sensitive to ciprofloxacin are also sensitive to other quinolones.
- Gram-negative organisms resistant to ciprofloxacin are resistant to all quinolones.
- Gram-positive organisms should generally be regarded as sensitive to linezolid.

- Gram-negative organisms sensitive to tetracyclines should be regarded as sensitive to tigecycline (except *Proteus* spp., *Morganella morganii* and *Providencia* spp.).
- Streptococci resistant to penicillin can be sensitive to cefotaxime and ceftriaxone but should be confirmed with MIC testing.
- Staphylococci and streptococci can be resistant to macrolides but sensitive to clindamycin. The lab should, however, first exclude the presence of the inducible MLS_B mechanism before reporting this phenotype.
- Ertapenem is more labile to AmpC than meropenem; therefore, if ertapenem is considered for use, then MIC testing should be performed in SPACE-M organisms.

CAUTIONS

- Rifampicin, ciprofloxacin and fusidic acid should never be given alone to *Staphylococcus aureus* as resistance will develop rapidly.
- Tigecycline should be avoided for bloodstream and urinary tract infections.
- Daptomycin was shown *in vitro* to be inactivated by pulmonary surfactant.
- The use of amoxicillin/clavulanate and piperacillin/tazobactam for treatment of ESBL infections other than urinary tract should be used with high caution.
- Tobramycin and amikacin are less active than gentamicin against gentamicin-sensitive *Enterobacterales*.
- In fact, *S. marcescens* can be gentamicin sensitive but resistant to amikacin and tobramycin.
- Gentamicin, on the other hand, is more nephrotoxic compared to other aminoglycosides.
- In contrast, tobramycin is more active than gentamicin against *P. aeruginosa*.
- Unlike ciprofloxacin and levofloxacin, moxifloxacin should not be given for urinary tract infections owing to low concentrations.
- Unlike ciprofloxacin and levofloxacin, moxifloxacin is not active against *P. aeruginosa*.

CLINICAL APPROACH

- For antimicrobials reported as sensitive: Verify if the reported susceptibility result is not in violation with known intrinsic resistance mechanisms.
- For antimicrobials reported as resistant: Consider any clinical or infection control implications and confirm whether confirmation testing is needed.
- For antimicrobials reported as intermediate sensitive: Consider the source of infection and consider using higher doses if no alternative agents are available.
- Generally avoid cephalosporins for SPACE-M bacteria reported as sensitive in the antibiogram.

BIBLIOGRAPHY

Andreassen S, Zalounina A, Paul M, Sanden L, Leibovici L. Interpretative reading of the antibiogram—A semi-naïve Bayesian approach. *Artif Intell Med*. November 2015;65(3):209–217.

Courvalin P. Interpretive reading of *in vitro* antibiotic susceptibility tests (the antibiogramme). *Clin Microbiol Infect*. February 1996;2(Suppl 1):S26–S34.

Leclercq R, Cantón R, Brown DF et al. EUCAST expert rules in antimicrobial susceptibility testing. *Clin Microbiol Infect*. February 2013;19(2):141–160.

Livermore DM, Winstanley TG, Shannon KP. Interpretative reading: Recognizing the unusual and inferring resistance mechanisms from resistance phenotypes. *J Antimicrob Chemother*. July 2001;48(Suppl 1):87–102.

MacDougall C. Beyond susceptible and resistant, Part I: Treatment of infections due to gram-negative organisms with inducible β-Lactamases. *J Pediatr Pharmacol Ther*. January–March 2011;16(1):23–30.

2.8 Understanding Microbiology Culture Results

Firza Alexander Gronthoud

CLINICAL CONSIDERATIONS

Proper use and interpretation of microbiology results is an integral part of diagnostic stewardship, antimicrobial stewardship and infection prevention and control. Requesting the right test and correct interpretation of microbiology results can avoid inappropriate antimicrobial treatment and promotes patient safety and care. The choice of microbiological test depends on the suspected infectious agent, specimen type and, in some cases, also on duration of illness. It is therefore worthwhile to consider the following.

MICROSCOPY

Gram Stain

Microbes can be directly visualized in bodily fluids and tissue samples with microscopy. The Gram stain is used for detection of bacteria. Bacteria can be classified as Gram positive or Gram negative based on their ability to retain crystal violet after decolourization with alcohol. Gram-positive bacteria retain crystal violet in their cell wall and have a purple colour. In contrast, in Gram-negative bacteria, the alcohol has removed the crystal violet (a process called decolourization) and a counterstain is used to make them visible and pink coloured. Counterstains used are safranin and carbol fuchsin. Counterstains are weaker stains than crystal violet and Gram-positive bacteria remain purple coloured. Gram stain can also be used to visualize common fungi such as *Candida* species, which are Gram positive.

Ziehl–Neelsen Stain

Mycobacteria can be detected using a Ziehl–Neelsen stain or a fluorescent auramine stain. Mycobacteria have a waxy mycolic acid in their cell wall which resists a Gram stain. A Ziehl–Neelsen stain was developed whereby carbol fuchsin is used as the initial stain and heat is applied to fixate the carbol fuchsin into the cell wall. Because of mycolic acid in their cell wall, the acid alcohol used in the decolourization is not able to remove carbol fuchsin from the cell wall, and consequently, they appear bright red. This is why mycobacteria are also called acid-fast bacilli. A sputum sample needs to contain at least 10^4 mycobacteria per millilitre before they can be detected with microscopy.

Nocardia bacteria can be detected using Gram stain or a modified Ziehl–Neelsen stain whereby no heat is used and the decolourization step with acid alcohol is shorter.

Intestinal parasites can be detected in stool using a direct wet preparation or an iodine stain (i.e. *Giardia lamblia*). With microscopy, trophozoites can be detected in the stool if either the stool is processed within 1 hour ('hot stool') or if the stool is fixated. A modified Ziehl–Neelsen stain can also be used to detect *Cryptosporidium* oocysts. A Giemsa stain is commonly used for microscopy of sterile samples, i.e. malaria parasites in blood. For moulds including *Aspergillus* spp., a lactophenol cotton blue stain or calcofluor-white stain is commonly used. India ink is used for *Cryptococcus* spp. in CSF. A rapid method to diagnose dermatophytes is a KOH test on skin scrapings (i.e. dermatophytes). Microscopy can also be performed on histology tissue sections with various stains including periodic acid-Schiff stain or a Grocott silver stain.

Microscopy rapidly detects the presence of organisms but is less sensitive than bacterial culture and molecular techniques such as PCR. In the cases of bacterial and mycobacterial infections, microscopy is less specific as it cannot identify to the species level. In non-sterile fluids, microscopy may not differentiate between infection and colonization. Lastly, microscopy cannot be used for antimicrobial drug susceptibility.

BACTERIAL CULTURE

- Bacterial and fungal culture is performed by inoculating different agar plates with clinical specimen and incubating at 37°C in an aerobic, CO_2 or anaerobic environment.
- Different plates are used to enable early differentiation between Gram-negative and Gram-positive bacteria.
- Blood agar is the main agar plate used for both Gram-negative and Gram-positive bacteria. Some bacteria produce haemolysins which partially (α-haemolytic) or completely (β-haemolytic) destroy red blood cells on blood agar plates. Streptococci can be α-haemolytic (also called viridans streptococci) or β-haemolytic. *Staphylococcus aureus* is β-haemolytic. Some coagulase-negative staphylococci can be β-haemolytic but most are non-haemolytic.
- Sensitivity of culture is significantly affected by prior antimicrobial use, transport time and specimen quality.
- Sensitivity of culture can be increased by using enriched broth or blood culture bottles. This is commonly done for sterile fluids and foreign bodies. The disadvantage is a lower specificity as contaminants are more easily cultured.
- Increased transport time allows overgrowth of commensal flora or reduces viability of bacteria.
- Identification and antimicrobial susceptibility testing can be performed on colony-forming units (CFUs) growing on the agar. One CFU amounts to 10^4 bacteria.
- Quantity of colony-forming units may help predict clinical significance.

IDENTIFICATION OF BACTERIA

- Preliminary identification is done through different growth properties on agar plates.
- Biochemical tests investigating metabolic properties of bacteria used to be the main method of identification. These biochemical tests were done by hand or using automated systems such as the ViTeK or Phoenix. These automated systems also can perform antimicrobial-susceptibility testing.
- Modern laboratories nowadays use Matrix Assisted Laser Desorption Ionization—Time of Flight or MALDI-ToF, whereby bacterial and yeast colonies are accelerated in a vacuum tube, and based on the acceleration patterns of proteins, a rapid diagnosis is available within minutes.
- Molecular techniques such as PCR and whole genome sequencing are increasingly used for a sensitive diagnosis (see Chapter 2.10).

BIOHAZARDS FOR LABORATORY WORKERS

- Organisms are classified in different hazard groups based on their level of risk to humans. Depending on the hazard group, different microbiological containment levels need to be used to minimize infection risk to laboratory staff. This means using extra precautions such as using personal protective equipment and processing specimens in biological safety cabinets.
- It is therefore important to notify the lab of a clinical suspicion of organisms belonging to hazard group 3 or 4 (see Table 2.8.1 for examples).

TABLE 2.8.1
Examples of Hazard Group Organisms

Hazard Group	Level of Risk	Examples
Hazard Group 1	Does not cause disease in humans	
Hazard Group 2	Cause disease in humans, hazard for employees. Effective prophylaxis or treatment available	*Campylobacter* spp., *C. diphtheriae, E. coli, Nocardia* spp.
Hazard Group 3	Causes severe disease in humans, serious hazard to employees, spreads into the community. Effective prophylaxis or treatment available	*Brucella* spp., *Burkholderia pseudomallei, E. coli* O157:H7, *Francisella tularensis* (Type A), *Rickettsia* spp., malaria, *M. tuberculosis*, rabies, *Salmonella* Typhi and Paratyphi, *Yesinia pestis*: MERS-CoV, SARS-CoV-1, SARS-CoV-2
Hazard Group 4	Cause severe disease in humans, serious hazard to employees. Likely to spread to the community and no effective prophylaxis or treatment available	Viral haemorrhagic viruses including Ebola virus and Marburg virus, simian B virus

CLINICAL PEARL

Mismatch between Gram stain and culture can indicate antibiotic effect or the need for extra plates and different incubation conditions. An abundance of Gram-negative rods in a sputum sample may indicate anaerobes compatible with aspiration pneumonia. Incubation of a blood agar plate containing gentamicin in an anaerobic environment is indicated.

TABLE 2.8.2
CSF Findings

Test	Bacterial	Viral	Fungal	Tuberculosis
Opening pressure	Elevated	Normal	Variable	Variable
White blood cell count/μL	$\geq$250	10–100	Variable	Variable
Cell differential	PMNs	Lymphocytes + monocytes	Lymphocytes	Lymphocytes
Protein	Elevated	Elevated	Elevated	Elevated
CSF-to-serum ratio	Decreased	Normal to low	Low	Low

CLINICAL APPROACH

SPECIMEN COLLECTION

- Clinical specimens should be collected from the suspected site of infection.
- Specimens from the respiratory tract, urine samples and wounds swab often grow colonizing bacteria. If there is a low suspicion of infection of these sites, avoid taking these samples.
- To avoid diagnosing bladder catheter colonization, the catheter should be removed or changed, after which a urine sample is collected.
- Specimens should be collected before antimicrobial treatment is started.

- Clinical information should be provided on the request form, as this will inform the laboratory if they need to use extra safety precautions, as well as decide on which laboratory techniques to use to increase likelihood of finding the cause of infection.
- Before tissue biopsies, surgical samples and difficult to obtain samples (i.e. CSF) are collected for microbiological investigation, it is useful to discuss with the clinical microbiologist how many specimens should be taken and which tests should be requested.
- Indicate the clinical likelihood of infectious aetiology to enable the laboratory to prioritize the tests in case limited specimen is received.

Once the microbiology results are available, interpretation of the results in the clinical context will further aid clinical management.

INTERPRETING GRAM STAINS

- Gram-positive cocci indicate presence of either staphylococci, streptococci or enterococci. Staphylococci are cocci in clusters. Streptococci and enterococci are cocci in chains whereby streptococci typically form long chains and enterococci short chains.
- Gram-negative rods indicate *Enterobacterales*, i.e. *E. coli*, or non-fermenters such as *Pseudomonas aeruginosa* or anaerobes.
- In sputum samples and intra-abdominal fluids, Gram-negative rods may also indicate the presence of anaerobes.
- An abundance of epithelial cells or respiratory squamous cells increases the likelihood that bacteria in the samples represent colonization rather than infection.
- White blood cells indicate signs of inflammation, not necessarily infection, and should be interpreted in clinical context.

INTERPRETATION OF BACTERIAL CULTURE RESULTS

- Culture remains the cornerstone of diagnosing bacterial and fungal infections.
- Quantity of bacteria may predict significance, but can be reduced by antibiotic use.
- Always compare quantities of potential pathogens to the quantity of commensal flora present.
- Differentiate between commensal flora and pathogens.
  - In non-sterile samples, coagulase-negative staphylococci, enterococci and α-haemolytic streptococci usually represent colonization.
  - Coliforms can be transient oropharyngeal colonizers. Their presence in sputum samples requires careful interpretation.
- Bacteria cultured from an aspirate are more likely to be clinically relevant compared to drain-fluid cultures, especially when the drain fluid has been sitting in the collection bag for a prolonged time.
- In the absence of intravascular catheters or foreign bodies, coagulase-negative staphylococci usually represent contamination.
- *Neisseria meningitidis* in a sputum or throat swab most likely represents colonization.

Below is a short overview of how to interpret common specimen types.

URINE SAMPLES

- A negative dipstick is useful for ruling out urinary tract infection (UTI). A positive dipstick, on the other hand, has a low positive predictive value, especially in the elderly and in the presence of an indwelling catheter.

- Pyuria is the presence of ten or more white blood cells (WBCs) per microlitre in urine and is a nonspecific finding.
- Pyuria with negative urine culture may indicate a sexually transmitted disease, malignancy, urethritis caused by *Ureaplasma urealyticum*, pyelonephritis, diabetes, renal tuberculosis or renal stones.
- Haematuria is the presence of red blood cells (RBCs) in urine and may be caused by non-infectious inflammation of the urinary tract, renal mycobacterial infection or *Schistosoma haematobium* infection in endemic areas.
- More than 10^3 colony-forming units (CFUs) per millilitre in the urine culture is associated with infection.
- True infection may occur in symptomatic patients with lower CFUs.
- *Staphylococcus aureus* is an uncommon uropathogen and should always be correlated to clinical picture as its presence in midstream urine could indicate bacteraemia.
- *Candida* spp. in urine most often represent colonization, especially after antibiotic use; the quantity is not correlated to clinical relevance. A low threshold for treatment should exist in immunocompromised individuals with UTI symptoms.
- Enterococci in midstream urine from immunocompetent individuals usually represents colonization.
- Common bacteria in uncomplicated UTI include *Escherichia coli*, *Klebsiella* spp., *Proteus* spp., and *Staphylococcus saprophyticus*. *Pseudomonas aeruginosa* and enterococci are more common in catheter-associated UTI.

BLOOD

- Gram stain results
  - Most Gram-negative rods in blood cultures are *E. coli* or *Klebsiella* spp.
  - Gram-negative coccobacilli in the aerobic bottle may indicate *Acinetobacter* spp. or *Moraxella catarrhalis*.
  - Slender Gram-negative rods in the aerobic bottle could indicate *Pseudomonas aeruginosa*.
  - Gram-negative rods in the anaerobic bottle could be coliforms, or anaerobes if after more than 2 days of incubation and pleiomorphic.
  - Gram-negative diplococci in the aerobic bottle indicate *Neisseria* spp.
  - Gram-positive cocci in clusters indicate staphylococci. If the bottle flags positive after more than 2 days, then usually it is a coagulase-negative *Staphylococcus*.
  - Gram-positive cocci in chains are either streptococci or enterococci. Small cocci in long chains are indicative of streptococci, whereas larger cocci in short chains could indicate enterococci.
  - Gram-positive cocci in pairs could indicate *Streptococcus pneumoniae*.
  - Gram-positive rods in the anaerobic botte could indicate *Clostridium* spp.
  - Large gram-positive rods in chains in the aerobic bottle could indicate *Bacillus* spp.
  - Small gram-positive, club-shaped rods could indicate corynebacteria.
- Coagulase-negative staphylococci, *Bacillus* spp. and *Corynebacterium* spp. in peripheral blood cultures often represent contamination, especially in the absence of clinical signs of infection. The clinical relevance is increased when multiple blood cultures are positive, especially in the presence of a intravascular catheters or foreign bodies.
- *Bacillus cereus* and *Corynebacterium jeikeium* are associated with central-line-associated bloodstream infections in immunocompromised individuals.
- Line sepsis is more likely if blood cultures from the line and peripheral stab or line tip grow the same organism and if the line set flags positive before the peripheral set 'time to positivity'.

- Intravascular catheter removal is indicated in cases of *S. aureus*, *Candida* spp. and *P. aeruginosa*.
- Prolonged incubation for members of the HACEK group is not necessary anymore.
- *Candida* spp. and *S. aureus* should be taken as true bacteraemias.
- α-Haemolytic streptococci could indicate contamination, translocation from the gastrointestinal tract or infective endocarditis. It is therefore important to assess how many blood culture sets flagged positive and correlate to clinical symptoms, presence of damaged valve or prosthetic valve, endocarditis stigmata. Source investigation should focus on dental examination, abdominal source and presence of mucositis in individuals receiving chemotherapy.
- α-Haemolytic streptococci are not associated with line sepsis.
- Type of organism can inform clinician regarding source of infection.
  - Coliforms and enterococci should prompt investigation of the urinary tract, biliary tract, translocation from gut (bowel obstruction, ischaemia) and peritonitis.
  - Endocarditis work-up is indicated when *S. aureus* and *Enterococcus faecalis* are isolated from blood cultures.
  - *S. aureus* and β-haemolytic streptococci require investigation of soft tissue.

RESPIRATORY TRACT

- Presence of epithelial cells in Gram stain indicates oropharyngeal contamination.
- Gram film of sputum sample should have less than 10 epithelial cells per low-powered field.
- Enterococci and *Candida* are a very rare cause of lower respiratory tract infections and almost always represent colonization.
- Sputum cultures can be difficult to interpret because the upper respiratory tract is colonized with bacteria; therefore, always correlate quantity of commensal flora to quantity of potential pathogen grown.

WOUND SWABS

- Wounds should only be swabbed if clinically infected as swabs from clean wounds may yield non-pathogenic colonizing bacteria such as coagulase-negative staphylococci and diphtheroids.
- *Staphylococcus aureus*, β-haemolytic streptococci and *Pseudomonas aeruginosa* are the most common causes of acute wound infections. Enterococci and coagulase-negative staphylococci most likely represent colonization.
- Anaerobes may be involved in infection of chronic wounds.
- Thrush is a clinical diagnosis and only requires swabbing if there is no clinical response to treatment.

CEREBROSPINAL FLUID

- CSF should be processed within 1–2 hours due to lysis of cells which occurs even at 4°C.
- Normal CSF is a clear fluid. Clouded CSF is caused by abundance of WBCs or RBCs, indicating trauma or infection (Table 2.8.2). Purulent CSF is thick and yellowish to greenish.
- Breakdown of RBCs in CSF releases bilirubin, resulting in a yellow, pink or orange discolouration termed xanthochromia.
- Red blood cells in CSF caused by a traumatic tap or a subarachnoid haemorrhage artificially increase the white blood cell count and protein level, thereby confounding the diagnosis.
- Opening pressures above 250 mm H_2O are diagnostic of intracranial hypertension. Opening pressure is elevated in cryptococcal meningitis.

- Fewer than 1 WBC per 500–700 RBCs indicates a traumatic tap.
- Pleocytosis refers to increased WBC in CSF: mild (5–50/mL), moderate (50–150/mL) or severe (150–3000/mL).
- The WBC count in normal adult CSF consists of 70% lymphocytes and 30% monocytes.
- Lymphocytosis is common in viral, fungal and tuberculous infections of the CNS, although a predominance of polymorphonuclear cells (PMNs) may be present in the early stages of these infections.
- CSF in bacterial meningitis is typically dominated by the presence of PMNs.
- However, more than 10% of bacterial meningitis cases will show a lymphocytic predominance, especially early in the clinical course and when there are fewer than 1000 WBCs per millilitre.
- Eosinophilic meningitis is defined as more than 10 eosinophils per millilitre or a total CSF cell count made up of more than 10% eosinophils. Parasitic infection should be suspected in this situation. Other possible causes may include tuberculosis and neurosyphilis.
- Neuroborreliosis shows a lymphocytic picture.
- Protein concentration is falsely elevated by the presence of RBCs in a traumatic tap situation.
- CSF glucose is about two-thirds of the serum glucose. Decreased glucose levels may be seen in 50% of bacterial CNS infections.
- Gram stain is positive in 60%–80% of bacterial meningitis.
- At least 6 mL of CSF is needed for tuberculosis (TB) culture.
- CSF to serum antibody testing can be performed for viral CNS infections.
- PCR can be negative in the first 2–3 days of HSV encephalitis.

BIBLIOGRAPHY

Jorgensen, JH et al. *Manual of Clinical Microbiology*, 11th ed. American Society of Microbiology, 2015.
Rahimi J, Woehrer A. Overview of cerebrospinal fluid cytology. *Handb Clin Neurol*. 2017;145:563–571.
http://www.hse.gov.uk/pubns/misc208.pdf
UK Standards for Microbiology Investigations: Investigation of urine. B 41i8.7, 11 January 2019.

2.9 Understanding Serology

Firza Alexander Gronthoud

CLINICAL CONSIDERATIONS

Proper use and interpretation of microbiology results is an integral part of diagnostic stewardship, antimicrobial stewardship and infection prevention and control. Requesting the right test and correct interpretation of microbiology results can avoid inappropriate antimicrobial treatment and promotes patient safety and care. The choice of serology test depends on the suspected infectious agent, specimen type and on duration of illness. It is therefore worthwhile to consider the following.

- Not all organisms can be easily detected directly using culture techniques, and it may then be useful to perform serology. Serology refers to the detection of antibodies and antigens in a variety of bodily fluids such as blood, respiratory samples, CSF and stool.
- After an infection has been established, it may take days to weeks before antibodies or antigens are detectable; this is called the window phase.
- Knowledge of the window phase of infections can guide timing of serology to avoid false-negative results.
- During the window phase, it may be more useful to request a molecular test such as polymerase chain reaction (PCR).
- As antibody titres may rise and fall, a convalescent serum sample may help determine whether there is an active infection or a past and resolved infection.
- Early antibiotic treatment can delay or prevent development of antibodies, causing false-negative titres, i.e. in Lyme disease.
- Antibodies show cross-reaction because organisms may have similar antigens. It can be useful to test for known cross-reacting pathogens and to repeat serology in 4 weeks.
- Serology is often used for viral infections, parasitic infections and bacteria which are difficult to culture, including *Borrelia burgdorferi* (Lyme disease), *Treponema pallidum* (syphilis), *Mycoplasma pneumoniae* and *Coxiella burnetii* (Q fever).
- Serology is commonly used for serotyping of *Salmonella* and *Shigella* species and differentiating among β-haemolytic streptococci.
- Antibody testing is part of pre-transplant screening protocols to guide antimicrobial prophylaxis post-transplant.
- Antibody testing is helpful in assessing response to vaccination.
- Antibody testing has a reduced sensitivity in immunocompromised individuals and reduced specificity in neonates and infants due to circulating maternal antibodies.
- False-positive test results are common in pregnant women and in haematological malignancies, including multiple myeloma.
- Although many serological assays exist (immunofluorescence, complement fixation, enzyme-linked immunosorbent assay [ELISA] also known as enzyme immunoassays [EIA] and Western Blot), nowadays automated analysers are used which mostly use EIA or chemiluminescent immunoassays. Because of the high sensitivity of these assays, false-positive results may occur. In such cases, the laboratory will confirm the result by using a second test, i.e. Western Blot. This two-step method is employed for Lyme disease and HIV.
- Serology is used to diagnose chronic or untreated infections such as Hepatitis B, Hepatitis C, HIV, syphilis.

- Serology can also be used to see if there is pre-existing immunity to infections i.e. pregnant patients, patients scheduled to undergo an organ or bone marrow transplant or sperm donors. These may include: varicella zoster, measles, rubella toxoplasma, CMV, EBV and parvovirus.

CLINICAL PEARL

Patients who have received blood products may have have false positive antibody test results due to owing to transfer of antibodies.

CLINICAL PEARL

IgG avidity testing can help determine whether an infection was recent. IgG avidity tests exist for toxoplasma and CMV. A low avidity (low binding strength of IgG to an antigen) indicates the infection occurred recently.

CLINICAL APPROACH

- Factors that determine the sensitivity of serology are the patient's immune status, the detection method used, the antigen preparation used in the test and timing of the test in relation to onset of illness and antibiotic treatment.
- In general, IgM indicates an acute infection whereas IgG indicates a past infection.
- IgM can be detectable for days–month after initial infection.
- Weak-positive results are difficult to interpret as they could indicate a very early infection or a false-positive result due to cross-reaction or due to a nonspecific reaction in the assay.
- It may then be useful to send a second sample 2–4 weeks later to monitor for titre dynamics.
- Common causes of false-positive results are organisms with similar antigens and rheumatoid factor.
- In contrast to IgG, IgM is prone to cross-reactivity, as can be seen between CMV, EBV and parvovirus, HSV and VZV, between the different arboviral flaviviruses (Zikavirus, Dengue and chikungunya) and between West nile Virus and St. Louis Encephalitis.
- For some organisms, multiple serological markers are tested, most notably hepatitis B and syphilis.
- A primary infection can be diagnosed by: 4 fold increase in IgG between serum taken in the acute phase and a convalescent serum sample taken 2 to 3 weeks later OR positive IgM OR IgG seroconversion.
- A re-infection may be diagnosed by a 4 fold increase in IgG.

Below are examples of interpretation of serological results of frequently requested tests.

HEPATITIS B

- *Hepatitis B surface antigen (HBsAg)*: A protein on the surface of the hepatitis B virus (HBV); it can be detected in high levels in serum during acute or chronic HBV infection. The presence of HBsAg indicates that the person is infectious. HBsAg is used in the hepatitis B vaccine.
- *Hepatitis B surface antibody (anti-HBs)*: Indicates either natural immunity after infection or immunity by vaccination.
- *Total hepatitis B core antibody (anti-HBc)*: Appears at the onset of symptoms in acute hepatitis B infection and persists for life.
- *IgM antibody to hepatitis B core antigen (IgM anti-HBc)*: Positivity indicates recent infection with HBV ($\leq$6 months). Indicates acute infection.

- *Hepatitis B e antigen (HBeAg)*: Found in serum during acute and chronic hepatitis B infection. Marker of active viral replication and high levels of HBV and infectiousness.
- *Hepatitis B e antibody (HBeAb or anti-HBe)*: Seroconversion from e antigen to e antibody predicts long-term clearance of HBV in patients undergoing antiviral therapy and indicates lower levels of HBV.

HEPATITIS B

Tests	Interpretation	Action
HBsAg positive **IgM anti-Hbc** positive **Anti-Hbc** positive **anti-HBs** negative	Acute hepatitis B infection	• Notify public health • Refer to hepatologist/infectious disease specialist • EDTA blood for PCR for viral load
HBsAg positive **anti-HBc** positive **IgM anti-Hbc** negative **anti-HBs** negative	Chronic hepatitis B infection	• Refer to hepatologist/infectious disease specialist • EDTA blood for PCR for viral load
HBsAg negative **anti-HBc** negative **anti-HBs** negative	Susceptible to hepatitis B infection	Consider hepatitis B vaccination
HBsAg negative **anti-HBc** negative **anti-HBs** positive	Immune due to hepatitis B vaccination	No action needed
HBsAg negative **anti-HBc** positive **anti-HBs** positive	• Immune due to natural infection • Hepatitis B can reactivate when immunosuppressed	Consider prophylaxis or monitor blood for viral reactivation using PCR during periods of immunosuppression
HBsAg negative **anti-HBc** positive **anti-HBs** negative	• Resolved infection (most common) • False-positive anti-HBc, thus susceptible • Low-level chronic infection • Resolving acute infection	• Add HBeAg and anti-HBe • Consider repeating serology in 4 weeks • Consider EDTA blood for PCR

HEPATITIS C

Test	Interpretation	Action
Anti-HCV negative	Susceptible to infection with hepatitis C	None
Anti-HCV positive	Ongoing infection with hepatitis C or past and resolved infection	EDTA blood for PCR

HEPATITIS E

Test	Interpretation	Action
HEV IgM negative **HEV IgG** negative	No prior contact with hepatitis E	None
HEV IgM positive **HEV IgG** negative	False-positive IgM or acute infection	• Repeat HEV serology in 4 weeks • EDTA blood and stool for PCR
HEV IgM positive **HEV IgG** positive	Acute infection, usually self-limiting	
HEV IgM negative **HEV IgG** positive	Past and resolved hepatitis E infection	Low risk of reactivation in individuals who become immunosuppressed after resolved infection

SYPHILIS

Test	Interpretation	Action

Syphilis Screen reactive
TPPA or TPHA reactive/
  indeterminate
RPR or VDRL reactive
  (varying dilutions)
	Consistent with recent or prior syphilis infection
	Consider:
	• Infectious syphilis (primary, secondary, early latent), especially if titre >1:8 and history of symptom(s), contact with an infected partner, other risk factors
	• Late latent syphilis or latent syphilis of unknown duration, especially if titre <1:8 and no history of treatment
	• Old treated syphilis
	• Cross-reaction with yaws, pinta or bejel
		Send convalescent sample in 2–4 weeks

Syphilis Screen reactive **TPPA or TPHA** reactive **RPR or VDRL** nonreactive	Consistent with recent or prior syphilis infection **Consider:** • Usually late latent syphilis or latent syphilis of unknown duration, with no history of treatment • Old treated syphilis • Incubating infectious syphilis (primary), especially if history of symptom(s), contact with an infected partner or other risk factors • Cross-reaction with yaws, pinta or bejel	Send convalescent sample in 2–4 weeks
Syphilis Screen reactive **TPPA or TPHA** indeterminate **RPR or VDRL** nonreactive	Inconclusive syphilis serology results **Consider:** • Incubating infectious syphilis (primary), especially if history of symptom(s), contact with an infected partner, or other risk factors • Old treated or untreated syphilis • False-positive screen	Send convalescent sample in 2–4 weeks
Syphilis Screen reactive **TPPA or TPHA** nonreactive **RPR or VDRL** nonreactive	Usually false-positive screen **Consider:** • Incubating infectious syphilis • Previously treated syphilis • Rarely, late latent syphilis	Send convalescent sample in 2–4 weeks
Syphilis Screen reactive **TPPA or TPHA** nonreactive **RPR or VDRL** reactive	Inconclusive syphilis serology results **Consider:** • Incubating infectious syphilis (primary), especially if history of symptom(s), contact with an infected partner, or other risk factors • Old treated or untreated syphilis • False positive	Send convalescent sample in 2–4 weeks
Syphilis Screen nonreactive **TPPA or TPHA** not performed **RPR or VDRL** not performed	Syphilis not present **Consider:** Early incubating syphilis can be nonreactive before antibodies develop	If clinical suspicion of early syphilis, send convalescents sample in 2–4 weeks to observe rise in titre or TPPA seroconversion

BIBLIOGRAPHY

Bennett JE, Dolin R, Blaser MJ. *Mandell, Douglas, and Bennett's Principles and Practice of Infectious Diseases: 2-Volume Set.* Vol. 1. Elsevier Health Sciences, 2014.

Janier M, Hegyi V, Dupin N et al. European guideline on the management of syphilis. *Acad Dermatol Venereol.* June 2015;29(6):1248.

Jorgensen JH, Pfaller MA, Carroll KC et al. *Manual of Clinical Microbiology,* 11th ed. American Society of Microbiology, 2015.

Landry ML Immunoglobulin M for acute infection: True or false? *Clin Vaccine Immunol.* 2016 Jul 5; 23(7):540–545.

2.10 Understanding Molecular Diagnosis

Firza Alexander Gronthoud

CLINICAL CONSIDERATIONS

Proper use and interpretation of microbiology results is an integral part of diagnostic stewardship, antimicrobial stewardship and infection prevention and control. Requesting the right test and correct interpretation of microbiology results can avoid inappropriate antimicrobial treatment and promotes patient safety and care. The choice to use a molecular test depends on the suspected infectious agent, specimen type and duration of illness. This chapter will provide a brief overview of important considerations when interpreting molecular microbiology results.

The most commonly used molecular test is PCR, which can rapidly detect microbial DNA or RNA within several hours, allowing a same-day result. An emerging role for PCR is rapid identification of bacterial causes of bloodstream infection and detection of common antimicrobial-resistance genes. Whole genome sequencing allows detection of known and unknown microbes and, similarly, known and unknown antimicrobial-resistance genes. Whole genome sequencing has also successfully been used in outbreak settings. PCR can also detect toxin production, which has been exploited for detection of *Clostridium difficile*.

Common uses for PCR are detection of blood-borne viruses, rapid screening for multidrug-resistant organisms to aid early decision-making for infection control precautions and screening for reactivation of CMV, EBV and adenovirus in bone marrow transplant recipients.

Multiplex PCR can detect multiple pathogens and is increasingly being used as part of a syndromic work-up for diagnosing meningitis, encephalitis, respiratory tract infection, infectious diarrhoea and sexually transmitted infections.

16S rRNA PCR is a pan-bacterial assay and useful when culture has remained negative; examples for its use are heart valves and sterile fluids such as joint fluid and CSF; similarly 18S and 28S rRNA genes are targets for panfungal PCR assays.

PCR is also used for genotyping of HIV and hepatitis viruses and antiviral-resistance testing. Another advantage of PCR is that new assays are fully automated, which increases laboratory capacity by allowing high throughput of multiple samples.

Quantitative PCR assays are used for assessing the microbial load which can be used to monitor response to treatment, i.e. HIV and blood-borne viruses, as well as help determine the clinical relevance, i.e. herpes viruses and BK virus.

PCR is a highly sensitive test but is unable to differentiate between viable and nonviable organisms (i.e. after successful treatment) or between colonization and infection. For some viral infections, the PCR test will only be able to detect the pathogen in the early phase of infection, most notably in the case of arboviral infection. For these pathogens, during later phases of infection, it may be more useful to request serology. On the other hand, PCR on CSF may be negative in the first 2–3 days of a herpes simplex I encephalitis. Furthermore, detection of herpes viruses in respiratory samples does not necessarily require treatment because these viruses can asymptomatically reactivate through life and be shed in bodily fluids. An exception are allogeneic stem cell recipients where pre-emptive treatment is started based on viral-load thresholds. Of note, after a traumatic tap, herpes viruses can be detected in CSF owing to spill over from the blood compartment into CSF. 16 s rRNA PCR is prone to false-positive results due to the use of universal primers and subsequent risk of detecting contaminating environmental DNA. PCR reactions may be inhibited in the presence of haemoglobin and blood culture media.

CLINICAL APPROACH

PCR is a very sensitive method; it can detect organisms that are present in clinical samples in very low quantities and which may just represent innocent bystanders. Defining quantitative thresholds and correlation with the clinical picture helps with assessing clinical significance of a positive PCR result.

CONSIDERATIONS WHEN INTERPRETING PCR RESULTS

False-positive results may occur owing to contamination with environmental DNA or carryover of previously amplified gene sequences. The use of less specific primers and probes may cause cross-reaction with other organisms.

False negative results may occur as a result of the timing of specimen collection or the sampling technique. Primers may not be able to bind to gene sequences which have undergone mutations.

Molecular techniques cannot differentiate between viable and nonviable organisms. Equally, these methods cannot differentiate between colonization and infection. However, detection of a pathogen in a sterile sample would support the diagnosis of infection. And finally, DNA and RNA may still be detectable weeks after the infection has cleared.

BACTERIAL INFECTIONS

- *Meningitis*: CSF for 16 s rRNA PCR or species-specific PCR for *Neisseria meningitidis* and *Streptococcus pneumoniae*.
- *Brain abscess*: 16 s rRNA PCR.
- *Pulmonary tuberculosis*: *Mycobacterium tuberculosis* in sputum and BAL. The GeneXpert is an example of a commercial PCR which can be used on respiratory samples and CSF. GeneXpert can also detect resistance to isoniazid and rifampicin.
- *Respiratory tract infection*: Multiplex PCR assays, either commercial or in-house assays, are commonly used for detection of *Mycoplasma pneumoniae*, *Legionella pneumophila*, *Chlamydia pneumoniae* and *Chlamydia psittaci*.
- PCR for diagnosis of atypical pneumonia is more useful than serology because
  - Mycoplasma antibodies are usually detectable 7–10 days after onset of illness.
  - Legionella antigen in urine may be negative in the first few days of infection. The sensitivity also depends on the severity of illness.
  - Chlamydia serology is not reliable due to a high rate of cross-reaction with other chlamydia species.
- *Culture negative endocarditis*: 16 s rRNA PCR on heart valve or EDTA blood for detection of DNA from *Bartonella* species and *Tropheryma whipplei*.
- *Septic arthritis*: 16 s rRNA PCR on joint fluid.
- 16 s rRNA on colonies which are not identifiable with neither biochemical tests nor MALDI-ToF.
- Multiplex PCR assays exist for bacterial gastroenteritis and bloodstream infections with commercial assays capable of detecting common antimicrobial-resistance genes.
- PCR has increasingly been used to detect toxin-producing *Clostridium difficile* and also to screen patients for carriage of multidrug-resistant organisms.

CLINICAL PEARL

Laboratories may use different PCR machines, techniques or primers. Some laboratories may also express viral load as copies/mL while other laboratories express viral load as International Units/mL. Comparing viral loads between different laboratories is therefore less useful.

VIRAL INFECTIONS

- Multiplex PCR assays exist for detection of viral meningoencephalitis, respiratory tract infection and gastroenteritis. For viral meningoencephalitis, it is important to inform the laboratory if the patient is immunocompromised, as additional viruses may need to be included in the PCR panel.
- Viral load of blood-borne viruses (HIV, HBV and HCV) for monitoring responses to treatment, genotyping and detection of antiviral resistance.
- Monitoring for reactivation of adenovirus, Epstein–Barr virus and cytomegalovirus in blood from allogeneic stem cell recipients.
- PCR can also detect resistance to acyclovir, ganciclovir and foscarnet in herpes viruses.
- Detection of BK virus in blood or urine from transplant recipients.

PARASITIC INFECTIONS

- Detection of malaria parasites *Trypanosoma cruzi* and *Leishmania* spp. in blood.
- Detection of *Giardia lamblia*, *Entamoeba histolytica* and *Cryptosporidium* spp. in stool,
- Detection of toxoplasma in blood or brain abscess.

FUNGAL INFECTIONS

- PCR has been used to detect moulds such as *Aspergillus* spp. and Mucorales.
- PCR for detection of *Pneumocystis jirovecii* pneumonia is more sensitive than microscopy. However, no official thresholds exist for distinguishing colonization from infection.
- PCR for *Pneumocystis jirovecii* should always be performed in combination with serum 1,3-β-D-glucan, A negative 1,3-β-D-glucan and a weak positive PCR is highly suggestive of colonization and other causes of infection should be explored.

BIBLIOGRAPHY

Jorgensen JH et al. *Manual of Clinical Microbiology*, 11th ed. American Society of Microbiology, 2015.

Messacar K, Parker SK, Todd JK, Dominguez SR. Implementation of rapid molecular infectious disease diagnostics: The role of diagnostic and antimicrobial stewardship. *J Clin Microbiol*. March 2017;55(3):715–723.

Millar BC, Xu J, Moore JE. Molecular diagnostics of medically important bacterial infections. *Curr Issues Mol Biol*. January 2007;9(1):21–39.

Section III

Treatment of Infections

3.1 Basic Principles of Antibiotic Treatment

Firza Alexander Gronthoud

CLINICAL CONSIDERATIONS

In managing patients with infections, very often, clinicians will need to initiate empirical antibiotics before definitive culture results become available. While the antimicrobial spectrum should be sufficiently broad so as to cover the most common pathogens involved, it is equally important to ensure that overly broad-spectrum antimicrobial agents are not being indiscriminately used, as this might create extensive 'collateral damage' to the resident flora and lead to emergence of multidrug-resistant pathogens. Once the infecting organisms are known, targeted antimicrobial therapy using the agent with the narrowest spectrum and the most favourable pharmacokinetic/pharmacodynamic profiles should be used to complete therapy. It is therefore worthwhile to consider the following.

WHAT IS THE CLINICAL DIAGNOSIS AND SITE OF INFECTION?

Different types of infections (e.g. pneumonia, intra-abdominal infections, etc.), as well as those occurring in different settings (e.g. community vs hospital-acquired), are typically caused by distinct groups of pathogenic organisms. In addition, the antibiotic chosen should achieve sufficient levels at the presumed site of infection.

WHAT IS THE HOST TYPE AND SEVERITY OF INFECTION?

Patients in different age groups, e.g. neonates versus adults, and those with normal versus compromised immune systems, e.g. neutropenic post-chemotherapy, functional/anatomical asplenia, etc., will have very different aetiologies for their infections. Patients with septic shock or who are deteriorating rapidly should receive broad-spectrum antibiotic coverage at the very beginning ('hit hard and hit early'), whereas stable patients may be observed for a period (typically 48–72 hrs) for their responses before considering any change or escalation in therapy.

DO WE HAVE ANY PRIOR MICROBIOLOGICAL DATA TO GUIDE OUR THERAPY? WHAT IS THE RISK OF DRUG-RESISTANT PATHOGENS?

Certain factors like recent hospitalization and prior antibiotic use within past 90 days will increase the risk of infections due to drug-resistant organisms. If the patient is known to be colonized by a specific pathogen, this should also be taken into account when considering empirical therapy. For patients hospitalized in specific units with nosocomial infections, data on the common pathogens encountered, as well as the hospital or unit-specific antibiogram, will be helpful in formulating the treatment regimen.

DO WE KNOW IF THERE ARE SPECIFIC CLASSES OF ANTIBIOTICS THAT SHOULD BE USED OR AVOIDED?

For serious and life-threatening infections, use of bactericidal agents (e.g. β-lactams) would generally be preferred over bacteriostatic agents (e.g. lincosamines). Drug allergy history must be carefully sought from patient and records prior to initiation of therapy. Certain classes of antibiotics may need to be avoided or used with caution in patients with underlying conditions (e.g. aminoglycosides in patients with renal failure).

Factors that may need to be considered when deciding on targeted antimicrobial therapy include the following.

SHOULD WE USE SINGLE OR COMBINATION THERAPY?

There are several reasons to combine antimicrobial therapy: to broaden spectrum, to achieve improved activity/synergy and to suppress the emergence of resistance.

In general, use a single agent with the narrowest spectrum to which the organism is susceptible whenever possible. Avoid combination therapy except for critically ill patients with documented infections due to *Pseudomonas aeruginosa* (anti-pseudomonal β-lactam plus an aminoglycoside), or for specific situations, e.g. ampicillin plus gentamicin for enterococcal endocarditis.

WHAT ABOUT THE SITE OF INFECTION AND ACTIVITY OF THE AGENT?

Choose agents with good tissue penetration for specific infections (e.g. fluoroquinolones for prostatic infections). Avoid agents which either penetrate poorly to the site of infection or are unlikely to be active locally, despite *in vitro* susceptibility; examples include cefazolin for meningitis due to methicillin-sensitive *S. aureus* (MSSA) (poor penetration to CNS), and aminoglycosides for treatment of intra-abdominal abscesses (inactivated in low PH and anaerobic conditions).

INTRAVENOUS-TO-ORAL SWITCH

Advantages: Lower treatment costs, decreased nursing time, reduced risk of infection from intravenous catheters, reduced length of hospital stay, higher patient satisfaction.

Indications
- Hemodynamic stability
- Patient is clinically improving (e.g., afebrile or reduction in temperature, normalizing WBC count)
- Functional GI tract (tolerating food, feeds, other oral medications)
- Ability to swallow or deliver drug via NG or feeding tube
- Patient is compliant

Exclusion Criteria
- Life-threatening or deep-seated infection* (e.g. severe sepsis or septic shock, CNS infections, endocarditis, endophthalmitis, bone and joint infections, vertebral or deep abscesses, necrotizing fasciitis, *Staphylococcus aureus* bacteraemia)
- Potential for malabsorption (e.g. continuous NG suction; severe or persistent nausea, vomiting, or diarrhoea; ileus or GI obstruction; active GI bleeding; short bowel syndrome; drug interactions that may affect absorption)

CLINICAL PEARL

Empirical therapy is the cornerstone for managing most patients with infections. The most important factors to consider are the clinical diagnosis and setting, the immune status of the host and severity of illness, as well as the risk of drug-resistant organisms. Prior microbiological results of the patient and unit-specific antibiogram should be taken into account when formulating the empirical regimen.

Once the infecting organism is known, targeted therapy using the narrowest-spectrum agent with good penetration and activity at the site of infection should be used for continuation of treatment.

CLINICAL APPROACH

- Does it cover the suspected organisms?
- Does it reach adequate concentration at site of infection?
- Does it require renal or hepatic dose adjustment?
- Does the patient have any underlying conditions, e.g. seizures, myasthenia gravis? (See Chapter 3.6.)
- Does it interact with any other medication the patient is on, e.g. SSRIs—linezolid (increases risk of serotonin syndrome), rifampicin—warfarin? (See Chapter 3.7.)
- Is the patient pregnant? (See Chapter 3.4.)
- Did the patient have any known reactions to antibiotics in the past, e.g. allergic reaction (most often β-lactam), Achilles tendinitis (quinolones), Stevens–Johnson (most often co-trimoxazole), heart failure or arrhythmias (macrolides and, to a lesser extent, quinolones)?
- Is the patient known to be colonized with *Clostridium difficile* (avoid quinolones, clindamycin and broad-spectrum β-lactam agents)?
- Does the patient have any previous positive culture results?
- Has the patient received antibiotic treatment in the past 3 months?
- Local practice patterns, local antibiotic resistance prevalence, product availability and costs.

BIBLIOGRAPHY

Bennett JE, Dolin R, Blaser MJ. *Mandell, Douglas, and Bennett's Principles and Practice of Infectious Diseases*. Philadelphia, PA: Elsevier/Saunders, 2015.
Grayson ML, Crowe SM, McCarthy JS, Mills J, Mouton JW, Norrby SR, Paterson DL, Pfaller MA. *Kucers' The Use of Antibiotics Sixth Edition: A Clinical Review of Antibacterial, Antifungal and Antiviral Drugs*. CRC Press, 29 October 2010.
Versalovic J, Carroll KC, Funke G, Jorgensen JH, Landry ML, Warnock DW. *Manual of Clinical Microbiology*, 10th ed. American Society of Microbiology, 2011.

3.2 Basic Principles of Antifungal Treatment

Firza Alexander Gronthoud

CLINICAL CONSIDERATIONS

Treatment of invasive fungal infections (IFIs) is often empirical and tailored to patient-specific risk factors as well as suspected fungal pathogens involved. It often involves a highly complex, specialized patient population in which, frequently, the only clinical finding is persistent fever not responding to antibiotics. Invasive fungal infections are associated with high morbidity and mortality; current diagnostic tools have suboptimal sensitivity and specificity, resulting in overuse or misuse of antifungal drugs. It is therefore worthwhile to consider the following.

BASIC COMPONENTS OF ANTIFUNGAL TREATMENT

- Choice of antifungal drug
- Avoid drug-drug interactions
- Clinical follow-up
- Source control
- Therapeutic drug monitoring
- Involvement of multidisciplinary team
- Local epidemiology

CHOICE OF ANTIFUNGAL

- Choice of antifungal depends heavily on the (suspected) fungal pathogen and site of infection
- Pathogen-drug empirical combinations
  - *Candida* spp.: Echinocandin or fluconazole
  - *Aspergillus* spp.: Voriconazole or isavuconazole; alternatively, liposomal amphotericin B
  - *Mucorales*: Amphotericin B; alternatively, isavuconazole (only licensed drug for mucormycosis, but less clinical data available)
  - *Pneumocystis jirovecii*: High-dose trimethoprim/sulfamethoxazole
  - *Cryptococcal meningitis*: Amphotericin B + flucytosine for induction, followed by fluconazole maintenance therapy
- Site of infection
  - *Urinary tract*: Fluconazole, conventional amphotericin B or flucytosine (short course)
  - *Eye*: Systemic fluconazole or voriconazole; may also require intravitreal injection with or without amphotericin B
  - *Brain*: Systemic azole or amphotericin B IV
  - *Biofilm infection*: Echinocandin or amphotericin B; requires removal of infected foreign body or catheters

CLINICAL PEARL

Treatment outcome depends also on the degree and course of immunosuppression in the patient, age, immunosuppressive drugs, underlying disease such as cancer or diabetes, malnutrition or co-infections, e.g. cytomegalovirus.

MINIMIZE DRUG-DRUG INTERACTIONS

Azoles are strong CYPP450 inhibitors and interact with vincristine, tacrolimus and cyclosporin. Rifampicin and phenytoin are strong CYP3A4 inducers which can increase clearance of azoles.

CLINICAL FOLLOW-UP

- Fever, clinical symptoms and inflammatory markers
- Monitor signs of drug toxicity
  - All antifungal drugs can cause hepatotoxicity, lowest risk seen with echinocandins.
  - *Azoles*: Prolonged QT interval. Visual disturbances and encephalopathy can be seen with voriconazole. IV voriconazole can result in renal toxicity.
  - *Echinocandins*: Low toxicity profile. Infusion-related reaction is a rare side effect.
  - *Amphotericin B*: Infusion-related reaction (lower with liposomal amphotericin B), renal toxicity, hypokalaemia, hepatotoxicity.
- Combination of imaging and biomarkers to start, stop or modify antifungal treatment
  - Imaging
    - High-resolution CT (HR CT) chest for pulmonary mould infection. Negative HR CT useful for ruling out pulmonary infection, but treatment may need to be started or continued as won't rule out extra-pulmonary infection.
    - Echocardiography should be considered when candidaemia. Endocarditis prompts surgical review and prolonged duration of treatment.
    - Dilated fundoscopy when candidaemia. If ocular infection and patient on echinocandin, then treatment should be switched to fluconazole or amphotericin B.
    - Ultrasound urinary tract if UTI. If fungus ball visible, should prompt for surgical review.
- Biomarkers
  - *1,3-β-D-glucan on blood (and CSF)*: High negative predictive value for ruling out PJP and candidaemia in all populations, high negative predictive value for ruling out IFI in haematological malignancy with profound neutropaenia (except Mucorales). Its main drawback is its low specificity.
  - *Galactomannan*: High sensitivity in BAL for detection of *Aspergillus* spp. but cannot rule out colonization. In blood: Low sensitivity in solid organ transplant recipients and non-neutropaenic patients.
  - Both galactomannan and 1,3-β-D-glucan are negative in infections caused by Mucorales and *Cryptococcus* spp.
  - *Cryptococcal antigen testing*: Can be performed in CSF and blood. High sensitivity and specificity.

SOURCE CONTROL

- Presence of infected intravascular lines or prosthetic devices increase duration and mortality of candidaemia.
- Pus collections should be drained, which allows for shorter duration of treatment.

Therapeutic Drug Monitoring (TDM)

- Optimize clinical effectiveness and minimize drug toxicity.
- Voriconazole, isavuconazole, itraconazole and posaconazole require TDM.
- Official recommendation for isavuconazole is 2–4 mg/L, but not established yet if this is the optimal clinical range.

Multidisciplinary Team

Management of fungal infections requires input from an experienced multidisciplinary team to optimize patient outcome:

- *Consultant infectious diseases and consultant microbiologist*: Diagnostic + treatment advice, diagnostic testing + interpretation of results, selection of antifungal drug
- *Antimicrobial pharmacist*: Antifungal drug dosages, PK/PD issues in specific patient populations, drug-drug interactions and therapeutic drug monitoring
- *Consultant haematologist, consultant anaesthetist (ICU) or transplant surgeon*: Risk stratification, assessing clinical signs and symptoms, antifungal drug prescribing, clinical management

Local Epidemiology

- The choice of empirical therapy is influenced by local antifungal resistance prevalence.
- In the UK for instance, the voriconazole resistance rate in *Aspergillus fumigatus* in clinical isolated in North West London is between 1 and 3% whereas in some parts of the Netherlands it may be as high as 20%.
- Voriconazole resistance in *Aspergillus* spp. may also show variation among different populations at risk (i.e. higher in haematology patients and lower in ICU patients).
- Because of widespread use of azoles, there is a global increase in infections caused by azole-resistant fungi such as Mucorales and *Candida auris*.

CLINICAL APPROACH

- Antifungals are prescribed in the context of prophylaxis, pre-emptive therapy, empirical treatment or targeted treatment (see Chapters 4.32, 4.34 and 4.48).
- Early antifungal treatment, when the fungal burden is lowest and the risk of dissemination to other organs is low, significantly improves patient outcome.

Prophylaxis

- The goal of prophylaxis is to prevent the development of infection and is indicated if there is a high risk of invasive fungal infections or high prevalence (i.e. >10%).
- Primary prophylaxis is indicated in individuals with severe and prolonged neutropaenia >10 days, as is seen with induction chemotherapy for acute myeloid leukaemia or in allogeneic HSCT recipients).
- In allogeneic HSCT recipients the antifungal agent should also be active against *Aspergillus* spp., i.e. posaconazole.
- If a mould infection has been cleared after treatment but the patient remains immunosuppressed, treatment should be continued until immune reconstitution (neutrophils count recovered, functional T cells, normal immunoglobulin levels and all immunosuppressive treatment stopped). This is called secondary prophylaxis.

Pre-Emptive Therapy

- In pre-emptive therapy, also called diagnostic-driven treatment, the trigger for starting antifungal treatment is a positive biomarker and/or positive CT thorax in the absence of clinical signs of infection in patients at risk of IFI.
- Diagnostic-driven treatment could potentially reduce the use of antifungal agents and improve outcome because biomarkers are positive several days before the onset of clinical symptoms. However, biomarkers have different sensitivities and specificities depending on the population at risk, background prevalence of fungal infections, previous antifungal treatment and false-positive results can occur.

CLINICAL PEARL

Symptoms of IFI are often nonspecific and current diagnostic tests have suboptimal test performance. Without antifungal stewardship, patients are exposed to unnecessary drug-related toxicities and higher costs, as well as providing an environment for the emergence of antifungal resistance.

Empirical Treatment

- The trigger to start antifungal treatment is persistent fever despite ≥ 36 hours antibiotic therapy in a patient at risk of invasive fungal infection.
- This approach is usually employed in critically ill patients at risk of invasive candidiasis or patients with severe and prolonged neutropaenia at risk for invasive mould infections.
- If a patient is on antifungal prophylaxis, an antifungal agent from a different class should be used for empirical therapy to avoid risk of cross-resistance.

Clinical Failure Despite Antifungal Therapy

- Has the antifungal agent been given adequate time to work?
  - It may take a week before *P. jirovecii* responds to treatment.
- Could there be another explanation for current signs and symptoms?
  - Invasive fungal infections predominantly occur in patients at high risk for bacterial and viral infections.
- Is the diagnosis correct?
  - A positive BDG with a negative CT chest and negative culture may indicate a false-positive result.
  - Conversely, a positive CT chest with negative biomarkers may indicate mucormycosis rather than aspergillosis or indicate bacterial/viral infection.
- Is the antifungal agent active against the (suspected) fungus?
  - Review antifungal susceptibility.
- Are there any medication-related factors?
  - Check the correct dose and route of administration.
  - Drug-drug interactions.
  - Check serum levels with therapeutic drug monitoring.
- Does the antifungal agent have adequate tissue penetration?
  - Echinocandins have poor penetration in the brain, eye and urinary tract.
  - In contrast to conventional amphotericin B, liposomal amphotericin B reaches low concentrations in the urinary tract.

- Has source control been achieved?
  - Remove any lines, catheters or devices.
  - Drain any abscesses.
  - Debride any necrotic lesions.
- If all of the above are not applicable, continue antifungal treatment and consider host factors: uncontrolled underlying disease or severely immunosuppressed state. Consider reducing any immunosuppressive agents or adding of granulocyte colony-stimulating factor in the case of neutropaenia.

BIBLIOGRAPHY

Kontoyiannis DP. Invasive Mycoses: Strategies for effective management. *Am J Med*. January 2012;125(1 Suppl):S25–138.

Kontoyiannis DP, Lewis RE. Treatment principles for the management of mold infections. *Cold Spring Harb Perspect Med*. 6 November 2014;5(4).

Nucci M, Perfect JR. When primary antifungal therapy fails. *Clin Infect Dis*. 1 May 2008;46(9):1426–1433.

Rautemaa-Richardson R, Rautemaa V, Al-Wathiqi F, Moore CB, Craig L, Felton TW, Muldoon EG. Impact of a diagnostics-driven antifungal stewardship programme in a UK tertiary referral teaching hospital. *J Antimicrob Chemother*. 1 December 2018;73(12):3488–3495.

Stevens DA, Zhang Y, Finkelman MA, Pappagianis D, Clemons KV, Martinez M. Cerebrospinal fluid (1,3)-beta-D-glucan testing is useful in diagnosis of coccidioidal meningitis. *J Clin Microbiol*. November 2016;54(11):2707–2710. Epub 2016 August 24.

3.3 β-Lactam Allergy

Firza Alexander Gronthoud

CLINICAL CONSIDERATION

β-Lactam allergy is frequently reported by patients, severely limiting treatment options for Gram-negative infections owing to risk of cross-reaction with other β-lactam agents. However, more than half of patients who self-report a β-lactam allergy (usually penicillin) are not allergic, and in non-severe allergies, other β-lactam antibiotics could still be used. It is therefore worthwhile to consider the following:

- Antibiotic allergy is a hypersensitivity to antimicrobials and can be classified based on the immunological nature of the reaction (see Table 3.3.1).
- Most of the β-lactam reported allergies are penicillin allergies because amoxicillin and amoxicillin/clavulanic acid are some of the most prescribed antimicrobials in the community and in hospitals.
- Patients who are allergic to penicillins have an increased likelihood of being allergic to other medication, including non-antibiotic medication.
- More than 90% of patients who report a penicillin allergy and subsequently receive a penicillin do not develop an allergic reaction because a significant proportion never had an allergic reaction to penicillin and also because IgE-mediated penicillin allergy wanes over time.
- The most common β-lactam allergy is a benign rash, which is tolerated well by patients.
- The cross-reaction between penicillin and β-lactam antibiotics is an IgE-mediated reaction and based on the similarity in the R1 and R2 sidechains of the β-lactam ring.
- Therefore, the rate of cross-reaction between penicillin and first-generation cephalosporins is higher than with third-generation cephalosporins (<3%) and carbapenems (<1%), with the exception being cefazolin, which has a very low cross-reactivity with penicillin.
- Obviously, these rates are lower in clinical practice because most patients with a reported β-lactam allergy are not allergic.
- Previous reported rates of 10% cross-reactivity between penicillins and cephalosporins is a myth because
  - Older cephalosporins were contaminated with penicillin.
  - Mixed definitions of allergic reaction were used in older studies.
- Aztreonam does not cross-react with penicillin, cephalosporins (except ceftazidime) and carbapenems.
- Chronic urticaria does not increase risk of penicillin allergy.

NEGATIVE CONSEQUENCES OF PENICILLIN ALLERGY LABELLING

- Use of less effective antimicrobials, i.e. vancomycin for treatment of *Staphylococcus aureus* bloodstream infections
- Use of broader-spectrum antimicrobials (i.e. meropenem) which leads to antimicrobial resistance or use of more toxic antimicrobials like aminoglycosides and glycopeptides

TABLE 3.3.1

Immunological Nature of Allergic Reactions

Type of Reaction	Reaction	Immune Mediators	Timing of Reaction
Acute IgE-mediated reaction	Pruritis, flushing, urticaria, wheezing, shortness of breath, bronchospasm, oedema, chest tightness and anaphylaxis	IgE on mast cells bind to allergens	Usually within 1 hour, sometimes 2 hours
Antibody-dependent cell-mediated cytotoxicity	Haemolytic anaemia, granulocytopaenia, thrombocytopaenia	IgM-, IgG-mediated cell lysis	After 72 hours
Immune complex-mediated hypersensitivity	Serum sickness-like syndrome	Ag/Ab complex formation and activation of complement	After 72 hours
T-cell-mediated reaction	Benign maculopapular rash, drug eruption or severe cutaneous adverse reactions (SCAR): Stevens–Johnson syndrome (SJS), toxic epidermal necrolysis (TEN) and drug reaction with eosinophilia and systemic symptoms (DRESS)	Activation of T cells, cytokine production, recruitment of effector cells	After 72 hours

CLINICAL APPROACH

Allergy history is important to assess the likelihood and severity of a β-lactam allergy based on described or documented allergic reaction. Key information:

- β-lactam agent used, signs and symptoms experienced, and interval between administration and occurrence of reaction
- Whether or not the patient took any other medication including antimicrobials
- Previously used antimicrobials which were tolerated

If a patient reports to have had diarrhoea and vomiting, dizziness, unknown reaction or a family member who developed a rash after administration of a β-lactam agent, then most likely the patient is not allergic.

If it is likely that the patient had a possible allergic reaction, then the type of allergic reaction needs to be classified as non-severe, moderate severe and very severe.

- *Non-severe*: Benign rash occurring days after administration
- *Moderate severe*: IgE-mediated reactions with exception of anaphylaxis
- *Very severe*: Anaphylaxis, SJS, TEN and DRESS, antibody-dependent cell cytotoxicity or immune-complex-mediated hypersensitivity

If the patient has an infection for which the optimal treatment is with a β-lactam agent, then obtain informed consent from the patient and perform β-lactam sensitivity testing unless the patient had a very severe allergic reaction. Patients should be directly observed for up to 1 hour when being challenged with a provocation test.

- *Non-severe reaction*: Perform β-lactam provocation test
- *Moderate severe reaction*: Skin test; if negative, perform β-lactam provocation test
- *Very severe reaction*: Penicillin allergy testing not indicted

TABLE 3.3.2

Alternative β-Lactam Treatment Options in Case of a True β-Lactam Allergy

β-Lactam Allergy	Severity of Allergy	Alternative β-Lactam
Penicillin	Non-severe rash	1st-, 2nd- or 3rd-Generation cephalosporin, aztreonam
Penicillin	Moderate severe reaction	3rd-Generation cephalosporin or aztreonam
Penicillin	Very severe reaction	Aztreonam or carbapenem
3rd-Generation cephalosporin	Non-severe rash or moderate severe reaction	Penicillin or aztreonam
3rd-Generation cephalosporin	Very severe reaction	Carbapenem or aztreonam
Carbapenem	Non-severe rash or moderate severe reaction	Penicillin; 1st-, 2nd- or 3rd-generation cephalosporin or aztreonam
Carbapenem	Very severe reaction	Aztreonam

Patients with a positive skin test result should be labelled allergic and do not need to undergo a provocation test. Negative penicillin skin testing has a high negative-predictive value for excluding a penicillin allergy (~95%) and approaching 100% if combined with a negative oral amoxicillin provocation.

β-LACTAM PROVOCATION DOSE OPTIONS

- Oral amoxicillin provocation doses: 250 or 500 mg
- Intravenous ceftazidime of ceftriaxone doses: 25, 100 or 500 mg

If a patient has a true moderate or very severe allergy, then either a desensitization procedure performed by an immunology specialist or referral to an allergy clinic can be considered, or treatment with alternative agents should be chosen (see Table 3.3.2 for alternative β-lactam agents).

PENICILLIN DESENSITIZATION

Patients are eligible for a desensitization procedure if they had one or multiple episodes of moderate or severe reactions to one or more β-lactams and are proven to be true allergic based on skin testing and/or oral antibiotic provocations. Desensitization is also indicated for patients who are unable to undergo skin testing.

BIBLIOGRAPHY

Blumenthal KG, Peter JG, Trubiano JA, Phillips EJ. Antibiotic allergy. *Lancet.* 12 January 2019;393(10167):183–198.

Mirakian R, Ewan PW, Durham SR, Youlten LJ, Dugué P, Friedmann PS, English JS, Huber PA, Nasser SM; BSACI. BSACI guidelines for the management of drug allergy. *Clin Exp Allergy.* January 2009;39(1):43–61.

Shenoy ES, Macy E, Rowe T, Blumenthal KG. Evaluation and management of penicillin allergy: A review. *JAMA.* 15 January 2019;321(2):188–199.

3.4 Antimicrobials in Pregnant Women

Firza Alexander Gronthoud

CLINICAL CONSIDERATIONS

Around 80% of all medications used in pregnancy are antibiotics. The most common indications for antibiotic treatment during pregnancy are asymptomatic bacteriuria, urinary tract infections and respiratory tract infections. Antimicrobial treatment in pregnant women is a dual-edged sword. Untreated infections are risk factors for maternal morbidity and, for the unborn child, associated with low birth weight, preterm birth, congenital defects and spontaneous abortion. Antibiotics have also been linked to altered gut microbiota with subsequent failure of maturation of the immune system and development of atopic disease in the newborn. Pregnancy also impacts pharmacokinetics and the effectiveness of antimicrobials. It is therefore worthwhile to consider the following.

PHYSIOLOGICAL CHANGES DURING PREGNANCY

Physiologic changes during pregnancy may lead to pharmacokinetic changes and impact antibiotic therapy. Pregnant women have decreased albumin. For highly protein-bound antibiotics, this means an increased volume of drug distribution and increased renal clearance. Further contributing to increased drug distribution is increased intravascular and extravascular volume. Increased renal clearance is further compounded by an increased glomerular filtration rate (GFR). Changes in gastrointestinal motility lead to reduced absorption and, consequently, reduced bioavailability of oral antibiotics.

SAFETY OF ANTIBIOTICS DURING PREGNANCY

- β-Lactam agents are generally safe to use. Ceftriaxone can cause kernicterus and should be used with caution.
- Glycopeptides are considered safe during pregnancy, although limited data exist on use during the first trimester.
- The lipoglycopeptides oritavancin and dalbavancin should be avoided unless benefits outweigh risks based on data from current animal studies.
- Daptomycin is generally considered to be safe during pregnancy.
- Oxazolidinones should be used with caution during pregnancy when potential benefits outweigh the risks. Fetal weight loss and bone and cartilage abnormalities were seen with tedizolid in animal studies.
- Streptomycin causes irreversible bilateral congenital deafness, especially during the first trimester of pregnancy, and is contraindicated. Other aminoglycosides have not been found to cause congenital deafness, and short courses may be used with caution.
- Colistin should be used with caution.
- Quinolones should be avoided during pregnancy because animal studies have demonstrated bone and cartilage damage in the fetus.
- Clindamycin and macrolides are generally considered to be safe.

- Tetracyclines cause permanent discolouration of bones and teeth of the fetus when administered beyond the second trimester and are therefore contraindicated past the fifth week of pregnancy. In rare cases, doxycycline may be considered in pregnant women who have life-threatening tick-borne illnesses.
- Nitrofurantoin, fosfomycin and systemic metronidazole are safe to use. However, nitrofurantoin is contraindicated within 30 days of delivery as it may cause neonatal haemolysis. Although fosfomycin is safe to use during the second and third trimesters, there is insufficient data regarding the use of fosfomycin in the first trimester.
- Trimethoprim and sulfamethoxazole are contraindicated in the first trimester owing to major congenital malformations. Sulfamethoxazole should be avoided after 32 weeks' gestation owing to risk of kernicterus.
- Acyclovir is safe to use in pregnancy whilst ganciclovir, cidofovir and foscarnet should be avoided during pregnancy because of their potential for teratogenic effects.
- Topical azoles for the treatment of superficial fungal infections are safe and effective.
- Continuous high-dose fluconazole in the first trimester of pregnancy is teratogenic.
- Itraconazole and amphotericin B are not linked to congenital defects and are safe to use during pregnancy.
- Griseofulvin, ketoconazole, voriconazole and flucytosine are contraindicated in pregnancy owing to a strong association with congenital defects.
- There are insufficient data to guide the use of echinocandins during pregnancy.

ANTIBIOTIC DOSING CHANGES DURING PREGNANCY

- High protein binding of penicillins may require a higher dosing.
- Cephalosporins have decreased plasma concentrations in pregnant patients because of increased renal elimination.
- Vancomycin requires therapeutic drug monitoring (TDM) in all patients. TDM may indicate higher doses are needed because of increased volume of distribution and increased renal clearance.
- Macrolides do not require dose adjustment owing to low protein binding, large volumes of distribution and hepatic metabolism.
- Clindamycin is widely distributed into most body tissues and is highly plasma protein bound (92%–94%). It is excreted in the urine as 10% active drug and metabolites, 3.6% in the feces, and the remainder excreted as inactive metabolites.

CLINICAL PEARL

β-Lactams, vancomycin, nitrofurantoin, metronidazole, clindamycin and fosfomycin are generally safe in pregnancy. Fluoroquinolones and tetracyclines are contraindicated in pregnancy.

CLINICAL APPROACH

- Confirm the indication for antibiotics.
- Determine which trimester in pregnancy the patient is in.
- Assess any antibiotic allergies.
- If antibacterial treatment is indicated, avoid quinolones, tetracyclines, voriconazole, flucytosine, ganciclovir, foscarnet and cidofovir. Aminoglycosides and fluconazole can be given for a short course. Safe to use are β-lactam, glycopeptides, daptomycin, nitrofurantoin,

fosfomycin, metronidazole and clindamycin, acyclovir and amphotericin B. Trimethoprim/
sulfamethoxazole may be used during the second trimester until 32 weeks' gestation.
* β-lactam agents with high protein binding may need higher doses owing to low albumin,
  increased volume of distribution and increased glomerular filtration rate.

BIBLIOGRAPHY

Bookstaver PB, Bland CM, Griffin B, Stover KR, Eiland LS, McLaughlin M. A review of antibiotic use in
pregnancy. *Pharmacotherapy.* November 2015;35(11):1052–1062

Lamont HF, Blogg HJ, Lamont RF. Safety of antimicrobial treatment during pregnancy: A current
review of resistance, immunomodulation and teratogenicity. *Expert Opin Drug Saf.* December
2014;13(12):1569–1581

Moudgal VV, Sobel JD. Antifungal drugs in pregnancy: A review. *Expert Opin Drug Saf.* September
2003;2(5):475–483.

Mylonas I. Antibiotic chemotherapy during pregnancy and lactation period aspects for consideration. *Arch
Gynecol Obstet.* January 2011;283(1):7–18.

3.5 Antimicrobial Agents and Liver Injury

Firza Alexander Gronthoud

CLINICAL CONSIDERATIONS

Antimicrobial agents can have severe side effects with organ-specific toxicity. Deranged liver function tests (LFTs) are a common occurrence during antimicrobial therapy. This may indicate an asymptomatic transient reaction or it may represent more severe liver injury which may or may not be induced or facilitated by antimicrobial therapy. It may therefore be worthwhile to consider the following.

LIVER INJURY

Although antimicrobials are the most common drugs associated with drug-induced liver injury, the incidence of liver injury is low and may be more likely to be directly related to infection rather than the antimicrobial agent used. Liver injury can be a result of a hypersensitivity reaction or an idiosyncratic liver injury based on molecular structure, i.e. hepatotoxic drug metabolites. Clues pointing towards an immunological reaction include rapid onset <72 hours and development of rash, fever or eosinophilia (see Chapter 3.3 for an overview of hypersensitivity reactions) and recurrent reaction upon re-exposure to the same agent.

RISK FACTORS

Impaired liver function or pre-existing liver disease, concurrent medications and excessive alcohol consumption may all increase likelihood of liver injury with or without involvement of antimicrobials. There may also be an association with the total daily antimicrobial dose. Previous hepatotoxic reaction to antibiotics further increases likelihood of liver injury. Liver injury usually manifests as a mild and transient reaction and rarely progresses to liver failure.

TIMING OF LIVER INJURY

The interval between antimicrobial treatment and occurrence of deranged LFTs and liver injury varies from immediately to within days or even weeks after antimicrobial treatment has finished. Close monitoring and assessment of potential causes for deranged LFTs are essential in preventing severe complications.

TYPE OF LIVER INJURY

Liver injury can present as:

- Hepatocellular injury— Increased alanine transferase (ALT) and aspartate aminotransferase (AST) with normal to mildly increased alkaline phosphatase (ALP) and gamma-GT
- Cholestatic injury
- Mixed hepatocellular-cholestatic injury

- Acute or chronic
- Granulomas
- Steatosis and steatohepatitis

HEPATOTOXIC PROFILE OF COMMONLY PRESCRIBED ANTIMICROBIALS

- *Ampicillin, amoxicillin, penicillin and benzylpenicillin*: Very rare; mainly, hepatocellular cholestasis has been described.
- *Flucloxacillin*: 1.8 per 100,000 prescriptions, or 2.6 per 100,000 users. Liver injury typically begins 20–30 days after starting the drug. Older patients and those receiving more than 2 weeks of treatment appear at increased risk. Liver damage associated with flucloxacillin was found to be cholestatic or mixed. Genotype HLA-B*5701, present in less than 4% of Europeans, carries an 80-fold increase risk of flucloxacillin liver injury. However, as this genotype will be infrequently encountered and the liver injury incidence of flucloxacillin is low, it is not necessary to routinely test patients for this genotype prior to starting a course of flucloxacillin.
- *Amoxicillin/clavulanic acid*: Most reported cause of drug-induced liver injury and mostly attributed to the clavulanic acid component. Risk of drug-induced liver injury is 1 per 2350 prescriptions. Liver injury can start during therapy or several days to weeks after cessation. Liver injury is cholestatic or mixed, but may be more hepatocellular in younger patients. The course is usually benign and symptoms resolve in a few weeks, but acute liver failure may occur. Amoxicillin/clavulanate is responsible for 13%–23% of drug-induced liver injury cases and is the leading cause of hospitalization for adverse hepatic events. Because symptom onset is usually delayed, early diagnosis is difficult. Prolonged or repeated courses or being >65 years of age increase the risk of developing liver injury. A significant association between the DRB1*1501-DRB5*0101-DQB1*0602 haplotype and cholestatic hepatitis related to amoxicillin/clavulanate has been demonstrated.
- *Sulfonamides*: Hepatotoxic drugs with an incidence of 1 per 1000 prescriptions. Trimethoprim/sulfamethoxazole usually induces mild cholestatic or mixed injury within a few days after initiation of treatment. Most cases of sulfonamide-induced liver injury are mild and patients usually recover within a few weeks of treatment discontinuation, but severe cases, including fulminant cases of necrosis and granulomatous hepatitis, have been described for the combination trimethoprim/sulfamethoxazole. The hepatotoxicity is thought to be due to an idiosyncratic reaction.
- *Cephalosporins*: Rarely implicated in liver injury. Cholestasis occurring within a few days is typical and appears immunologically mediated. Ceftriaxone has been associated with hepatocellular damage with eosinophilia and high IgE levels, but the typical adverse effect is biliary sludge formation because this agent can precipitate in bile as a calcium salt.
- *Macrolides*: Liver injury is seen in less than 4 cases per 100,000 patients prescribed erythromycin. The latency period is between 6 and 20 days, is usually cholestatic or mixed and can resemble acute cholecystitis. Liver injury is accompanied by a hypersensitivity reaction in half of the cases (fever, rash or peripheral eosinophilia). Symptoms and biochemical abnormalities resolve within 2–5 weeks of treatment discontinuation; very occasionally, cholestasis persists for 3–6 months. Clarithromycin liver injury is similar to that of erythromycin, but with a slightly higher risk of severe injury. Liver injury is rare in azithromycin.
- *Quinolones*: Mild rises in liver enzymes occur in a minority of cases, 2%–3%, and are reversible.
- *Tetracyclines*: Low oral doses of tetracyclines rarely cause liver injury: 1 per 18 million doses to 1.5 cases per 100,000 prescriptions, representing one of the lowest rates for any antibiotic with an established liver injury risk. When it does occur, it can induce

hepatocellular, cholestatic or mixed injury in similar proportions. Microvesicular steatosis is the characteristic feature of treatment with intravenous or large oral doses of tetracycline, whereas cholestasis is the predominant clinicopathological pattern with oxytetracycline and minocycline. Doxycycline does not seem to be associated with liver injury.

- *Linezolid*: Prolonged treatment with linezolid has been associated with severe liver failure and lactic acidosis. Liver biopsy may show microvesicular steatosis.
- *Rifampicin*: Fewer than 2% of patients administered rifampicin develop increased serum transaminase levels. Severe liver injury occurs in 0%–0.7% of patients. Liver injury attributed to rifampicin itself is rare; it may contribute to increased liver injury when co-administered with isoniazid and, especially, pyrazinamide.
- *Azoles*: Azoles have also been associated with liver injury, in particular, ketoconazole, voriconazole and, to a lesser extent, fluconazole. Liver injury has also been documented for amphotericin B.

CLINICAL APPROACH

Clinical signs and symptoms of liver injury cannot be used to differentiate between antimicrobial induced injury or other aetiology, and no specific test exists.

Drug-induced liver injury is diagnosed by ruling out other possibilities and deciding whether clinical signs and symptoms, biochemical findings, time between drug administration and onset of symptoms could be explained by any current or recent antimicrobial treatment.

To rule out other causes of liver injury, it is essential to take a sexual history, history of blood transfusions, intravenous drug use, excessive alcohol intake and determine if the patient might have an undiagnosed chronic liver disease such as chronic hepatitis, liver cirrhosis or hepatocellular carcinoma.

Delayed onset of liver impairment up until weeks after completely a course of antimicrobials has been described and makes it further challenging.

It is also useful to do an ultrasound of the liver and biliary tract, request a consult from the gastroenterology team and, if clinically indicated, obtain a liver biopsy.

CLINICAL PEARL

Excluding other potential causes, withholding the suspected culprit and closely monitoring the patient is the definitive method to ascertain whether or not the suspected antimicrobial agent is the true cause of the liver injury.

ALGORITHM/DIAGNOSING DRUG-INDUCED LIVE INJURY

- The onset after starting the drug: Time to onset
- The recovery after stopping the drug: Time to recovery
- What is the biochemical picture? Hepatocellular injury is more seen in nitrofurantoin whilst mixed injury is seen with amoxicillin/clavulanic acid and sulfonamides. A mixed pattern fits more with drug-induced liver injury rather than a viral hepatitis or a cholangitis, for example.
- Are there any clinical symptoms? For example, hypersensitivity reaction indicates a drug reaction and fever with jaundice and right upper quadrant pain fits with a cholangitis.
- Are there any other potential causes of liver injury? For example, other medication or a history of intravenous drug use or sepsis-driven liver injury.
- Is the antimicrobial agent a known cause of liver injury?
- Has the patient tolerated this antimicrobial in the past without any issues?

CLINICAL PEARL

Hepatocellular injury may indicate a viral hepatitis. It is useful to take a sexual history, travel history and intravenous drug history to ascertain risk factors for hepatitis A, B, C and E.

BIBLIOGRAPHY

Andrade RJ, Tulkens PM. Hepatic Safety of Antibiotics Used in Primary Care. *J Antimicrob Chemother.* July 2011;66(7):1431–1446.

Devarbhavi H, Andrade RJ. Drug-Induced Liver Injury Due to Antimicrobials, Central Nervous System Agents, and Nonsteroidal Anti-Inflammatory Drugs. *Semin Liver Dis.* May 2014;34(2):145–161.

LiverTox: Clinical and Research Information on Drug Induced Liver Injury [Internet]. Bethesda (MD): National Institute of Diabetes and Digestive and Kidney Diseases, 2012. Clinical Course and Diagnosis Of Drug Induced Liver Disease. [Updated 2019 May 4].

3.6 Antimicrobial Agents and Neurotoxicity

Firza Alexander Gronthoud

CLINICAL CONSIDERATIONS

One of the adverse events that antibiotics are linked to is neurotoxicity, with seizures being the most reported neurological adverse event. However, based on current evidence, it is unclear how strong this association is and avoiding use of a particular antibiotic because of a potential risk of neurotoxicity leads to use of more broad-spectrum antibiotics or antibiotics with inferior effectiveness. This ultimately increases risk of antimicrobial resistance and compromises patient safety and outcome. Neurotoxicity, on the other hand, can have severe complications, and some may go unrecognized for a prolonged time. It is therefore worthwhile to consider the following.

LIKELIHOOD AND MECHANISM OF NEUROTOXICITY

Evidence for neurotoxic effects of antibacterials, such as seizures and encephalopathy, is based on low-quality evidence (i.e. case reports), with adverse events occurring at a low frequency. Increased CNS drug concentration has been suggested to contribute to development of seizures and can result from impaired renal function and/or a disrupted blood–brain barrier (i.e. due to brain lesions). Peripheral neuropathy and optic neuritis are other adverse antimicrobial drug events directly caused by antimicrobials. Pre-existing neurological diseases also increase the risk of neurotoxicity. For instance, there are reports of epileptic insults elicited by quinolones, and aminoglycosides should be avoided in patients with myasthenia gravis. Drug-drug interactions also play a role as demonstrated by carbapenems which decrease the concentration of valproic acid which is an antiepileptic drug, and linezolid should be used with caution in individuals on certain antidepressants as it increases the risk of serotonin syndrome.

CLINICAL MANIFESTATIONS OF ANTIBIOTIC-INDUCED NEUROTOXICITY

- Central nervous system effects, such as convulsive or nonconvulsive seizures and encephalopathy (altered mental status, psychosis, hallucinations)
- Optic neuropathy, which presents as vision loss
- Peripheral neuropathy affecting sensory nerves, motor nerves and autonomic nerves (symptoms are muscle weakness, altered or loss of sensation, pain in affected areas and, if autonomic nerves are affected, orthostatic hypotension, altered sweating, bladder dysfunction, gastroparesis)
- Ototoxicity caused by aminoglycosides, polymyxins

ANTIMICROBIALS LINKED TO NEUROTOXICITY

The following adverse events linked to antimicrobials are rare but have been reported:

- *Seizures*: β-Lactams (penicillins, cefepime, imipenem), quinolones and isoniazid
- *Encephalopathy*: Voriconazole, β-lactams, gentamicin, metronidazole

- *Optic neuropathy*: Ethambutol and linezolid
- *Peripheral (poly)neuropathy*: Metronidazole, linezolid, isoniazid, daptomycin, dapsone, quinolones and triazoles
- *Neuromuscular blockade*: Aminoglycosides, fluoroquinolones; macrolides may disrupt neuromuscular transmission and should be avoided in patients with myasthenia gravis

DRUG-DRUG INTERACTIONS

- Erythromycin and clarithromycin are strong inhibitors of CYP450 enzymes whereas rifampicin is a strong inducer.
- Azithromycin is not linked to seizure-inducing effects mainly because it does not inhibit CYP3A4.
- Concomitant use of antiepileptic agents metabolized by CYP450 enzymes may lead to an increase or decrease in the antiepileptic drug serum level.
- Antiepileptic drugs which are metabolized by CYP450 enzymes are carbamazepine, phenytoin and phenobarbital.
- Carbapenems reduce the half-life valproic acid, increasing drug clearance and subtherapeutic plasma levels.
- Concomitant use of nephrotoxic drugs may potentiate risk of antibiotic-induced seizures owing to reduced clearance and higher antimicrobial drug concentrations in the CNS.

ANTIMICROBIAL-SPECIFIC NEUROTOXIC PROPERTIES

β-Lactam Agents in General

Antibiotic-related symptomatic seizures are mainly reported in association with β-lactams, especially benzylpenicillin, cefepime and imipenem, whereby the risk is elevated in high-dose therapy, renal dysfunction and underlying brain diseases. A disrupted blood–brain barrier, for example, in meningitis, further increases risk of seizures.

Penicillin

- Penicillins interact with the neurotransmitter γ-aminobutyric acid (GABA) and thereby lower the seizure threshold.
- Penicillins are thought to be less neurotoxic than cephalosporins.
- There are no data regarding amoxicillin/clavulanic acid.

Cephalosporins

- Cephalosporins lower the seizure threshold by antagonistic binding at the GABA receptor.
- Cefepime is more frequently reported to cause seizures compared to other cephalosporins.

Carbapenems

- There is a structural resemblance of the β-lactam ring with the GABA neurotransmitter, enabling carbapenems to interact at the GABA receptor and act as a GABA antagonist.
- Imipenem is more seizure-inducing than meropenem because it has a higher affinity to the GABA receptors than other carbapenems.

Quinolones

- Fluoroquinolones inhibit GABAergic transmission by blocking the intracerebral $GABA_A$ receptors.
- Although quinolones such as ciprofloxacin are often cited as associated with seizures, seizures are a rare event.

- Evidence for seizures is mainly based on case reports with seizures described in patients with renal failure and underlying CNS disease or status epilepticus with additional administration of theophylline.
- Levofloxacin seems to have a very low CNS toxicity, with even fewer cases reported compared to other quinolones and lower CNS penetration compared to other quinolones.

Aminoglycosides

- The main neurotoxic effect of aminoglycosides is ototoxicity.
- The main risk factors for ototoxicity are large doses, high blood drug levels and a long duration of therapy.
- Other risk factors include the following: Elderly, renal insufficiency, pre-existing hearing problems, a family history of ototoxicity and concomitant use of loop diuretics or other ototoxic or nephrotoxic medications.
- Aminoglycosides should be avoided in individuals with the mitochondrial m.1555A>G mutation, which causes progressive hearing loss.
- Hearing loss caused by aminoglycosides is irreversible.
- Vestibular toxicity can also occur and is duration dependent.
- Vestibular injury is dose or concentration independent and even topical inhalation and eardrop administration have been associated with vestibular injury.
- Vestibular toxicity is reversible.
- Less commonly reported are encephalopathy, peripheral neuropathy and neuromuscular blockade.
- Gentamicin is the drug in this class for which cases of encephalopathy and polyneuropathy have been described.
- Several aminoglycosides, including neomycin, streptomycin, kanamycin, tobramycin, gentamicin, amikacin and netilmicin, have been implicated in determination of neuromuscular blockade, mimicking myasthenia gravis, renal disease, neuromuscular disease, botulism and hypocalcaemia, or with the concomitant administration of muscle relaxants (i.e. d-tubocurarine, succinylcholine chloride or similar anaesthetic agents).
- Aminoglycosides have been found to inhibit the presynaptic release of acetylcholine and to prevent the internalization of calcium into the presynaptic region of the axon.
- These findings explain why administration of calcium gluconate may reverse the blockade and why it is the treatment of choice for this critical adverse event.

Metronidazole

Mainly peripheral neuropathy and encephalopathy have been reported.

Linezolid

Linezolid is a reversible inhibitor of monoamine oxidase A and increases risk of serotonin syndrome when other serotonergic medications are co-administered.

Risk of serotonin syndrome is highest for concomitant selective serotonin reuptake inhibitors (SSRIs) and serotonin norepinephrine reuptake inhibitor.

Isoniazid

Isoniazid inhibits formation of pyridoxine, resulting in peripheral neuropathy and seizures.

Ethambutol

Optic neuropathy is dose and duration dependent with risk highest in dosages of ≥25 mg/kg/day and a duration of ≥2 months.

Triazoles

Polyneuropathy occurs in 10% of patients receiving triazole therapy for more than 4 months, with risk highest in itraconazole > voriconazole > posaconazole.

ANTIBIOTICS WITHOUT EVIDENCE FOR EPILEPSY

The following antibiotics seem to have no risk for seizures: trimethoprim/sulfamethoxazole, aminoglycosides, glycopeptides, lipopeptides, nitrofurantoin, fosfomycin, clindamycin and tetracyclines.

CLINICAL PEARL

As most seizures associated with cephalosporins are nonconvulsive, continuous EEG should be considered in patients with altered levels of consciousness.

CLINICAL APPROACH

GENERAL POINTS TO CONSIDER BEFORE STARTING ANTIMICROBIAL THERAPY

- Avoid high-dose antimicrobial therapy in patients with renal impairment, brain disease or a disrupted blood–brain barrier; if used, carefully monitor for seizure activity.
- If patients are on antiepileptic drugs and concomitant antimicrobial therapy, drug serum levels of antiepileptic drugs should be performed to avoid the risk of toxicity or inadequate antiepileptic therapy.
- If seizures are under control with antiepileptic drugs, the benefits may outweigh the risks.
- Individuals with malnutrition, chronic alcohol dependence or diabetes are at increased risk for peripheral neuropathy.
- Antimicrobials that can cause peripheral neuropathy should be used with caution and individuals receiving isoniazid should receive pyridoxine.
- Therapeutic drug monitoring is essential in avoiding toxic doses. Therapeutic drug monitoring consists of measuring trough levels in serum to prevent toxic drug accumulation in the brain. Measuring cerebrospinal fluid levels is less informative as it is not representative of drug concentration in brain tissue.

IF SEIZURES OCCUR

- Assess known risk factors: renal impairment, drug-drug interactions, underlying brain disease.
- Investigate alternative causes, i.e. infections can cause epilepsy, hepatic encephalopathy.
- If no other cause found, stop antibiotic and monitor neurological changes.
- Measure concentration of antimicrobial and drugs that interact with the antimicrobial such as antiepileptics.
- Status epilepticus should be managed as in other circumstances.
- Long-term treatment with antiepileptic agents is usually not needed.
- Short-term treatment with antiepileptic drugs should be discussed with the neurologist if multiple seizures occur.
- Perform EEG for ongoing encephalopathy. Start antiepileptic agent for nonconvulsive epilepsy.
- Consider haemofiltration if there is persistent neurotoxicity, even after antibiotic has been stopped, especially if toxic levels have been detected.

PERIPHERAL NEUROPATHY

- Measure glucose, vitamin B/folate status, thyroid function and paraproteinaemia.
- Look for non-medication related causes: diabetes, vitamin B/folate deficiency, paraproteinaemias, autoimmune disease, renal failure, and hypothyroidism.
- Screen drug chart for non-antibiotic drugs which are associated with neuropathy, i.e. chemotherapy.
- Consider EMG, MRI and CT.
- Drugs used to treat neuropathic pain are NSAIDS, tricyclic antidepressants, gabapentin and pregabalin.

SEROTONIN SYNDROME

- Monitor for symptoms of serotonin syndrome in patients receiving linezolid and SSRIs.
- Symptoms are mental changes, tachycardia, hypertension, loss of muscle coordination, muscle twitching, excessive sweating, shivering or shaking, diarrhoea, trouble with coordination and/or fever.
- Immediately discontinue linezolid.
- Provide supportive care.
- Sedate with benzodiazepines.
- It may take several days for serotonin syndrome to resolve.
- In severe cases, administration of serotonin antagonists is indicated.

CLINICAL PEARL

Carbapenems decrease the concentration of valproic acid, and this combination should be avoided. Combination of (val)ganciclovir and imipenem should be avoided as it increases risk of seizures.

BIBLIOGRAPHY

Bhattacharyya S, Darby R, Berkowitz AL. Antibiotic-induced neurotoxicity. *Curr Infect Dis Rep.* December 2014;16(12):448.

Bhattacharyya S, Darby RR, Raibagkar P, Gonzalez Castro LN, Berkowitz AL. Antibiotic-associated encephalopathy. *Neurology.* 8 March 2016;86(10):963–971.

Chui CS, Chan EW, Wong AY, Root A, Douglas IJ, Wong IC. Association between oral fluoroquinolones and seizures: A self-controlled case series study. *Neurology.* 3 May 2016;86(18):1708–1715.

Cock HR. Drug-induced status epilepticus. *Epilepsy Behav.* August 2015;49:76–82.

Esposito S, Canevini MP, Principi N. Complications associated with antibiotic administration: Neurological adverse events and interference with antiepileptic drugs. *Int J Antimicrob Agents.* July 2017;50(1):1–8.

Grill MF, Maganti RK. Neurotoxic effects associated with antibiotic use: Management considerations. *Br J Clin Pharmacol.* September 2011;72(3):381–393.

Sutter R, Rüegg S, Tschudin-Sutter S. Seizures as adverse events of antibiotic drugs: A systematic review. *Neurology.* 13 October 2015;85(15):1332–1341.

3.7 Antimicrobial Agents and Drug Interactions

Firza Alexander Gronthoud

CLINICAL CONSIDERATIONS

If a patient is clinically not improving despite a clear diagnosis, positive culture and sensitivity result, it could be due to a drug interaction affecting the effectiveness of the antibiotic. In addition, antimicrobial agents can influence drug metabolizing enzymes, posing a risk for a possibly serious drug-drug interactions (DDIs). It may therefore be worthwhile to consider the following.

ENVIRONMENTAL FACTORS INFLUENCING ANTIMICROBIAL EFFECTIVENESS

- Precipitation of drugs in a central line.
- Physical interaction such as degradation of meropenem at room temperature.
- Some antimicrobials such as voriconazole sequester in the extracorporeal circuit membrane oxygenation (ECMO) circuit.
- Vancomycin cannot be administered in the same intravenous line as β-lactam, and moxifloxacin and other medications such as propofol, methylprednisolone and furosemide owing to physical and or chemical incompatibilities.

Drugs can increase or decrease each other's effect when administered together. This is called pharmacodynamic interaction.

- *Synergism*: Penicillins + gentamicin or amoxicillin + cephalosporin for treatment of endocarditis.
- *Antagonism*: *In vitro* antagonism has been demonstrated for clindamycin, linezolid and macrolides as they bind to the same subunit of the ribosome. This has not been replicated *in vivo*.
- *Additive*
  - Cisplatin and aminoglycosides should not be administered together as the nephrotoxicity of each drug is increased.
  - The renal function should be closely monitored when aminoglycosides, polymyxins and vancomycin are administered together.
  - The combination of vancomycin with piperacillin/tazobactam has also been shown to increase nephrotoxicity.
  - There may be an increased risk of cardiotoxicity and arrhythmias when macrolides and quinolones are administered together.

The absorption, distribution, metabolism and excretion (ADME) of antimicrobials can be influenced by food and other medication. These are called pharmacokinetic interactions.

ABSORPTION

- Antacids and proton-pump inhibitors decrease gastric pH, which in turn decreases the absorption of oral itraconazole and oral penicillin.

- Absorption of quinolones is reduced when given within 2 hours of mineral antacids (magnesium, aluminium or calcium), zinc or iron preparations or after concomitant intake with aluminium-containing drugs.
- Moxifloxacin does not interact with calcium supplements.
- Milk decreases the absorption of antibiotics such as tetracycline or ciprofloxacin.

P-GLYCOPROTEIN (P-GP)

- P-glycoprotein is a drug efflux pump and is found in the intestine, liver, kidneys and brain. Its main function is to prevent absorption or uptake of drugs.
- Clarithromycin and ketoconazole are inhibitors of P-glycoprotein whilst rifampicin is an inducer.

DISTRIBUTION

- Ceftriaxone precipitates with calcium and should not be infused together with solutions that contain calcium such as Ringer's solution, Hartmann's solution or total parenteral solution. The risk of precipitation is highest in neonates.
- Diclofenac causes an increase in ceftriaxone biliary excretion and some decrease of the drug's urinary excretion.

METABOLISM

The main mode of altered drug metabolism is by inhibition or induction of cytochrome P450 enzymes, which are found in the liver and gut. CYP3A4 is responsible for the metabolism of more than 50% of medicines.

Cytochrome P450 enzymes are mainly expressed in the liver, but they are also found in the small intestine, lungs, placenta and kidneys.

Owing to genetic differences in CYP450 enzymes some people are rapid drug metabolizers or conversely poor metabolizers.

Drugs can be both metabolized by and inhibit by the same CYP450 enzyme (e.g., erythromycin and doxycycline), or they can be metabolized by one enzyme and inhibit or induce another enzyme (terbinafine).

Drugs may be intentionally combined to take advantage of CYP450 inhibition. Ritonavir is added to boost lopinavir levels for treatment of HIV.

- Potent inhibitors of CYP3A4 include clarithromycin, erythromycin, diltiazem, itraconazole, ketoconazole, ritonavir, verapamil, goldenseal and grapefruit (intestinal CYP3A4).
- Potent inducers of CYP3A4 include rifampicin phenobarbital, phenytoin, rifampicin, St John's wort and glucocorticoids.
- Drugs which are metabolized by CYP450 are theophylline, cyclosporin, carbamazepine and phenytoin, terfenadine, warfarin and oral contraceptives.
- Ciprofloxacin is the only quinolone which inhibits CYP450 (CYP1A2) and significantly reduces theophylline level and significantly increases caffeine half-life.
- Compared to other macrolides, azithromycin does not inhibit CYP450 enzymes.
- Clarithromycin inhibits intestinal as well as hepatic cytochrome P450 isoenzymes, interaction potential is greatest with orally administered drugs which are metabolized by intestinal CYP3A4.
- Rifabutin is a less potent CYP450 inducer than rifampicin and may potentially be used instead.
- Although linezolid is not metabolized by CYP450 enzymes; linezolid levels are decreased when rifampicin is co-administered.

CLINICAL PEARL

Serum levels of drugs such as mycophenolate mofetil which undergo enterohepatic circulation and are metabolized by intestinal microflora should be monitored when co-administered with broad-spectrum antibiotics that affect the gut microbiome, i.e. amoxicillin/clavulanic acid and ciprofloxacin.

EXCRETION

- Probenecid competes for renal tubular secretion and significantly increases serum levels of renally cleared β-lactams such as penicillins and cefotaxime.
- Penicillin G half-life may be prolonged by probenecid aspirin, phenylbutazone, sulfonamides, indomethacin, thiazide diuretics, furosemide and ethacrynic acid by competition for renal tubular secretion.

CLINICAL PEARL

Cytokines, such as IL-6, can affect drug metabolism by reduced expression of CYP3A4, CYP2B and CYP2C. Immunotherapy that alters cytokine response may therefore have an effect on antibiotic therapy.

CLINICAL APPROACH

If a patient is experiencing side effects or if there is a lack of clinical response to an antibiotic, drug-drug interaction should be considered. The first step is to check if the antibiotic administered to the patient requires therapeutic drug monitoring. If this is the case, verify if levels have been adequately monitored and if the level is within therapeutic range. The second step is to check the drug chart to determine if there could be any drug-drug interaction. Third step is to investigate the patient's dietary plan as milk, grapefruit and nutritional feeds can affect drug absorption and metabolism.

CLINICAL PEARL

If a drug interaction occurs, the responsible drug should be replaced with an alternative drug that is not likely to cause the side effect. In general, it cannot be expected to avoid a drug-drug interaction by simply increasing the time period between the administration of the interacting drugs. Several studies have shown that changes in the cytochrome activity can last for ≥24 h.

The following antimicrobials deserve special attention.

RIFAMPICIN

Rifampicin is a very potent inducer of CYP450 enzymes and has many drug interactions, including warfarin. Rifampicin has excellent biofilm penetration and is often used as part of endocarditis or foreign-body infections. Linezolid is increasingly used as an oral stepdown for these infections as well. If the combination of linezolid and rifampicin is needed, consider increasing linezolid dose to 600 mg TDS and monitoring the trough level, which should be between 2 and 7 μg/mL.

MACROLIDES

- Erythromycin and clarithromycin increase levels of cyclosporin, digoxin, midazolam, simvastatin and tacrolimus and increase half-life of theophylline. Erythromycin and clarithromycin increase risk of bleeding in patients on warfarin.
- Clarithromycin and, to a lesser extent, erythromycin are inhibitors of intestinal and renal P-glycoprotein.

AZOLES

- Azoles are substrates and potent inhibitors of CYP450, predominantly CYP3A4.
- Voriconazole is mainly metabolized by CYP2C19 and, to a lesser extent, by CYP3A4.
- Fluconazole is a strong inhibitor of CYP2C9. The CYP3A4 inhibitory potential is lower than for ketoconazole and itraconazole but may be higher at higher doses.
- Unlike other azoles, voriconazole is neither a substrate nor an inhibitor of P-glycoprotein.
- H2 antagonists or proton-pump inhibitors reduce the absorption and oral availability of the itraconazole capsule by ~30%–60%. Voriconazole and fluconazole are not affected.
- If there is no alternative to itraconazole, then the itraconazole oral suspension should be used. If the capsule form is used, itraconazole serum concentrations should be repeatedly monitored.
- Rifabutin and voriconazole coadministration not only leads to decreased voriconazole levels but also increases rifabutin concentrations to toxic levels, and so the concomitant use of these anti-infectives is contraindicated. A similar two-way interaction occurs with voriconazole and phenytoin, which is a CYP2C9 substrate and CYP inducer. Phenytoin decreases voriconazole levels, but repeated dose administration of voriconazole can increase the area under the curve (AUC) of phenytoin by 80% by competing for the CYP2C9 enzyme (See Chapter 3.8 for more information on AUC). Therefore, during coadministration of voriconazole and phenytoin, monitoring of plasma phenytoin concentrations and appropriate dose adjustments are recommended.
- If concomitant treatment with an azole and tacrolimus or ciclosporin is necessary, the dose of the immunosuppressant should be reduced, and renal function parameters and serum concentrations of the immunosuppressant should be closely monitored.
- Azoles and warfarin should not be administered together. If this combination cannot be avoided, then prothrombin time needs to be monitored and warfarin dose needs to be adjusted accordingly.

BIBLIOGRAPHY

Li X, Yan Z, Wu Q et al. Glucocorticoid receptor contributes to the altered expression of hepatic cytochrome P450 upon cigarette smoking. *Mol Med Rep.* December 2016;14(6):5271–5280.

Lynch T, Price A. The effect of Cytochrome P450 metabolism on drug response, interactions, and adverse effects. *Am Fam Physician.* 1 August 2007;76(3):391–396.

Raverdy V, Ampe E, Hecq JD, Tulkens PM. Stability and compatibility of vancomycin for administration by continuous infusion. *J Antimicrob Chemother.* May 2013;68(5):1179–1182.

Shakeri-Nejad K, Stahlmann R. Drug interactions during therapy with three major groups of antimicrobial agents. *Expert Opin Pharmacother.* April 2006;7(6):639–651.

3.8 Pharmacokinetic and Pharmacodynamic Considerations

Firza Alexander Gronthoud

CLINICAL CONSIDERATIONS

Effectiveness of antimicrobial therapy depends on both the drug movement in the human body (pharmacokinetics) and pathogen-specific antimicrobial activity (pharmacodynamics). Pharmacokinetics (PK) is determined by drug absorption, tissue distribution, metabolism and elimination. Pharmacodynamics (PD) is mostly determined by the minimum inhibitory concentration (MIC), minimum bactericidal concentration (MBC), post-antibiotic effect (PAE) and killing rate. Knowledge of PK and PD is essential to achieve optimal effectiveness of antimicrobial efficacy. It is therefore worthwhile to consider the following.

FACTORS INFLUENCING PHARMACOKINETICS

The following pharmacokinetic factors determine if the antimicrobial reaches effective concentration at the site of infection:

- *Drug absorption*: Influenced by bioavailability, drug-food interactions, gastrointestinal conditions, first/second pass metabolism
- *Drug distribution*: Influenced by lipid solubility, blood flow, protein binding, regional blood flow
- *Drug metabolism*: Influenced by linear pharmacokinetics, drug-drug interactions, once enzymes saturated, small dose increase causes disproportionately increased serum levels
- *Drug excretion*: Influenced by renal clearance, biliary/GI clearance

SPECIFIC PATIENT GROUPS AND PHARMACOKINETIC ALTERATIONS

- *Patients with renal insufficiency*: Decreased clearance
- *Neonates*: Decreased clearance
- *Children*: Increased clearance

CRITICALLY ILL

- Altered pharmacokinetics include increased volume of distribution (Vd), hypoalbuminaemia, delayed gastric emptying, augmented (increased) renal clearance, acute kidney injury (AKI), interstitial fluid shifts and changes in regional blood flow.
- Multiorgan failure can result in alterations to the absorption, distribution, metabolism and excretion of a drug.
- Alterations in protein binding, fluid shifts into the interstitium and pH affect drug distribution. These are most relevant for hydrophilic drugs that have a relatively low Vd.
- For concentration-dependent agents, an increase in volume of distribution will reduce the ability for a standard dose to achieve a high C_{max}.

- Higher proportions of unbound drug owing to low serum protein concentrations result in temporarily high drug concentrations, but as hypoalbuminaemia is associated with increased Vd, the free drug is diluted over the total body water.
- Augmented renal clearance increases risk of subtherapeutic concentrations with time-dependent antimicrobials.
- Where patients have AKI, the impact of altered PK depends on the proportion of antimicrobial that is renally excreted.

OBESITY

- Obesity results in increased body mass (lean and fat), increased cardiac output and blood volume, increased renal clearance, hepatic metabolic changes, changes in serum protein levels, reduced tissue penetration, shorter mean T1/2, increased volume of distribution (Vd).
- Fixed regimens can lead to underdosing. In contrast, total body weight (TBW)-based dosing leads to overdosing and toxicity.
- Blood flow in fat is poor and accounts for 5% of cardiac output compared to 22% in the lean tissue.
- As well as increased percentage of fat per kg of body weight, obese individuals have a larger absolute lean body mass (LBM), with lean components accounting for 20%–40% of excess body weight.

PREGNANCY AND PHARMACOKINETICS

- Potential altered pharmacokinetics include increased clearance, increased Vd, increased maternal fat and total body water, reduced plasma protein levels, delayed gastric emptying, increased gastric pH, increased cardiac output and renal blood flow and altered activity of hepatic metabolizing enzymes.
- Serum levels of many drugs are lower in pregnancy, largely due to the increased renal clearance and expanded intravascular volume.

ANTIMICROBIAL DRUG PROPERTIES AND PHARMACOKINETICS

- Hydrophilic versus lipophilic and relationship with type of organism and site of infection
  - Hydrophilic agents (β-lactams, glycopeptides, aminoglycosides) are unable to passively diffuse through the cytoplasmic membrane and are inactive against intracellular organisms. They have a limited extracellular distribution and are often excreted renally.
  - Lipophilic agents (macrolides, tetracyclines, fluoroquinolones) freely cross membranes and consequently are against intracellular organisms. They also have a wide distribution, accumulate intracellularly and often undergo hepatic metabolism.
- Protein binding; only the unbound portion is active

CLINICAL PEARL

- Important predictors of clinical success.
- *In vitro* susceptibility breakpoint.
- Resistance mechanisms.
- Site of infection and dosing regimen.
- The MIC predicts the serum concentrations but may not necessarily correlate to clinical outcome; concentrations at the site of infection may be more important.
- Underdosing is associated with insufficient treatment and increased risk of resistance, and overdosing is associated with toxicity.

PHARMACODYNAMIC PROPERTIES OF ANTIMICROBIALS

- *Time-dependent drugs*: β-Lactams, nitrofurantoin, erythromycin, tigecycline and oxazolidinones. *In vivo* efficacy is determined by time between doses with antibiotic concentration exceeding the MIC (T > MIC).
- *Concentration-dependent drugs*: Aminoglycosides, quinolones, fosfomycin and semisynthetic macrolides. The *in vivo* efficacy is determined by either the ratio between peak concentration (C_{max}) and MIC (C_{max}/MIC) or ratio between the area under the plasma concentration curve (AUC) and the MIC (AUC/MIC).

THE MINIMUM INHIBITORY CONCENTRATION (MIC)

- MIC is the *in vitro* concentration needed to prevent visible growth.
- The goal of MIC testing is to determine antimicrobial susceptibility by growing microorganisms in various antibiotic concentrations.
- The MIC is a PD predictor of antimicrobial efficacy. It is important to realize that:
  - The observed MIC is dependent on the bacterial inoculum used and the incubation time.
  - *In vivo*, the antibiotic concentration may also fluctuate and decrease over time at the site of infection.
  - MIC is measured in broth and not in the range of physiological environments found in the human body. Bacterial growth conditions in the 'test tube' differ from those *in vivo*.
  - Because MIC results are not 100% accurate, antibiotic concentration in the human body changes over time and may show interhuman variability despite administration of the same dose, and bacteria may show different growth characteristics *in vivo*; *in vitro* susceptibility may not always accurately predict *in vivo* response.

PITFALLS WHEN INTERPRETING MICs

- Most laboratories are not capable of performing a sufficiently accurate and reproducible determination of an MIC value owing to the inherent assay variation in the MIC test and interobserver interpretation.
- There may often be a twofold dilution step difference between two test methods (i.e. E-test versus microbroth dilution) or within the same method if the MIC test is repeated multiple times with the same test strain and the same test method.
- If the same strain–antimicrobial combination is tested in a range of laboratories, the log2 standard deviation might increase to 0.5–1 twofold dilution and more when media obtained from several manufacturers are used.
- This may lead to significant dosing adjustment errors, which could ultimately be harmful to patients.

DOSE-DEPENDENT TOXICITY

- *Colistin*: Nephrotoxicity, neurotoxicity
- *Aminoglycosides*: Nephrotoxicity, ototoxicity
- *Fluoroquinolones*: Neurotoxicity (seizures)
- *Imipenem/cilastatin and penicillin*: Neurotoxicity (seizures)
- *Linezolid*: Myelosuppression, lactic acidosis (hyperventilation, low bicarbonate), peripheral/optic neuropathy
- *Trimethoprim/sulfamethoxazole*: Myelosuppression
- *Chloramphenicol*: Myelosuppression
- *Daptomycin*: Musculotoxicity (increased CPK, myalgia, rhabdomyolysis)

CLINICAL APPROACH

To optimize clinical success, the following strategies should be used:
- Antimicrobial susceptibility testing and determining of the MIC.
- Therapeutic drug monitoring to ensure adequate levels are achieved.
- Renal function monitoring as this can significantly alter antimicrobial level and increase drug toxicity.
- Pharmacokinetics are altered in the critically ill and obese, and alternative dosing should be used.

INCREASING LIKELIHOOD OF ATTAINMENT OF PK-PD TARGET

- Prolonging the infusion rather than increasing the dose increases killing rate of time-dependent antimicrobials.
- Increasing the dose increases the killing rate of concentration-dependent antimicrobials.

AUGMENTED RENAL CLEARANCE

- *Concentration-dependent antimicrobials*: C_{max}/MIC is maximized by prolonging dosing interval without changing the dose.
- *Time-dependent agents*: T > MIC is maximized by reducing the dose while maintaining the dosing interval maximizes T > MIC.

SEVERE HYPALBUMINAEMIA

- Increased loading and maintenance doses may be necessary when using highly bound hydrophilic antibiotics.

OBESITY

- Loading doses should be based on ideal body weight (IBW) when the distribution of a drug is restricted to lean tissues.
- For drugs distributed mostly in lean mass and partly fat tissue, a calculation of loading dose should be performed with IBW plus a percentage of excess body weight (EBW = TBW − IBW), and loading dose for drugs equally distributed in fat tissues should be TBW.
- Hydrophilic antibiotics distribute well in water but not adipose tissue. As the water content of adipose tissue approximates 30%, the Vd for hydrophilic drugs may be only 0.3 of the Vd in other tissues. This distribution into the water component of adipose tissue may warrant increasing the dose in proportion to the EBW using the dosing weight correction factor (DWCF).

THERAPEUTIC DRUG MONITORING

- Therapeutic drug monitoring (TDM) is used to optimize antibiotic use with the overall aims of improving exposure and outcomes, minimizing toxicity and ultimately reduce antimicrobial resistance.
- It is most commonly employed for drugs with a narrow therapeutic range and is likely to be beneficial in populations where there is profound PK variability such as critical illness.
- TDM is used to ensure that target exposures are being achieved, as previously discussed.
- Certain patient populations may be expected to have altered PK such that the recommended dose from the drug manufacturer may not be sufficient to achieve therapeutic targets.

- The MIC of the organism can also impact on the dose necessary to achieve target concentrations.
- For certain antimicrobials, the outcomes of certain infections correlate with the AUC/MIC ratio, which in turn correlates with serum trough levels such that the trough level is a surrogate PK measure.
- For example, when treating MRSA infections with vancomycin, a trough concentration of 15 mg/L will result in an AUC/MIC ratio of >400 and is therefore a suitable target for therapy.

BIBLIOGRAPHY

2019 Antibiotic therapy as personalized medicine - General considerations and complicating factors – APMS How to optimize antibiotic Pk Pd for Gram-negative infections in critically ill patients. *Curr Opin Infect Dis.* 2018;31:555–565.

Mouton JW, Muller AE, Canton R, Giske CG, Kahlmeter G, Turnidge J. MIC-based dose adjustment: Facts and fables. *J Antimicrob Chemother.* 1 March 2018;73(3):564–568.

Pharmacokinetic and Pharmacodynamic principles of anti-infective dosing. *Clin Ther.* September 2016;38(9):1930–1947.

3.9 Source Control

Firza Alexander Gronthoud

CLINICAL CONSIDERATIONS

In clinical practice, the situation may occur that despite a clear diagnosis and appropriate antimicrobial therapy, patients are not improving or are even deteriorating. It is then often worthwhile to revisit the source of infection. Source control also plays an important role in identifying the causative pathogens and guiding antimicrobial therapy as is explained later in this chapter. It is therefore worthwhile to consider the following factors.

PERSISTENT FOCUS OF INFECTION

When there is a persistent focus of infection such as an infected foreign body or intestinal perforation with ongoing leakage and abscess formation, it is often more effective to anatomically control or even remove the source of infection whereby antimicrobial agents act as supportive therapy.

INSUFFICIENT ANTIMICROBIAL DRUG ACTIVITY AT SOURCE OF INFECTION

To prevent further spread of infection to healthy tissue, our immune system can form an abscess. An abscess is a walled-off collection of pus containing a mixture of dead tissue, host inflammatory cells and bacteria, fungi or parasites. An abscess can shield pathogens from antimicrobial agents and it may get larger and more painful as the infection continues and more pus is produced. Certain antimicrobial classes such as aminoglycosides are less active in pus owing to the anaerobic and acidic conditions. Similarly, the ability to penetrate necrotic tissue and reach therapeutic concentration exceeding the MIC is also a key determinant for clinical effectiveness and varies among different antimicrobial classes.

URGENCY

There is a time delay between administration of antimicrobial agents and clinical effectiveness, and in immediate life-threatening infections, resection of the source can dramatically improve patient survival (Table 3.9.1).

CLINICAL APPROACH

DRAINAGE OF COLLECTIONS

- *What to drain*: Liquefied pus collections, abscesses and infected haematomas.
- *Rationale*: Reduction of bacterial load leads to improved healing and reduces risk of spread of infection.
- *When*: Size of collection and location dictate timing of drainage.
- *How*: Drainage can be performed percutaneously, endoscopically or surgically.

TABLE 3.9.1
Urgency of Source Control

Level 1 Urgency: Emergent Source Control	Level 2 Urgency: Urgent Source Control	Level 3 Urgency: Delayed Source Control
To be performed within 1–2 hours after diagnosis	As soon as patient is haemodynamically stable, cultures for microbiology have been taken and empiric antibiotic therapy has been initiated	When demarcations between healthy and necrotic tissue is clearly visible (3–6 weeks)
Necrotizing fasciitis	Pleural empyema	Necrotizing pancreatitis
Intestinal ischaemia	Acute cholecystitis/cholangitis	
	Gastrointestinal perforation	

CLINICAL PEARL

If a patient is clinically not improving or even deteriorating despite targeted antimicrobial therapy and drainage, assess whether the drain is adequately draining. It may need to be repositioned or resized or multiple drains may be required. In these cases, it can be useful to request imaging studies such as ultrasound or CT.

RESECTION OF INFECTED OR NECROTIC TISSUE

- *What to resect*: Infected and/or necrotic tissue (also called debridement) or perforated or necrotic bowel.
- *Rationale*: Prevention of further spread of infection or complete removal of the source of infection and improving the healing potential of remaining healthy tissue.
- *When*: Timing of resection varies per infection. For example, in the early stages of necrotizing pancreatitis, healthy tissue is not clearly demarcated from necrotic tissue and blood vessels may not be clearly visible. Debridement, if performed too soon, may result in considerable bleeding. Conversely, necrotizing fasciitis is a rapidly spreading infection in which early necrosectomy dramatically improves patient survival.
- *How*: Surgical resection using a blade or laser, wash-outs, chemical solutions, autolytic using specific dressings and by maggot therapy for necrotic tissue.

CLINICAL PEARL

Necrotic tissue provides a favourable environment for bacteria to proliferate as host inflammatory cells and antimicrobial drugs are unlikely to reach significant concentrations in the absence of local blood supply.

REMOVAL OF A COLONIZED FOREIGN BODY

- *What to remove*: Intravascular catheters, urinary catheters, ventricular drains or shunts, prosthetic valves, pacemakers, vascular grafts and prosthetic joints.
- *Rationale*: Prosthetic devices act as a permanent source of infection and can maintain an infection or significantly increase the risk of recurrence.

- *When*: Different criteria exist for different catheter- or device-associated infections, but typically rests on a combination of clinical symptoms, a positive culture or PCR result and radiological findings compatible with infected device (e.g. valve vegetations).

CLINICAL PEARL

Bacteria and yeasts can form a biofilm on foreign bodies which not only allows them to adhere to the surface, but also enables them to evade host defence mechanisms and antibiotics.

CLINICAL PEARL

Some prosthetic materials are not easily removable due to (1) their location (e.g. prosthetic joint), (2) the function they serve (e.g. port-a-cath) or (3) a combination of 1 and 2 (e.g. prosthetic valve and a vascular graft). These infections typically require a longer treatment duration (weeks–months) using drugs that have the best biofilm-penetrating abilities.

The clinical vignettes below illustrate how source control can aid in the microbiological diagnosis and guidance of antimicrobial therapy. As you can see, sometimes multiple source control measures are needed.

CLINICAL VIGNETTES

The surgical team is wondering if antibiotic treatment needs to be escalated for a 24-year-old male who is being treated for a necrotizing fasciitis of his right lower leg. He remains in septic shock despite treatment with piperacillin/tazobactam, clindamycin and gentamicin. He was admitted yesterday for urgent debridement and antibiotic therapy. The surgical plan is to perform a second debridement soon. You advise to continue current antibiotic regime, perform debridement as soon as possible and send debrided tissue to the microbiology laboratory for culture.

- Necrotizing fasciitis is a rapidly spreading infection, almost always complicated by severe sepsis or septic shock and associated with high mortality.
- Early and aggressive debridement should be performed and carried out until the wound margins bleed readily. Multiple debridements are frequently needed.
- Debrided tissue sent to the microbiology laboratory can help identify the involved pathogens and guide antimicrobial therapy.

The junior doctor on the surgical ward wants to know which oral antibiotics can be prescribed and for how long for a patient who had an urgent colectomy for a perforated diverticulitis with secondary peritonitis. He is being treated with ceftriaxone and metronidazole. As he is improving, the surgical team feels there is no need for drainage of a 3 ×4 cm pelvic collection. You advise to drain the collection to guide antibiotic treatment.

- Perforation causes abdominal microbial spillage, potentially leading to an ongoing peritonitis with intra-abdominal pus collections.
- Depending on the extent of the perforation and the presence of collections, source control can be achieved through resection of perforated part of the bowel, primary closure of the perforation and drainage of any collection.

- Secondary peritonitis due to intestinal perforation often involves a polymicrobial flora. It is therefore important that drain fluids are sent for culture to help rationalize antimicrobial therapy.
- If source control is achieved and the patient is clinically and biochemically improving, antimicrobial therapy can often be discontinued within 4–10 days.

A 56-year-old male is on amoxicillin/clavulanic acid IV for a community-acquired pneumonia with empyema. He has a chest drain which is still producing pus. No samples have been sent to the microbiology laboratory. He is clinically improving, and the house officer asks you how long to continue antibiotic therapy. You advise to send drain samples for culture, continue antibiotics for at least 3 weeks post-drainage and then review. Oral stepdown depends on culture results or response to intravenous therapy.

- Complication of pneumonia, trauma or, less commonly, as a complication of thoracic surgical procedures.
- In the early stages, empyema is liquid and drainage via placement of a chest tube allows removal of pus and expansion of the lung.
- Percutaneous catheters have a failure rate of up to 20% when collections are extensive or multiloculated.
- If tube thoracostomy fails (e.g. in a later stage of the empyema when a thick fibrous peel has formed), video-assisted thoracic surgery (VATS) can be performed, allowing for decortication of empyema.

BIBLIOGRAPHY

Birkenkamp K, O'Horo JC, Kashyap R, Kloesel B, Lahr BD, Daniels CE, Nichols FC 3rd, Baddour LM. Empyema management: A cohort study evaluating antimicrobial therapy. *J Infect*. May 2016;72(5):537–543.
De Waele JJ. Early source control in sepsis. *Langenbecks Arch Surg*. June 2010;395(5):489–494.
Eckmann C. The importance of source control in the management of severe skin and soft tissue infections. *Curr Opin Infect Dis*. April 2016;29(2):139–144.
Miura F et al. TG13 flowchart for the management of acute cholangitis and cholecystitis. *J Hepatobiliary Pancreat Sci*. January 2013;20(1):47–54.
Marshall JC. Principles of source control in the early management of sepsis. *Curr Infect Dis Rep*. September 2010;12(5):345–353.

3.10 Antibiotic Treatment Failure

Firza Alexander Gronthoud

CLINICAL CONSIDERATIONS

Slow or absence of response to antibiotic treatment is a relatively frequent problem faced by the clinician. There are several factors causing a slow or even stagnating response to treatment. It might therefore be worthwhile to consider the following.

EVALUATION OF CLINICAL PARAMETERS IN THE FIRST 48–72 HOURS

- Symptoms and signs (i.e., a decrease in fever, tachycardia, respiratory rate or confusion)
- Laboratory values (i.e. decreasing leukocyte count, PCT [procalcitonin] or CRP), organ function markers (reduction or cessation of vasopressors, improvement of hypoxemia, increasing urine output)
- Radiologic findings (i.e. size reduction of an abscess, improvement in lung opacities)

CLINICAL PEARL

- Radiographic infiltrate, amount and quality of secretions, fever and high white cell count (WCC) are poor predictors of clinical response to therapy.
- Specific physiologic variables, such as a PaO_2-to-FiO_2 ratio, can much more accurately differentiate between antibiotic responders and non-responders.
- Several weeks or even months may be required before chest radiography or CT scan shows complete resolution of an infiltrate.

GENERAL FACTORS TO BE CONSIDERED WHEN THERE IS PARTIAL OR NO RESPONSE TO ANTIBIOTICS

- Non-infectious aetiology
- Comorbidities such as immunocompromise, COPD, alcoholism, diabetes, chronic kidney disease, malignancy or use of immunosuppressive drugs may delay or slow down rate of recovery
- Persistent source of infection: Ongoing perforation with intraabdominal leakage, abscess that needs draining, intravascular catheter or indwelling catheter, hydronephrosis, obstructed biliary flow
- Development of complications from the initial infection: Septic emboli to other organs (i.e. endophthalmitis with candidaemia), meningitis complicated by ventriculitis or brain abscess, pneumonia complicated by lung abscess or empyema, endocarditis
- Development of a hospital-acquired infection
- Unrecognized sacral sore developing into an abscess
- Drug fever

CLINICAL PEARL

Sustained defervescence, clinical stability, reduction of sequential organ failure assessment (SOFA) score comparing the day of re-assessment with the day antibiotic treatment is started in a 48–72-h timeframe better reflects clinical response.

ANTIBIOTIC THERAPY-SPECIFIC FACTORS CAUSING A PARTIAL OR ABSENT CLINICAL RESPONSE

- Misdiagnosis of the pathogen or the presence of a resistant pathogen: Current antibiotic regimen is not (or partially) treating the infection.
- Drug penetration: Suboptimal antibiotic tissue penetration reduces antibiotic effectiveness.
- Dose and route: Suboptimal dose or low bioavailability of certain oral drugs.
- Drug-drug interactions: May lead to increased antibiotic clearance and reduced antibiotic concentrations at target site.
- Therapeutic drug monitoring: Subtherapeutic antibiotic levels impair antibiotic killing.

CLINICAL APPROACH

Assessment of response should be performed early enough to allow successful rescue therapy, but not too early, to allow evidence of clinical response. Usually this means giving antibiotics 48–72 hours to work. If there is partial or no response after 48–72 hours, consider the following strategies:

If a patient is clinically not improving despite a clear diagnosis, positive microbiology culture and sensitivity results, check if:

1. Patient is receiving correct dose and frequency.
   a. Check compliance if outpatient.
   b. Check drug chart if inpatient.
2. Check for drug-drug interaction.
   a. Discuss with pharmacist if there could be a drug-drug interaction, e.g. Cytochrome P450 (CYP450) enzyme induction/inhibition.
   b. Direct interaction antibiotics with other medication or fluids and check if they need to be given at separate times.
3. Check if the old diagnosis is correct.
   a. Confirm with clinical team how the original diagnosis was made and if there was enough evidence to support it. Review documented symptoms, biochemistry, imaging and microbiology and histology.
4. Check if there is a new source of infection.
   a. Repeat diagnostic work-up.

CLINICAL PEARLS

Microbiology results are frequently misinterpreted, leading to a wrong diagnosis, i.e. a positive dipstick and positive urine culture, actually representing asymptomatic bacteriuria rather than urinary tract infection or a sputum culture with +coliforms and +++respiratory flora indicating colonization rather than pneumonia.

ON ANTIBIOTIC THERAPY, REMAINS FEBRILE, BUT INFLAMMATORY MARKERS FALLING

1. Investigate if there could be persistent source of infection.
   a. Antibiotics are holding infection and patient needs source control (i.e. drainage, debridement, line removal, stent removal, nephrostomy removal).
2. Consider if the source of infection could have a polymicrobial flora that the current antibiotics may only be partially covering.
   a. Review old culture results and see if there are any bacteria that are resistant to the current antibiotic therapy. This could be clinical cultures or screening cultures.
3. Antibiotics are partially treating the bacteria and there may be a resistant bacteria as well.
   a. Check if the *in vitro* sensitivity is correct.
   b. Check if the MIC is borderline sensitive.
   c. Check if the bacteria is an AmpC. Remember that tazobactam may only cover some AmpC enzymes. Ertapenem is less stable than other carbapenems against AmpC.
4. Check if there could be other sources of fever.
   a. Cancer may be component of fever.
   b. Drug fever.

CLINICAL PEARL

Escalating antibiotics based exclusively on PCT or CRP results should be avoided as it is not associated with a better outcome.

ON ANTIBIOTIC THERAPY, REMAINS FEBRILE, CLINICALLY STABLE, INFLAMMATORY MARKERS STATIC NOW

1. Check if there could be persistent source of infection.
   a. Antibiotics are holding infection and patient needs source control (drainage, debridement, line removal, stent removal, nephrostomy removal).
2. Antibiotics are partially treating the bacteria and there may be a resistant bacteria as well.
   a. Check if the *in vitro* sensitivity is correct.
   b. Check if the MIC is borderline sensitive.
3. Is there a drug-drug interaction? Induction of CYP450 for example can lead to increased clearance of antimicrobials.

CLINICAL PEARL

- Systemic corticosteroids are often used in combination with antibiotics for treatment of bacterial meningitis, tuberculous meningitis and pneumocystis pneumonia in patients with AIDS.
- Temporary discontinuation or dose reduction of immunosuppressive agents may be required in transplant recipients or patients with rheumatologic disorders.
- Intravenous immunoglobulin therapy can be used, in addition to surgical debridement and antimicrobial therapy, in the treatment of necrotizing fasciitis caused by group A streptococci and severe toxic shock syndrome.

Recurrent Episodes of Fever, Responding to Courses of Antibiotic Therapy, Unknown Source

- Fever of unknown origin: Think brain abscess, sinusitis, otitis media, lung abscess, endocarditis, osteomyelitis, vertebral osteomyelitis, spondylodiscitis, epidural abscess, abdominal abscess, subphrenic abscess.
- If travel history, think *Brucella*, and other tropical endemic infections (see Chapter 6.1).
- Animal exposure (see Chapter 2.2).

BIBLIOGRAPHY

Bassetti M, Montero JG, Paiva JA. When antibiotic treatment fails. *Intensive Care Med.* January 2018;44(1):73–75.

Bennett JE, Dolin R, Blaser MJ. *Mandell, Douglas, and Bennett's Principles and Practice of Infectious Diseases: 2-Volume Set*, vol. 1. Elsevier Health Sciences, 2014.

Section IV

Special Problems

4.1 Acute Streptococcal Pharyngitis

Firza Alexander Gronthoud

CLINICAL CONSIDERATIONS

STREPTOCOCCUS PYOGENES OR GROUP A STREPTOCOCCUS (GAS)

GAS is the main cause of bacterial pharyngitis and causes up to 30% of all cases of acute pharyngitis in children and up to 10% in adults. Patients with pharyngitis spread GAS via the respiratory route. GAS pharyngitis has an incubation period of 2–5 days and symptoms can last up to 5 days. Antimicrobial therapy reduces duration and severity of symptoms by 1–2 days (when begun within 48 hours of illness). Its main goal is to prevent transmission to others and reduce risk of rheumatic fever. Some guidelines recommend routine treatment of GAS pharyngitis. GAS bacteraemia is rarely associated with uncomplicated pharyngitis or nonsuppurative complications of pharyngitis.

RISK OF POSTSTREPTOCOCCAL COMPLICATIONS

The rate of poststreptococcal complications is generally low. Risk factors are:

- Individuals at increased risk of severe infections such as the immunocompromised.
- Valvular heart disease
- History of rheumatic fever
- Of note, pharyngitis in male patients aged 21–40 years who are smokers is more frequently complicated by peritonsillar abscess

COMPLICATIONS OF STREPTOCOCCAL PHARYNGITIS

Complications of streptococcal pharyngitis can result from extension of infection beyond the oropharynx, termed suppurative complications, or as immune phenomena, termed nonsuppurative complications.

NONSUPPURATIVE COMPLICATIONS OF GAS TONSILLOPHARYNGITIS

- *Acute rheumatic fever (ARF)*: Develops 2–3 weeks after initial pharyngitis. Clinical manifestations are arthritis, carditis, chorea, subcutaneous nodules and erythema marginatum. Low incidence in industrialized countries.
- *Poststreptococcal reactive arthritis (PSRA)*: Occurs within 1 month following pharyngitis and involves ≥1 joint.
- *Scarlet fever or 'scarlatina'*: Diffuse erythematous eruption occurring in association with pharyngitis and caused by skin reactivity to pyrogenic exotoxin produced by GAS.
- *Streptococcal toxic shock syndrome*: See Chapter 4.33.
- *Acute glomerulonephritis*: Infection with specific nephritogenic strains of GAS. Ranges from microscopic haematuria to acute nephritic syndrome. Renal failure can occur. In contrast to PSRA, only glomerulonephritis is linked with skin infections due to GAS.

- *Paediatric autoimmune neuropsychiatric disorder associated with group A streptococci (PANDAS)*: Development of obsessive-compulsive disorder or tic disorders following GAS infection.

CLINICAL PEARL

- The rash of scarlet fever is a diffuse blanchable erythema. Raised papules give a rough texture like 'sandpaper'.
- Starting in the groin and armpits, followed by rapid expansion to the trunk and extremities with sparing of palms and soles before desquamation sets in.
- Accompanied by circumoral pallor and a strawberry tongue.
- Pastia's lines or Pastia's signs appear before the rash and persist after desquamation. These are confluent petechiae in a linear pattern found in skin creases, i.e. groin, axilla, neck folds.
- Children may return to school or day care 24 hours after initiation of antibiotics.

SUPPURATIVE COMPLICATIONS OF GAS

- *Otitis media*: GAS causes a minority of all cases of acute otitis media (AOM), but incidence of AOM due to GAS is increased during the winter months
- *Sinusitis*
- *Peritonsillar abscess, also called quinsy*: Often polymicrobial flora involved

PREVENTION OF TRANSMISSION AND COMPLICATIONS

Penicillin decreases risk of rheumatic fever by about two-thirds with greatest risk reduction in children 5–15 years living in geographical areas with highest incidence of rheumatic fever. The effect of penicillin on risk reduction of other nonsuppurative complications is not well known.

GAS can spread among close contacts, leading to clusters of cases and recurrent infections in households or other close contact settings. The rate of GAS transmission from an infectious case to close contacts is estimated to be between 5% and 50%. Antibiotics eliminate GAS from the oropharynx in about 80%–90% of cases after 24 hours of therapy. About half of patients with untreated streptococcal pharyngitis are shedding GAS in the oropharynx for 3–4 weeks after resolution of symptoms.

CLINICAL APPROACH

The diagnosis of GAS pharyngitis is supported by a positive microbiologic test (throat culture or rapid antigen detection test [RADT] for GAS), symptoms consistent with pharyngitis and either a negative viral respiratory PCR or absence of signs and symptoms of viral infections (e.g. coryza, conjunctivitis, cough, hoarseness, anterior stomatitis, discrete ulcerative lesions or vesicles, diarrhoea).

The likelihood of a GAS pharyngitis can be predicted with the Centor or FeverPAIN criteria. Criteria are less sensitive in young children who often have aspecific symptoms (see Table 4.1.2).

WHOM TO TEST

A throat swab or rapid test is indicated if there is an acute tonsillopharyngitis or scarlatiniform rash and viral causes have been excluded (Table 4.1.1).

TABLE 4.1.1

Differential Diagnosis of Pharyngitis

Pathogen	Clinical Syndrome	Comments
Respiratory viruses (influenza A&B, parainfluenza, rhinovirus, adenovirus)	Cough, coryza, conjunctivitis, rhinorrhoea	May or may not have pharyngeal exudate Enteroviral infection is more common in summer and autumn
Herpes viruses: CMV, EBV, HSV	Sore throat, lymphadenopathy, general malaise, extreme tiredness	Mononucleosis (CMV or EBV) accompanied by lymphadenopathy and splenomegaly
Lemierre's syndrome caused by *Fusobacterium necrophorum*	Pharyngitis with jugular thrombophlebitis, neck swelling, with bloodstream infection and risk of septic emboli to other organs	
M. pneumoniae and *C. pneumoniae*	Similar to respiratory viruses	
Vincent's angina or trench mouth	Acute onset of bad breath, severe oral pain, and necrotizing ulcerations of the gingiva	
Tularaemia	Ulcerations and exudates in pharynx	History of eating meat from undomesticated animals May mimic diphtheria Unresponsive to penicillin therapy
Diphtheria	Grey membrane in nose and throat that bleeds when dislodged	Rare outside low- and middle-income countries due to DTP vaccines
Sexually transmitted disease: acute HIV, gonorrhoea, *Chlamydia*	Acute primary HIV infection: associated adenopathy, rash, fever and splenomegaly	
Candida infection	Oral thrush	Immunocompromised individuals, including those undergoing chemotherapy or oropharyngeal irradiation for cancer

CLINICAL PEARL

A positive culture or rapid antigen test in the presence of viral symptoms may indicate asymptomatic carrier, especially in the presence of a positive respiratory viral PCR result, and may lead to unnecessary antibiotic treatment. Especially in adults, the rapid antigen test has a low positive predictive value.

MICROBIOLOGY TESTS

- Throat swab and/or streptococcal rapid test. If initial testing with RADT is negative in a child or adolescent, do standard throat culture because RADT may miss as many as 30% of cases of GAS pharyngitis. Sensitivity of a well-performed throat culture is 95% whilst sensitivity of RADT is 70%–90%.
- Throat culture also can identify other bacteria that cause pharyngitis less commonly than GAS (e.g. group C and group G streptococci, *Arcanobacterium haemolyticum*).
- *Streptococcus pyogenes* is a Gram-positive coccus in chains. It produces β-haemolytic colonies and due to its capsule colonies, may appear mucoid. GAS can be typed based on its M protein.

TABLE 4.1.2
Clinical Prediction Rules for GAS Pharyngitis

Centor Criteria	FeverPAIN Criteria
• Tonsillar exudate	• Fever (during previous 24 hours)
• Tender anterior cervical lymphadenopathy or lymphadenitis	• Purulent exudate
	• Attend rapidly (within 3 days after onset of symptoms)
• History of fever (over 38°C)	• Severely inflamed tonsils
• Absence of cough	• Absence of cough or coryzal symptoms

Notes: Centor criteria: Each item is 1 point. A score of 0, 1 or 2 has a predictive value of 3%–17%. A score of 3 or 4 has a predictive value of 32%–56%.

FeverPAIN criteria: Each item is 1 point. A score of 1 has a predictive value of 13%–18%. A score of 2 or 3 has a predictive value of 34%–40%. A score of 4 or 5 has a predictive value of 62%–65%.

- Both tonsils or tonsillar fossae in patients who have undergone tonsillectomy and the posterior pharynx should be swabbed. Avoid contact with the tongue or the buccal mucosa.
- For Lemierre's syndrome, throat swab, blood cultures, ultrasonography jugular veins.
- HIV test.
- Antistreptolysin titres should be determined if suspicion of acute rheumatic fever or glomerulonephritis and recent history of a sore throat.

MANAGEMENT OF GAS TONSILLOPHARYNGITIS

- Supportive care measures such as non-steroidal anti-inflammatory drugs (NSAIDs) or acetaminophen may be administered to relieve fever and pain.
- Antibiotic treatment, if indicated, consists of amoxicillin or penicillin V for 10 days. If penicillin IgE-mediated allergy, consider clindamycin, a macrolide. Azithromycin has a long half-life and can be given for a 3- or 5-day course.
- A third-generation cephalosporin can be used in case of IgE-mediated allergic reaction unless there is a history of anaphylaxis.
- If non-IgE-mediated allergy, consider an oral cephalosporin, i.e. cefalexin.
- Fever and constitutional symptoms typically resolve within 1–3 days of starting treatment.
- Most patients can return to work or school after 24 hours of antibiotic treatment, provided they are afebrile and otherwise well.

TEST OF CURE

Only indicated in individuals at risk for complications, recurrent infection or transmission to others:

- Patients with a history of acute rheumatic fever
- Patients who acquired infection during an outbreak of acute rheumatic fever or poststreptococcal glomerulonephritis
- Patients who acquired infection during a cluster of cases in their household or other close-contact setting

If positive, repeat 10-day course with amoxicillin/clavulanic acid or a third-generation oral cephalosporin.

TREATMENT CAVEATS

- There is increasing resistance to macrolides and clindamycin.
- *Staphylococcus aureus*, *Haemophilus influenzae*, *Moraxella catarrhalis* and anaerobes may produce β-lactamases rendering penicillin or amoxicillin inactive.
- Penicillin and amoxicillin also decrease the quantity of α-streptococci in the oropharynx, which naturally protect against GAS infection.

If persistent or recurrent infection after a 10-day course of antibiotics, consider the following:

- Nonadherence with the prescribed antimicrobial regimen
- Recurrent infection: Suspect if clusters of GAS infections are occurring in the area
- Infection with a different pathogen
- Presence of a suppurative complication, such as a peritonsillar abscess
- Treatment failure: Persistent infection is rare but most often occurs in children, particularly those under age 5

For patients with frequent, mild-to-moderate recurrent infections, delaying the start of antibiotic therapy by 2–3 days is an alternate approach. Delaying therapy may allow the development of immunity against the infecting strain, resulting in higher eradication rates without increasing the risk of acute rheumatic fever.

For patients with frequent, severe episodes of GAS pharyngitis that recur despite appropriate antibiotic treatment, consider discussing tonsillectomy with an ENT surgeon.

CLINICAL PEARL

A persistent, severe sore throat accompanied by fever, trismus or a muffled voice suggests a local complication such as peritonsillar cellulitis or abscess.

PREVENTING GAS INFECTION

- *Hand hygiene*: Cornerstone of preventing transmission to others.
- *Post-exposure prophylaxis*: Testing and treatment of asymptomatic persons who have been exposed to a patient with GAS pharyngitis are not routinely recommended, except for patients with a history of acute rheumatic fever, during outbreaks of acute rheumatic fever and/or poststreptococcal glomerulonephritis or when GAS infections are recurring in households or other close contact settings.

Patients with a history of acute rheumatic fever are at high risk for recurrent rheumatic fever and the development of chronic valvular heart disease with any subsequent GAS infection.

Recommend long-term antibiotic prophylaxis for all. Intramuscular penicillin G benzathine is the treatment of choice, although other options are also available. Duration of prophylaxis is not defined. Treat all household contacts when the patient or any household member develops GAS pharyngitis to prevent recurrence.

TREATMENT OF CHRONIC CARRIERS

Consider treating carriers during outbreaks of acute rheumatic fever and/or poststreptococcal glomerulonephritis or when GAS infections are recurring in households or other close-contact settings. Oral options for treatment of chronic carriage include clindamycin, amoxicillin/clavulanate and penicillin plus rifampin. Intramuscular benzathine penicillin plus oral rifampin is a rarely used alternative. When used with either oral or parenteral penicillin, rifampin is typically given only during the last 4 days of therapy.

BIBLIOGRAPHY

Alho OP, Koivunen P, Penna T, Teppo H, Koskela M, Luotonen J. Tonsillectomy versus watchful waiting in recurrent streptococcal pharyngitis in adults: randomised controlled trial. *BMJ*. 2007;334(7600):939.

Beggs S, Peterson G, Tompson A. Antibiotic use for the prevention and treatment of rheumatic fever and rheumatic heart disease in children. Report for the 2nd Meeting of World Health Organization's subcommittee of the Expert Committee of the Selection and Use of Essential Medicines. *Second Meeting of the Subcommittee of the Expert Committee on the Selection and Use of Essential Medicines* Geneva, 29 September to 3 October 2008.

BMJ Best Practice. https://bestpractice.bmj.com/topics/en-gb/5

Centor RM, Atkinson TP, Ratliff AE et al. The clinical presentation of *Fusobacterium*-positive and streptococcal-positive pharyngitis in a university health clinic. *Ann Intern Med*. 2015;162:241–247.

Pelucchi C, Grigoryan L, Galeone C et al. Guideline for the management of acute sore throat. *Clin Microbiol Infect*. 2012;18(Suppl. 1):1–27.

4.2 Animal Bites

Firza Alexander Gronthoud

CLINICAL CONSIDERATIONS

Animals bites are common reasons people seek medical attention. The most common animal bites worldwide are dog and cat bites and are estimated to be around 5%–25% and 30%–50%, respectively. Monkey bites are especially prevalent in India. Depending on the nature of the bite, the type of animal and geographical location, there is a risk of deadly complications such as rabies and tetanus. It is therefore worthwhile to consider the following.

RISK OF INFECTION

Deep and contaminated wounds and wounds in hands, feet, joints or sites with poor perfusion carry higher risk of infection. Also, infection is more likely in children younger than 2 years, diabetic patients, persons with prosthetic heart valves and those having immunocompromised conditions.

MICROBIOLOGY

Animal bites can cause a local soft tissue infection which may spread haematogenously. Often a polymicrobial flora is involved. Animal bites are usually polymicrobial with respect to the oral flora of the biting animal, consisting of staphylococci, streptococci and anaerobes. *Staphylococcus intermedius* is a coagulase-negative *Staphylococcus* that is associated with dog bites. The following bacteria are typically associated with cat and dog bites.

CAPNOCYTOPHAGOSIS

The genus *Capnocytophaga* (capno depicts its dependence on carbon dioxide to grow) consists of fastidious organisms commonly associated with dog bites. The representative species is *Capnocytophaga canimorsus*, which can cause septicaemia, endocarditis and meningitis. Alcoholics and immunocompromised individuals, especially those who have undergone a splenectomy, are particularly prone to complicated infections.

CAT SCRATCH DISEASE

Cats are the main reservoir of *Bartonella henselae*, which causes cat scratch disease. It can be transmitted via cat scratches or bites. Clinical presentation can range from lymphadenopathy to fulminant infections. Like capnocytophagosis, people with a compromised immune system, classically in those who develop acquired immunodeficiency syndrome (AIDS), are at risk of serious infections.

PASTEURELLOSIS

The disease is caused by *Pasteurella multocida*, a Gram-negative coccobacillus found in mammals and birds. Many domestic mammals (i.e. cats, dogs, rabbits and small rodents) carry *P. multocida* as part of their normal flora. Human infections typically result from bites and scratches. Pasteurellosis can present as painful skin and wound infections. In severe cases, it may result in bacteraemia, endocarditis, meningitis and osteomyelitis.

RABIES

Rabies is an RNA virus belonging to the genus *Lyssavirus* in the family *Rhabdoviridae*, order *Mononegavirales*. Rabies remains the most lethal infectious disease associated with animal bites. Dog bites are the predominant route of rabies transmission worldwide. Most cases of rabies (95%) occur in Africa and Asia, mainly in India. There has been a significant decrease in dog rabies cases in Latin America and the Caribbean. In Western Europe, Canada, the United States, Japan and some Latin American countries, dog rabies has been eliminated. Bats account for the predominant route of transmission in the Americas. In Europe, rabies is mostly found in bats and foxes. Australia, the United Kingdom and parts of Western Europe are considered free of rabies in terrestrial animals due to wildlife vaccination programmes, together with the availability of effective commercial vaccination for domestic animals.

Rabies is transmitted through saliva of an infected animal by a bite or scratch, or when saliva from an infected animal comes into contact with broken skin or mucous membranes (eyes, nose or mouth). Rabies virus then migrates to the central nervous system via the peripheral nerves, where it causes a fatal encephalitis. The virus replicates in the brain and disseminates to many different tissues. The incubation period of rabies is usually between 1 and 2 months; in rare cases, it can be as short as 4 days or up to 19 years. Most cases occur within a year. Bites in sites with many peripheral nerves such as the head, neck and hands have shorter incubation periods. The incubation period is also influenced by inoculum size. Infection with rabies manifests as furious rabies or, less commonly, paralytic rabies.

Furious rabies is characterized by laryngeal spasms, which occur in response to attempts to drink water; these can be accompanied by a feeling of terror, followed by deterioration, coma and death. Paralytic rabies causes paraesthesia and weakness at the bite site and an ascending paralysis which results in respiratory failure, inability to swallow and death.

TETANUS

Tetanus is caused by a neurotoxin produced by *Clostridium tetani*, an anaerobic spore-forming, Gram-positive rod. *Clostridium tetani* can be present in the intestines and feces of horses, sheep, cattle, dogs, cats, rats, guinea pigs, chickens and other animals. The spores are widespread in the environment, including in soil, and can survive hostile conditions for long periods of time. Infection is acquired when tetanus spores are inoculated into wounds.

The highest incidence occurs in individuals >65 years old. The incubation period of the disease is usually between 3 and 21 days, although it may range from 1 day to several months, depending on the character, extent and localization of the wound. Poor prognosis is associated with incubation <4 days or when the time between first symptom and first spasm is <2 days.

Tetanus has four presentations:

- *Generalized tetanus*: Most common. Usually starts with trismus (lockjaw), with progression to the rest of the muscles of the body leading to tonic contractions, spasms, dysphagia, opisthotonus and a rigid abdomen.
- *Localized tetanus*: Sometimes toxin only tracks up the nerves of an affected limb, and in these cases, only that limb may be affected. Localized tetanus may progress to generalized tetanus.
- *Cephalic tetanus*: A form of local tetanus affecting the head, face or neck.
- *Neonatal tetanus*: Caused by contamination of the umbilical stump of a child born to a mother with no immunity to tetanus. Initially manifests as inability to feed, but classical generalized tetanus soon sets in.

Simian Herpes B Virus (B Virus)

Simian herpes B virus is a is a double-stranded DNA *Cercopithecine herpesvirus* 1 similar to herpes simplex virus (HSV)-1 and HSV-2. The important reservoir is the macaques. Like the HSV in humans, macaques can asymptomatically shed B virus throughout life, making any macaque bite high risk for infection with B virus. The incubation period for infection in humans ranges from 2 days to 5 weeks, with most cases presenting 5–21 days after exposure. Infection with B virus in humans is characterized by herpetic skin lesions, sensory changes near the exposure site, fever and flu-like symptoms. Lymphadenopathy may develop proximal to the site of inoculation. Simian B virus travels to the central nervous system, causing encephalomyelitis and eventually death.

The risk of a monkey bite resulting in B virus infection seems very low as the main reservoir is the macaque, nearly all known infections in humans occurred in biomedical research employees and about 2% of macaques are shedding B virus at any given time.

CLINICAL PEARL

Following the primary tetanus series, immunity persists for 10 years after the fourth dose and for at least 20 years after the fifth dose.

CLINICAL APPROACH

History

- The type of animal involved, if it was a pet or a wild animal, any unusual behaviour by the animal that could point towards rabies
- If the animal attack was provoked
- Nature and mechanism of the bite
- Tetanus and rabies vaccination status
- Antibiotic allergies
- Medical comorbidities (i.e. diabetes or immunosuppressive medication)

Physical Examination

- Monitor temperature, blood pressure and heart rate and look for signs of sepsis
- Location, size, extent and depth of the bite (may be useful to take any photographs or drawings)
- The type of wound (i.e. laceration, puncture, abrasion, crush, fracture)
- Signs of soft tissue infection, i.e. redness, swelling, pus, lymphadenopathy
- Presence of any foreign body like teeth from the animal, abscess or haematoma
- The degree of crush injury, devitalized tissue, nerve or tendon damage and any involvement of muscle, bone, joint or blood vessel

Wound Cleaning

All open wounds should be thoroughly cleaned, using soap and water, followed by disinfection using 70% alcohol or iodine solution when available. The wounds should be kept primarily open.

The general approach for animal bites is wound cleaning of the exposed area by thoroughly washing and scrubbing the area or wound with soap, concentrated solution of detergent, povidone-iodine, or chlorhexidine and water and then irrigating the washed area with running water for 15–20 minutes. Surgical debridement of devitalized tissue in high-risk tetanus-prone wounds is crucial for prevention of tetanus.

ANTIBIOTIC PROPHYLAXIS

Antibiotic prophylaxis is not routinely indicated unless:

- Cat bites (long teeth likely to cause deep puncture wounds)
- Bites on hands, feet, face or genitals
- Contaminated wound
- Significant tissue damage
- Deep wound involving bone, joint, tendon or vascular structures
- Comorbidities such as diabetes, immunocompromised, prosthetic valve or joint
- Age: neonates, infants and the elderly

If prophylactic antibiotic is indicated, it should cover the oral flora of the animal. Oral amoxicillin/clavulanic acid 625 mg 8-hourly for 3–5 days can be given. Alternatively, doxycycline 100 mg 12-hourly + metronidazole 500 mg (400 mg in the UK) 8-hourly can be given.

For heavily contaminated wounds that may contain environmental tetanus spores, antibiotics are thought to prevent further production of tetanus toxin by killing the *C. tetani*.

TETANUS POST-EXPOSURE PROPHYLAXIS (PEP)

The following acts as a basic approach to tetanus PEP, but it is recommended to consult national guidelines as there may be some differences in definitions of tetanus-prone wounds, immunization schedule and indications for the active tetanus vaccine and passive immunoglobulins.

Wounds are prone to be contaminated with tetanus spores if:

- Systemic sepsis
- Wounds containing foreign bodies (especially wound splinters)
- Compound fracture
- The animal has been rooting in soil or lives in an agricultural setting and therefore its saliva may contain tetanus spores
- Deep penetrating wounds or extensive tissue damage
- Wound is heavily contaminated with soil or horse manure
- Wound requires surgical intervention that is delayed for more than 6 hours

Patients with clean wounds not meeting the aforementioned criteria do not require tetanus prophylaxis. However, they may require a booster if the last dose was more than 5–10 years ago. Tetanus-prone wounds require immunization (see Table 4.2.1). The tetanus immunoglobulins and tetanus vaccine should not be given at the same site. The dose of intramuscular tetanus immunoglobulins is 250 IU, or 500 IU if more than 24 hours have elapsed or there is risk of heavy contamination. Peak levels are achieved 4 days after an IM dose. The tetanus vaccine is based on tetanus toxin extract and can be given to pregnant women and immunocompromised individuals.

TABLE 4.2.1
Tetanus Vaccination

History of Tetanus Immunization	Tetanus-Prone Wounds	
	Tetanus Immunoglobulin	Tetanus Vaccine
Has completed full rabies immunization in the past	NO	YES if >5–10 years since last immunization
Not fully immunized, uncertain or unimmunized	YES	YES + full immunization course

It is advised to look up national guidance for recommendations on the type of vaccine and how to administer it.

It is advised to contact public health authorities if the patient has had an anaphylaxis to a previous dose of a tetanus-containing vaccine, or to neomycin, streptomycin or polymyxin B (which may be present in trace amounts). Contact the local public health authorities if in any doubt.

Rabies Post-Exposure Prophylaxis (PEP)

Risk of rabies depends on the country where the bite took place, the animal involved and nature of the bite.

High risk considerations for rabies:

- See section 'Rabies' under 'Clinical Considerations' for a general overview on geographical risks. Links to websites with more detailed information can be found in the 'Bibliography'.
- Nature of the bite: Bites with broken skin, contamination of mucous membranes or skin lesions with animal saliva or bodily fluid, and bites in head or neck are high risk.
- Provoked animal bites are higher risk than unprovoked bites.
- Bats are universally high risk for rabies. The risk of dog rabies depends on the country. Domesticated pets are less likely to have rabies than wild dogs on the streets in developing countries.

Rabies PEP consists of rabies vaccine +/− human rabies immune globulin. A patient with a previous history of rabies vaccination should only receive the rabies vaccine. If the animal is available for 10 days of confinement and observation and exhibits normal behaviour during that time, prophylaxis can be withheld. Prophylaxis should be instituted immediately if the animal develops clinical signs of rabies. At this point, the animal should be euthanized, and the brain should be forwarded to a laboratory for definitive diagnosis.

If rabies, prophylaxis is then human rabies immune globulin (HRIG) given on day 0, plus a series of human rabies vaccines (HRVs) on days 0, 3, 7 and 14 (immunocompromised patients should receive fifth dose on day 28 and subsequent titre check).

Simian B Post-Exposure Prophylaxis

PEP is indicated for macaque monkey bites and should ideally be given within 72 hours: Valacyclovir 1 gram 8-hourly for 14 days or acyclovir 800 mg 5 times daily for 14 days. Administration of B virus–specific immunoglobulin, if available, may be effective.

PEP is not indicated for skin exposure in which the skin remains intact.

BIBLIOGRAPHY

Abrahamian FM, Goldstein EJ. Microbiology of animal bite wound infections. *Clin Microbiol Rev.* 2011 April;24(2):231–246.

Cohen JI, Davenport DS, Stewart JA, Deitchman S, Hilliard JK, Chapman LE; B Virus Working Group. Recommendations for prevention of and therapy for exposure to B virus (*Cercopithecine herpesvirus* 1). *Clin Infect Dis.* 2002 November 15;35(10):1191–1203. Epub 2002 Oct 17.

Dendle C, Looke D. Review article: Animal bites: An update for management with a focus on infections. *Emerg Med Australas.* 2008 December;20(6):458–467.

Hemachudha T, Ugolini G, Wacharapluesadee S, Sungkarat W, Shuangshoti S, Laothamatas J. Human rabies: Neuropathogenesis, diagnosis, and management. *Lancet Neurol.* 2013 May;12(5):498–513.

https://travelhealthpro.org.uk/countries.

https://www.gov.uk/government/publications/rabies-risks-by-country/rabies-risks-in-terrestrial-ani mals-by-country.

Riesland NJ, Wilde H. Expert review of evidence bases for managing monkey bites in travelers. *J Travel Med.* 2015 July–August;22(4):259–262.

4.3 Asymptotic Bacteriuria

Firza Alexander Gronthoud

CLINICAL CONSIDERATIONS

Bacteria in the urine in a patient without any symptoms is often mistaken for UTI, leading to unnecessary antibiotic treatment with increased risk of adverse events and antimicrobial resistance. To prevent unnecessary antibiotic treatment of asymptomatic bacteriuria, it is worthwhile to consider the following.

WHAT IS ASYMPTOMATIC BACTERIURIA?

Asymptomatic bacteriuria is the presence of bacteria in an appropriately collected urine specimen obtained from an individual without signs or symptoms of urinary tract infection.

Asymptomatic bacteriuria is most common in elderly women or individuals with diabetes or indwelling catheters. The prevalence of bacteriuria among young women is strongly associated with sexual activity. Asymptomatic bacteriuria is rare in healthy young men. Patients with short-term indwelling urethral catheters acquire bacteriuria at the rate of 2%–7% per day. Patients undergoing haemodialysis have a prevalence of asymptomatic bacteriuria of 28%.

MICROBIOLOGICAL CRITERIA FOR ASYMPTOMATIC BACTERIURIA

- Midstream urine in men: Presence of 10^5 colony-forming units (CFU)/mL
- Midstream urine female: 2 urine samples containing 10^5 CFU/mL of the same bacteria
- Catheter urine: 10^2 CFU/mL is consistent with bacteriuria for both men and women

SCREENING FOR ASYMPTOMATIC BACTERIURIA

Screening for asymptomatic bacteriuria should only be performed in pregnant women and individuals undergoing urological procedures as they are at increased risk of urinary tract infections.

Screening for asymptomatic bacteriuria should otherwise not be performed as, in itself, it is not associated with any long-term adverse outcomes, such as hypertension, chronic kidney disease, genitourinary cancer or decreased duration of survival. Treatment of asymptomatic bacteriuria neither decreases the frequency of symptomatic infection nor prevents further episodes of asymptomatic bacteriuria. In addition, treatment of asymptomatic bacteriuria may itself be associated with emergence of antimicrobial resistance, adverse drug effects and cost.

PYURIA

Pyuria is the presence of white blood cells in the urine and may indicate an inflammatory process in the urinary tract. Pyuria in the presence of bacteriuria therefore does not automatically indicate urinary tract infection, especially in asymptomatic bacteriuria. Even in cystitis, persistent pyuria may have another cause, i.e. renal tuberculosis and sexually transmitted diseases, or be non-infectious, such as interstitial nephritis. Thus, by itself, the presence of pyuria is not sufficient to diagnose bacteriuria, and the presence or absence of pyuria does not differentiate symptomatic from asymptomatic urinary infection. Pyuria accompanying asymptomatic bacteriuria is not an indication for antimicrobial treatment.

CLINICAL APPROACH

SCREENING FOR ASYMPTOMATIC BACTERIURIA

Screening for asymptomatic bacteriuria is only recommended in pregnant women and individuals who are to undergo a urological procedure. Pregnant women should be screened for bacteriuria at least once in early pregnancy. Screening for pyuria has a low sensitivity—only ~50% for identification of bacteriuria in pregnant women.

UROLOGICAL INTERVENTIONS

Patients with asymptomatic bacteriuria who undergo urological procedures associated with mucosal bleeding have a high rate of post-procedure bacteraemia and sepsis. Bacteraemia occurs in up to 60% of bacteriuric patients who undergo transurethral prostatic resection. Insertion or replacement of an indwelling bladder catheter is associated with a low risk of bacteraemia, and antimicrobial treatment is not beneficial.

TREATMENT OF ASYMPTOMATIC BACTERIURIA IN PREGNANT WOMEN

Antimicrobial treatment of asymptomatic bacteriuria during pregnancy significantly decreases the risk of subsequent pyelonephritis and decreases the frequency of low-birth-weight infants and preterm delivery. The duration of antimicrobial therapy should be 3–7 days. It is recommended to periodically screen recurrent bacteriuria after completion of therapy.

TREATMENT OF INDIVIDUALS UNDERGOING UROLOGICAL PROCEDURES

The appropriate timing for initiation of antimicrobial therapy is not well defined. Although 72 hours before the intervention has been suggested, this is likely to be excessive and allows the opportunity for superinfection before the procedure. Initiation of therapy the night before or immediately before the procedure is effective.

An assessment for the presence of bacteriuria should be obtained so results will be available to direct antimicrobial therapy prior to the procedure.

Antimicrobial therapy should be initiated shortly before the procedure. Antimicrobial therapy should not be continued beyond the procedure unless an indwelling catheter remains in place.

INDIVIDUALS WITH INDWELLING CATHETER

Asymptomatic bacteriuria or candiduria should not be screened for or treated in patients with an indwelling urethral catheter.

CLINICAL VIGNETTE

You receive a phone call from the haematology registrar, who is seeing one of his patients who is 2 months post-allogeneic transplant and on tacrolimus, cyclosporine and acyclovir. A urine culture grows an E. coli, *resistant to amoxicillin and trimethoprim. The patient is asymptomatic. The registrar is wondering how to treat this* E. coli. *You advise not to start treatment and monitor.*

- There is no association between asymptomatic bacteriuria and graft survival.
- Transplant recipients with urinary infection and poor graft outcome are characterized by urologic abnormalities and are identified by episodes of symptomatic urinary infection, rather than bacteriuria.
- There are no official guideline recommendations for screening for bacteriuria in solid-organ transplant recipients or bone marrow transplant recipients.

BIBLIOGRAPHY

Cai T, Koves B, Johansen TE. Asymptomatic bacteriuria, to screen or not to screen – And when to treat? *Curr Opin Urol*. 2017 March;27(2):107–111.

Cormican M, Murphy AW, Vellinga A. Interpreting asymptomatic bacteriuria. *BMJ*. 2011 August 4;343:d4780.

Cortes-Penfield NW, Trautner BW, Jump RLP. Urinary tract infection and asymptomatic bacteriuria in older adults. *Infect Dis Clin North Am*. 2017 December;31(4):673–688.

Nicolle LE. Asymptomatic bacteriuria. *Curr Opin Infect Dis*. 2014;27:90–96.

Nicolle LE, Gupta K, Bradley SF et al. Clinical practice guideline for the management of asymptomatic bacteriuria: 2019 update by the Infectious Diseases Society of America. *Clin Infect Dis*. 2019 May 2;68(10):1611–1615.

4.4 Atypical Pneumonia

Firza Alexander Gronthoud

CLINICAL CONSIDERATIONS

Atypical pneumonia refers to any type of community acquired pneumonia (CAP) not caused by common pathogens such as *Streptococcus pneumoniae* and *Haemophilus influenzae* and radiological images appear 'atypical', characterized by neither a lobar nor consolidating appearance. The most common atypicals are *Mycoplasma pneumoniae*, *Legionella pneumophila*, *Chlamydia pneumoniae* and *Chlamydia psittaci*. This chapter discusses atypical pneumonia caused by *M. pneumoniae* and *L. pneumophila*, as they are most commonly encountered in patients who present in the hospital.

LEGIONELLA PNEUMOPHILA

- Aerobic, Gram-negative intracellular organism.
- Transmitted via aerosols from contaminated water sources and soil.
- High infectious dose required, person-to-person transmission very rare.
- Incubation period 2–10 days, median 4 days.
- Acute self-limiting disease 'Pontiac fever' occurring within 6 hours thought to be toxin mediated.
- Severe pneumonia is called 'Legionnaires' disease'.
- Legionnaires' disease has nonspecific clinical findings and hyponatraemia may occur.
- Tetracyclines are least active *in vitro* against *Legionella* compared to macrolides and fluoroquinolones.
- Azithromycin is the most active macrolide against *Legionella*.
- Clarithromycin is bacteriostatic against *Legionella*.
- Rifampicin is active, but clinical effectiveness and survival rates are not well characterized.
- Levofloxacin and moxifloxacin are very active and potentially more active than macrolides.
- The duration of therapy is based on consensus.
- Treatment duration is 7–10 days but may be extended for patients with lung abscesses, empyema, endocarditis and extrapulmonary infection or immunosuppressed patients with prolonged illness.
- In addition to the slowly resolving or residual radiographic abnormalities, patients may experience generalized weakness and fatigue for months. Residual abnormalities on pulmonary function testing may be seen as long as 2 years later.
- Patients presenting late in the course of disease with bilateral infiltrates usually do poorly.
- *Legionella* antigen test in urine may be negative in the first 72 hours, and its sensitivity depends on the bacterial burden and severity of illness.
- *Legionella* antigen can be excreted for 42 days or longer after onset of treatment.

MYCOPLASMA PNEUMONIAE

- The most common cause of atypical pneumonia.
- Slow-growing organism and incubation period of 2–3 weeks.
- *M. pneumoniae* (MP) is one of the most common causes of community-acquired pneumonia (CAP), causing about 10%–40% of all CAP in children and young adolescents.
- Most common presentation is upper respiratory tract infection.
- *M. pneumoniae* infections show an endemic transmission pattern, with cyclic epidemics every 3–5 years.

- Usually mild self-limiting upper respiratory disease, but can cause severe pneumonia.
- Onset is insidious, with patients first presenting with low-grade fever, malaise, headache and non-productive cough.
- The findings on chest X-rays may vary considerably in patients with *M. pneumoniae* pneumonia, although there are some common and recognizable features.
- Common chest X-ray patterns include bronchopneumonia, plate-like atelectasis, nodular infiltration and hilar adenopathy.
- May mimic pneumococcal pneumonia with lobar consolidation with or without parapneumonic effusion.
- *Mycoplasma* species have high mutation rates, macrolides are commonly used antibiotics, and there is increasing macrolide resistance in various organisms including *M. pneumoniae*.
- Options include tetracyclines or fluoroquinolones, which are not recommended as a first-line antibiotic choice as they have age-related contraindications in children.
- No reports on naturally occurring resistance to tetracyclines against *M. pneumoniae*.
- Minocycline and doxycycline both have good activity against *M. pneumoniae*.
- Traditionally, diagnosis of MP infection relied on detecting a rise of IgG titre in paired sera or detection of MP IgM in acute-phase serum. However, antibodies may not appear until 7 days after the onset of symptoms and may thus provide a diagnosis only retrospectively in many cases.
- PCR is a more sensitive and practical method for detecting *M. pneumoniae*.
- However, PCR cannot differentiate between asymptomatic carriage and symptomatic infection.
- This may also mean that in patients with respiratory symptoms, *M. pneumoniae* may be an innocent bystander.
- Potentially, there is a risk for false-negative results due to inhibitory factors in the samples, in which case a new sample should be sent.
- The time interval between onset of illness and first sample is essential for the sensitivity of serology. In a community outbreak of *M. pneumoniae* infection (n=48), PCR detected all but one patient in the first 3 weeks since onset of disease.
- In contrast, in the first week of onset of disease, only 21% of the patients were detected by serology.
- Transmission occurs through droplets from the nose and throat of infected people, especially when they cough and sneeze.
- Human-to-human transmission requires prolonged close contact with an infected person.
- Spread in families, schools and institutions occurs slowly.

CLINICAL PEARL

- Rate of *M. pneumoniae* carriage in healthy people is 0%–13.5%.
- Prolonged *M. pneumoniae* colonization in the respiratory tract during the exposure to antibiotics for various indications may also contribute to emerging macrolide resistance seen worldwide.

Mycoplasma pneumoniae, *Chlamydia pneumoniae* and *Chlamydia psittaci* are not involved in hospital-acquired pneumonia. Routine testing and empirical treatment for these organisms should not be performed. Equally, hospitals have a *Legionella* control programme, and in the absence of any *Legionella* control issues, *Legionella* should not be considered.

CLINICAL PEARL

Mycoplasma pneumoniae also has extrapulmonary manifestations: meningoencephalitis and Stevens–Johnson syndrome are known complications. *Mycoplasma pneumoniae* infection can lead to development of autoantibodies in cold agglutinin disease, leading to haemolytic anaemia. In individuals with immune deficiencies, septic arthritis has been described. Finally, *M. pneumoniae* may cause pericarditis, myocarditis and blood culture-negative endocarditis.

CLINICAL APPROACH

- Lower respiratory tract sample for microscopy, culture and sensitivity testing, a PCR for *Mycoplasma pneumoniae*, *Legionella* and *Chlamydia pneumophila*.
- Especially in the winter months, a viral PCR for respiratory viruses is recommended as well. Many laboratories nowadays will have a respiratory panel which includes the atypicals and respiratory viruses.
- Urine for pneumococcal antigen and *Legionella* antigen. Rapid turnaround time. Negative result does not rule out infection with these organisms.
- *Mycoplasma* serology may be considered if the duration of illness is more than a week.
- Start empirical antibiotic treatment with a β-lactam with either levofloxacin, azithromycin or clarithromycin.
- Stop the β-lactam antibiotic once atypical infection is confirmed.

CLINICAL PEARL

- Combination therapy of clarithromycin and rifampin for treatment of *Legionella* has no additional benefit compared with clarithromycin monotherapy.
- Length of hospital stay is increased with duration of rifampin treatment owing to adverse drug events.
- Combination of rifampicin, clarithromycin and erythromycin should be avoided as rifampicin is a strong CYP3A4 inducer and clarithromycin is a strong CYP3A4 inhibitor, and antibiotic serum levels and levels of other drugs will be significantly affected.

BIBLIOGRAPHY

Hagel S, Schmitt S, Kesselmeier M, Baier M, Welte T, Ewig S, Pletz MW. *M. pneumoniae* and *C. pneumoniae* are no relevant pathogens in critically ill patients with hospital-acquired respiratory tract infections. *Infection*. 2019 June;47(3):471–474.

Pedro-Botet ML, Yu VL. Treatment strategies for *Legionella* infection. *Expert Opin Pharmacother*. 2009;10(7):1109–1121.

Waites KB, Xiao L, Liu Y, Balish MF, Atkinson TP. *Mycoplasma pneumoniae* from the respiratory tract and beyond. *Clin Microbiol Rev*. 2017 July;30(3):747–809.

4.5 Bacterial Skin and Soft Tissue Infections

Firza Alexander Gronthoud

CLINICAL CONSIDERATIONS

Bacterial skin and soft tissue infection (SSTI) is a common infection and has a wide clinical spectrum ranging from mild forms to life-threatening diseases. Besides antibiotic treatment, surgical procedures may sometimes be needed. SSTIs have a high rate of treatment failure of up to 30%. It is therefore worthwhile to consider the following.

RISK FACTORS

Cardiovascular disease, diabetes mellitus, peripheral vascular disease, post-operative wounds and chronic lymphoedema are important risk factors for SSTIs.

CLINICAL SPECTRUM

Bacterial skin and soft tissue infections include wound infections, impetigo, cellulitis/erysipelas and cutaneous abscess. Fournier's gangrene and necrotizing fasciitis are life-threatening soft tissue infections requiring early and aggressive debridement and broad-spectrum antibiotic treatment. If *Streptococcus pyogenes* is involved, then often intravenous immunoglobulins are administered as well.

CLINICAL SYMPTOMS

SSTIs can be accompanied by local, regional and systemic involvement. A wound infection can be discharging pus with surrounding redness and swelling. A cellulitis/erysipelas is a painful, red and swollen local inflammation which may be accompanied by regional lymph node enlargement. Systemic signs include fever and, in severe infections, patients present septic with tachycardia, rigors and hypotension.

It should be noted that cellulitis and erysipelas are generally unilateral infections. The non-infectious differential diagnosis is: varicose eczema, deep venous thrombosis, acute liposclerosis, lower leg oedema with secondary blistering, erythema nodosum, other panniculitis or vasculitis and pyoderma gangrenosum.

BACTERIAL AETIOLOGY

Skin and soft tissue infections are mainly caused by *Staphylococcus aureus* and β-haemolytic streptococci such as *Streptococcus pyogenes* (GAS). Depending on local epidemiology, methicillin-resistant *S. aureus* (MRSA) is frequently present with a previous history of MRSA infection, advanced age, chronic open wounds, underlying chronic disease and repeated contact with a healthcare facility.

Community-acquired MRSA tends to be more virulent than hospital-acquired MRSA, may carry genes that encode the Panton–Valentine leucocidin (PVL) and is more common in the United States than in Europe. Gram-negative and anaerobic bacteria can be found in surgical-site infections and SSTIs in the perianal and inguinal area. Polymicrobial flora can be found in diabetic ulcers. In immunocompromised patients, Gram-negative bacteria should also be considered in cellulitis/ erysipelas.

LESS COMMON CAUSES

Fungi (*Cryptococcus* spp., *Fusarium* spp., *Aspergillus* spp.), *Nocardia* spp., *Actinomyces* spp., *Mycobacterium tuberculosis* and nontuberculous mycobacteria.

CLINICAL PEARL

Breaks in the skin, such as leg ulcers, burns and surgical or traumatic wounds, allow colonization with not only skin flora, but also Gram-negative organisms such as *Pseudomonas aeruginosa*, *Proteus mirabilis* and yeasts, and these organisms may initially only represent colonization not requiring treatment.

ANTIBIOTIC TREATMENT

The majority of patients can be treated effectively as outpatients with or without surgical intervention. Patients without systemic signs of infection can be treated with oral antibiotics. Generally antibiotic therapy is targeted against Gram-positive bacteria. Intravenous-to-oral antibiotic switch is indicated for patients who have had no fever for more than 24 hours, improving inflammatory markers and can take oral medication. Patients who are afebrile for at least 48 hours and physically independent are ready to be discharged.

CLINICAL RESPONSE

Clinical response should be evaluated 48–72 hours after initiation of therapy as it can take a few days for cellulitis/erysipelas to start responding to appropriate antibiotic therapy. Conversely, patients whose conditions deteriorate despite empiric antibiotic therapy should be treated more aggressively on the basis of Gram staining, culture and antibiotic susceptibility. Worsening of acute bacterial skin and skin structure infection (ABSSSI) may indicate the presence of MRSA or Gram-negative organisms.

CLINICAL PEARL

A 48-hour delay in starting appropriate antibiotic therapy is an independent risk factor for treatment failure.

CLINICAL APPROACH

The basic approach to every skin and soft tissue infection is source control via debridement and/or drainage, deep wound culture with susceptibility testing and early and appropriate empiric antibiotic therapy.

DIAGNOSTIC WORK-UP

Microbiologic investigations often have limited values. Blood cultures have low sensitivities and are only positive in up to 10% of cases, and surface wound cultures usually represent colonizing bacteria and yeasts. However, wound cultures are highly recommended in patients with severe local infection and those who have failed on antibiotic treatment. The best specimens, if indicated, are tissue biopsies after debridement (e.g. necrotic tissues) and pus specimens after drainage of any abscesses. If a wound is discharging pus, it is best to irrigate the wound, gently press the area around the wound and take a swab of any discharge. Ultrasonography is an easy and fast method to detect any abscesses and can be used to guide therapeutic aspiration of deeper abscesses.

Computed tomography or magnetic resonance imaging scans can be used to determine the extent of tissue involvement and whether an infection is necrotizing.

In immunocompromised patients who are systemically unwell and who have one or multiple necrotic lesions, the differential diagnosis is ecthyma gangrenosum lesions caused by *Pseudomonas aeruginosa* or localized or disseminated infection with life-threatening moulds such as *Fusarium* spp. and Mucorales. It is essential to take multiple blood cultures and biopsies of the lesions.

ANTIBIOTIC TREATMENT

Recommended treatment duration is at least 5 days and then continue until clinical resolution of symptoms. Cellulitis can usually be treated with 1–2 weeks of antibiotics. For antibiotic choices, see Table 4.5.1.

SOURCE CONTROL

Inadequate or absence of drainage is often a reason for failure of an initial outpatient antibiotic regimen. Patients with large and deep abscesses that require extensive debridement may require hospitalization for operative treatment and more intensive therapies (see Chapter 3.9).

ANTIBIOTIC PROPHYLAXIS FOR RECURRENT CELLULITIS

Up to a third of patients who have had a hospital admission with cellulitis develop a recurrence within a mean of 3 years. Lymphoedema and venous insufficiency are significant risk factors. Antibiotics may reduce the risk of leg cellulitis by 66% in adults who have had at least two previous episodes. Therefore, antibiotic prophylaxis for 1 or 2 years can be considered for patients with predisposing conditions who have had at least 2 episodes of cellulitis. Options for antibiotic prophylaxis are penicillin V 250 mg twice daily or erythromycin 250 mg twice daily. For patients who are allergic to these antibiotics, other options are clarithromycin 250 mg daily, clindamycin 150 mg daily, cefalexin 125 mg daily or doxycycline 50 mg daily.

TABLE 4.5.1
Treatment Options for Cellulitis and Erysipelas

Aetiology	Intravenous Regimen	Oral Regimen
MSSA and streptococci	Flucloxacillin 1–2 g 6-hourly	Clindamycin 600 mg 8-hourly or Clindamycin 450 mg 6-hourly
Penicillin allergy	Ceftriaxone 2 g once daily OR Cefazolin 1–2 g 8-hourly non-severe penicillin allergy	
MRSA	Vancomycin (dosing according to local policy) Teicoplanin 6 mg/kg, 3 loading doses every 12 hours, thereafter 6 mg/kg once daily Daptomycin 4–6 mg/kg once daily Clindamycin 600 mg 8-hourly or 450 mg 6-hourly	Clindamycin 600 mg 8-hourly or 450 mg 6-hourly Linezolid 600 mg 12-hourly Doxycycline 100 mg 12-hourly Co-trimoxazole 960 mg 12-hourly

TABLE 4.5.2
Dose Regimens of Newer Agents for SSTIs

Antibiotic	Regimen	Licenced Duration
Tedizolid	200 mg IV/PO once daily	6 days
Dalbavancin	1 g IV followed 1 week later by 500 mg IV OR	2 weeks
	1500 mg IV	1 dose
Oritavancin	1200 mg IV	1 dose

There is no cross-reaction between erythromycin and clarithromycin. Cefalexin should be avoided in severe penicillin allergy but may be considered in individuals who developed a non-severe rash to penicillin.

NEW AGENTS ON THE MARKET LICENSED FOR SSTIs

Tedizolid is the second-generation oxazolidinone. It has been found to be statistically non-inferior to linezolid with a more favourable toxicity profile. Dalbavancin and oritavancin are new glycopeptides with a long half-life and ideal candidates for outpatient parenteral antibiotic therapy (see Table 4.5.2 for dose regimens).

BIBLIOGRAPHY

British Lymphology Society, 2016. Consensus document on the management of cellulitis in lymphoedema. https://www.lymphoedema.org/wp-content/uploads/2020/01/cellulitis_consensus.pdf.
Dryden MS. Complicated skin and soft tissue infection. *J Antimicrob Chemother.* 2010 November;65(Suppl 3):iii35–iii44.
Navarro-San Francisco C, Ruiz-Garbajosa P, Cantón R. The what, when and how in performing and interpreting microbiological diagnostic tests in skin and soft tissue infections. *Curr Opin Infect Dis.* 2018 April;31(2):104–112.
Poulakou G, Lagou S, Tsiodras S. What's new in the epidemiology of skin and soft tissue infections in 2018? *Curr Opin Infect Dis.* 2019 April;32(2):77–86.
Russo A, Concia E, Cristini F et al. Current and future trends in antibiotic therapy of acute bacterial skin and skin-structure infections. *Clin Microbiol Infect.* 2016 April;22(Suppl 2):S27–S36.
Stevens DL, Bisno AL, Chambers HF et al. Practice guidelines for the diagnosis and management of skin and soft tissue infections: 2014 update by the Infectious Diseases Society of America. *Clin Infect Dis.* 2014 July 15;59(2):e10–e52.

4.6 Bloodstream Infections

Firza Alexander Gronthoud

CLINICAL CONSIDERATIONS

Bloodstream infections (BSIs) are characterized by the presence of bacteria or fungi in the bloodstream and, untreated, can lead to high morbidity and mortality. Once in the bloodstream, microbes can disseminate to other organs or foreign bodies and cause further disease. Infected foreign bodies or intravascular devices, on the other hand, can cause persistent BSI, and removing the infected source is key. Not all positive blood cultures represent true infection. It is therefore worthwhile to consider the following.

SOURCES OF BSIs

Sources of BSIs can be divided into:

- *Anatomical tract*: Urinary tract, respiratory tract infections, biliary tract and intra-abdominal, cardiac and bones and joints
- *Foreign bodies*: Central lines, peripheral inserted central catheters, port-a-cath (port) and bladder catheter, prosthetic joints and prosthetic valves

Some of these sources can cause persistent positive blood cultures despite appropriate antibiotic therapy: any intravascular device, infected thrombus, intravascular graft and endocarditis.

FACTORS PROMOTING BSI

Patients who undergo surgery are at risk of developing BSI because normal anatomical barriers are disrupted (see Chapter 2.1), and during surgery, a bladder catheter or central venous catheter may be inserted which is not removed. Malnutrition and diabetes impair the immune system.

CLINICAL PEARL

Candida spp. and *S. aureus* in blood culture should always be considered relevant, and endocarditis needs to be ruled out.

MICROBIAL FLORA

Most BSIs are caused by bacteria. This is also called bacteraemia. Most community-acquired bacteraemias are caused by *Escherichia coli*, *Klebsiella* spp. and *Staphylococcus aureus*, and are most often caused by a urinary tract infection, soft tissue infection or cholangitis. An important cause of urinary tract infection is dehydration and lack of proper bladder catheter care. Community-acquired pneumonia caused by *Streptococcus pneumoniae* is accompanied by a bacteraemia in 80% of the cases. Hospital-acquired bacteraemias are caused by a much broader range of bacteria for several reasons. During admission, patients become colonized with hospital flora and many patients undergo invasive procedures such as surgery or have central venous catheters (CVCs) predisposing them to bloodstream infections. Bacteria involved in hospital-acquired bacteraemia are *Pseudomonas aeruginosa*, *Enterobacter cloacae* complex, *Serratia marcescens* and *Acinetobacter baumannii*.

Fungi are another cause of BSI. This is called fungaemia. The most common causes of fungaemia are yeasts. The most common yeasts involved are *Candida albicans* and non-albicans species such as *C. glabrata*, *C. parapsilosis*, *C. krusei* and *C. tropicalis*. *Candida auris* is an emerging multidrug-resistant *Candida* of international concern. Blood cultures are only positive in 50% of candidaemia. To rule out a candidaemia, it is useful to test the fungal biomarker (1–3)-β-D-glucan (BDG). A negative BDG has a high negative predictive value (see Chapter 4.32). Other yeasts involved are *Cryptococcus* spp. and *Histoplasma capsulatum*. *Cryptococcal* fungaemia is strongly associated with HIV. Most moulds do not grow in blood cultures; exceptions are *Fusarium* spp. and, less commonly, *Aspergillus terreus*.

ORGANISMS USUALLY REPRESENTING CONTAMINATION

A positive blood culture does not always represent infection. Especially if the blood culture was not aseptically collected, contamination can easily occur. Common blood culture contaminants are skin flora such as coagulase-negative staphylococci, diptheroids, *Bacillus* spp. and *Propionibacterium acnes*. Less commonly, viridans streptococci can be found as contaminants.. To audit blood culture collection practices in hospitals, a generally accepted rule is that contaminants should be cultures in less than 3% of all blood cultures collected.

HAEMATOGENOUS SPREAD

Bacteria such as *Salmonella* or *Treponema pallidum* (syphilis or lues) have the ability to invade the blood vessel and cause an aortitis, for example. Other bacteria such as *S. aureus* and *Candida* spp. have a high propensity to disseminate to other organs. In patients with positive blood cultures with these two organisms and a diagnosis of splenic abscess/discitis/brain abscess/lung emboli, an endocarditis should always be ruled out.

CLINICAL APPROACH

KEY PRINCIPLES

Blood Culture Collection

For adults, take at least two sets of blood cultures, with each set containing an aerobic bottle and an anaerobic bottle. For children, one paediatric bottle is sufficient. To diagnose CVC BSI, take one set from the CVC and one peripheral set. A diagnosis of BSI can be made based on time to differential where the CVC blood culture set flags positive before the peripheral set, whereby each grows the same organism. The timing of taking blood cultures is less important.

A common myth is that blood cultures should be collected when a patient has a fever. By this time, the bacteria may have already left the bloodstream. Volume of blood culture is more important, 20–30 mL per blood culture set. For a paediatric bottle, 5 mL should be collected. This is because, often during BSI, the number of pathogens in the blood can be as low as 1 CFU/mL. If endocarditis is suspected, then three sets of blood cultures should be taken in 24 hours' time.

Blood cultures for clearance of BSI are usually not needed. Exceptions are *S. aureus* and *Candida* species as this determines the duration of treatment.

Transport of Blood Culture

Ideally, blood cultures should be transported to the microbiology laboratory immediately, where they are incubated at 37°C. If this is not possible, then blood cultures may be stored at room temperature for 12–16 hours.

Time to Result

For most bacteraemias, the blood culture flags positive in the first 2 days. For *Candida* spp., it can be 3 days or sometimes more. Blood cultures are usually incubated for 5–7 days before they are regarded as negative. Organisms belonging to the HACEK group do not require prolonged incubation anymore. Positive blood cultures are always phoned out by the microbiology laboratory, so it is not necessary to chase blood culture results.

Empirical Treatment

The choice of empirical antibiotics is based on suspected source, previous positive microbiology culture, local antibiotic-resistance prevalence and if there is an ongoing outbreak of certain bacteria. Antibiotic resistance rates can show local, regional and national differences. It is therefore recommended to follow local hospital antibiotic guidelines.

Source Investigation and Source Control

Locating the source of infection is important as it determines the duration of treatment and helps choose an antibiotic which reaches high local concentrations. Furthermore, although there may be one type of bacteria in the blood culture, the infection at the source may be polymicrobial, and source control enables microbiological sampling at the site of infection. Generally, urosepsis and pneumosepsis are monomicrobial whilst intra-abdominal infections are polymicrobial.

Source control is essential (see Chapter 3.9). This entails removing or changing the bladder catheter. A CVC should always be removed in case of an *S. aureus*, *Candida* spp. or *P. aeruginosa* CVC-associated bacteraemia. In all other cases, CVC removal is indicated if persistent fever and/or persistent positive blood cultures.

Duration of Treatment

Duration of treatment depends on the source of the BSI. General rules are: a pneumosepsis with an *S. pneumoniae* can be treated for 5–7 days, a hospital-acquired pneumonia with bacteraemia and urosepsis can be treated for 7 days. For cholangitis, the duration of treatment depends on source control. If there is adequate biliary drainage, depending on clinical response, duration of treatment can be as short as 3 days. Bloodstream infections with *S. aureus* or *Candida* species require at least 14 days from first negative blood culture. For CVC-associated BSI with coagulase-negative staphylococci, the antibiotics can be stopped if the CVC has been removed. If the CVC has been retained, then duration can be 3–5 days and extended to 10–14 days for immunocompromised individuals.

Antibiotic courses should be as short as possible to minimize risk of resistance and toxicity. Parameters that can be used to justify short courses are: immunocompetent, high antibiotic concentrations at site of infection, appropriate antibiotic therapy, no persistent source of infection (i.e. infected foreign bodies or undrained abscesses) and rapid clinical improvement.

What to Do When Specific Organisms Are Found in Blood Cultures

Staphylococcus aureus

The most common sources are skin and intravascular devices. Organisms can easily disseminate to other organs. Always look for endocarditis stigmata and signs of spondylodiscitis, septic arthritis and osteomyelitis. Perform echocardiography and funduscopy and repeat blood cultures after 72 hours. Duration of treatment is at least 14 days from first negative blood culture. Duration is 4–6 weeks of intravenous antibiotics if dissemination to other organs has occurred. Intravascular devices always require removal. Preferred treatment options are intravenous flucloxacillin 2 g four times a day. If MRSA, then vancomycin IV or daptomycin IV. If vancomycin-sensitive but MIC ≥1 mg/L or if severe infection, then pre-dose level should be 15–20 mg/L.

Candida Species

The most common sources are intra-abdominal and intravascular devices. Intravenous drug use is also an important risk factor. *Candida* UTI is rarely associated with bloodstream infection. *Candida* spp. can disseminate to other organs such as the eye, heart valves, kidneys and, less often, the central nervous system. Always perform funduscopy and echocardiography and have a low threshold to perform imaging of the renal tract. If confusion or other neurological signs, perform CT with contrast or MRI of the brain. Duration of treatment is at least 14 days from the first negative blood culture. In critically ill and immunocompromised patients, start with an echinocandin. In other cases, fluconazole can be considered if no previous fluconazole exposure and not colonized with fluconazole-resistant *Candida* spp.

Enterococcus faecalis

The most common sources are intestines or urinary tract. Around 27% of the cases can be complicated by an endocarditis. Look for endocarditis stigmata and perform echocardiography. In the absence of endocarditis or other deep seated infections, general treatment is with amoxicillin 1 g four times a day IV and, depending on source, can be stepped down to oral amoxicillin 1 gram 3 times a day.

Viridans Streptococci

This can be colonization, transient bacteraemia or endocarditis. If streptococci from the milleri group are isolated (*S. anginosus*, *S. intermedius* and *S. constellatus*), then look for abscesses such as intra-abdominal abscess or liver abscess.

Skin Flora

Coagulase-negative staphylococci, diphtheroids, *Bacillus* spp., *Corynebacterium* spp. and *Propionibacterium acnes* are usually blood culture contaminants. If multiple blood culture sets are positive, then have a high suspicion of infected central venous catheter or any other foreign bodies such as a prosthetic joint or prosthetic heart valve. *Bacillus cereus* and *Corynebacterium jeikeium* are associated with central venous catheter bloodstream infections in immunocompromised individuals.

Enterobacterales (e.g. *E. coli, Klebsiella* spp. or *Enterobacter cloacae* Complex)

Most common sources are urinary tract, intra-abdominal, biliary tract and, in hospitalized patients, also the respiratory tract. Not typically associated with endocarditis. *Enterobacter cloacae* complex should not be treated with cephalosporins owing to chromosomal production of AmpC enzyme, unless it is fully sensitive, including to amoxicillin/clavulanic acid and cefuroxime (see Chapters 2.6 and 5.1).

Anaerobes

Consider odontogenic source or intra-abdominal source. If *Fusobacterium necrophorum* is isolated, perform ultrasound duplex neck and throat inspection for Lemierre's syndrome (throat infection with peritonsillar abscess and infectious thrombophlebitis of the internal jugular vein).

Polymicrobial Flora

If the multiple skin flora are isolated, then this most likely represents colonization. If multiple Gram-negatives with or without enterococci or streptococci are isolated, then consider an intra-abdominal source such as a liver abscess, fistula or biliary source.

WHAT TO DO WHEN THERE ARE PERSISTENT POSITIVE BLOOD CULTURES

Review the drug chart to ensure the correct dose and frequency are administered and no doses have been missed. For glycopeptides, aminoglycosides and some azoles, ensure the pre-dose level is in range. Review the antibiogram to ensure the organism is not resistant to the antibiotic. Some bacteria may appear *in vitro* sensitive but become resistant rapidly to certain antibiotics (see Chapter 2.7).

Another explanation could be that there is a persistent source of infection. This can be a persistent intravascular source such as a central venous catheter, an infected thrombus, endocarditis or an infected vascular graft. Extravascular sources could be undrained abscesses, indwelling bladder catheter, infected prosthetic devices or osteomyelitis. This differential diagnosis is broad and liaison with an infection specialist is highly recommended.

CLINICAL PEARL

It is often difficult to ascertain whether or not an intravascular thrombus is infected. Discuss with the radiologist if the appearance on imaging could fit with an infected thrombus or if a PET/CT would be of additional value. The decision to treat for 6 weeks or to stop antibiotics and clinically monitor with repeat blood cultures should be decided on a per-case basis.

WHAT TO DO WHEN A PATIENT DOES NOT HAVE ANY SPECIFIC CLINICAL SYMPTOMS AND A POSITIVE BLOOD CULTURE

Sometimes no clear source is found. Bacteria can translocate from the gut when there is increased pressure, i.e. ileus, reduced intestinal blood flow, during surgery or after surgery when an ischaemic bowel has developed or from chemotherapy-induced mucositis. Another explanation could be that a patient has received a previous antibiotic course and other clinical specimens such as urine are culture negative as a result. Patients with HIV are at increased risk of bloodstream infections with nontyphoidal *Salmonella*. Patients without a spleen are at increased risk of infections caused by encapsulated bacteria, typically *Streptococcus pneumoniae*, *Neisseria meningitidis* and *Haemophilus influenzae*. Alcohol dependence is another risk factor for pneumococcal infections.

It may be worthwhile to repeat biochemistry; deranged liver function tests may indicate a biliary source. It may be worthwhile to repeat a chest X-ray or order an abdominal ultrasound or CT abdomen to look for hidden sources such as fistula, liver abscess or subphrenic abscess, or consider an infected thrombus at an old central venous line site.

BIBLIOGRAPHY

Bennett JE, Dolin R, Blaser MJ. *Mandell, Douglas, and Bennett's Principles and Practice of Infectious Diseases*. Philadelphia, PA: Elsevier/Saunders, 2015.

Jorgensen JH, Pfalle MAr, Carroll KC, Funke G, Landry ML, Richter SS, Warnock DW. *Manual of Clinical Microbiology*, 11th Edition, American Society of Microbiology, 2015.

Miller JM, Binnicker MJ, Campbell S et al. A guide to utilization of the microbiology laboratory for diagnosis of infectious diseases: 2018 Update by the Infectious Diseases Society of America and the American Society for Microbiology. *Clin Infect Dis*. 2018 August 31;67(6):e1–e94.

4.7 *Bordetella pertussis*

Firza Alexander Gronthoud

CLINICAL CONSIDERATIONS

Despite mass pertussis vaccination strategies and a 95% uptake rate in infants in developed countries, cyclic epidemics continue to occur every 2–5 years. Increasing incidence of individual cases suggests that current vaccines do not prevent circulation of pertussis, making pertussis arguably the least-well-controlled vaccine-preventable disease. Diagnosis is often late, increasing likelihood of transmission in the community. It is therefore worthwhile to consider the following.

- *Bordetella pertussis* and *Bordetella parapertussis* are the causative agents of pertussis or whooping cough, and infections caused by *B. parapertussis* tend to be somewhat milder.
- The bacteria are transmitted by droplets.
- In susceptible contacts, the *B. pertussis* transmission rate is close to 90%.
- In highly vaccinated European countries, the basic reproduction number (R_0) is estimated to be around 6.
- Pertussis continues to circulate in populations where high vaccination coverage of infants and children is achieved because the protection after natural infection and vaccination wanes after several years.
- Therefore, the epidemiology has shifted whereby pertussis circulates in adults, whereas in the pre-vaccination era, pertussis occurred in infants and children.
- In patients with longer-lasting coughs, a diagnosis of pertussis should be entertained irrespective of their vaccination status.
- A carrier state does not exist in pertussis; however, in outbreaks, *Bordetella* DNA may be detected by PCR in asymptomatic patients.
- Most hospitalizations and deaths occur in infancy, and in this age group, deaths may not even be diagnosed as pertussis.

INCUBATION PERIOD

- 7–10 days (range: 4–28 days)

SYMPTOMS

- *Catarrhal phase*: (lasts 1–2 weeks) rhinorrhoea, sneezing and non-specific coughs.
- *Paroxysmal phase*: (lasts 3–6 weeks) in primary infections of unvaccinated children, typical symptoms of pertussis are coughing spasms, whooping and vomiting.
- *Convalescent phase*: (lasts 1–12 weeks) paroxysms may recur whenever the patient suffers any subsequent respiratory infection but, in adolescents and adults, are milder in nature.
- Pertussis is still transmissible in the convalescent phase.
- Cases in neonates and unvaccinated young infants often present with apnoea as the only symptom.
- In older children, adolescents and adults, the symptoms can vary widely.
- Adult pertussis is associated with a long persistent cough which is sometimes paroxysmal, usually worsens at night and has a mean duration of approximately 6 weeks.

- Symptoms tend to be less severe in reinfections.
- Atypical pertussis is becoming increasingly common, and often a persistent cough is the only sign of the disease.

DIAGNOSIS

- Early diagnosis of pertussis allows for prompt treatment with antibiotics, which helps to control spread of the disease.
- Pertussis should be strongly suspected in cases with cough existing for 2 weeks with one or more of paroxysmal cough, inspiratory whoop and/or vomiting immediately after coughing.
- In unvaccinated infants, the white blood count often shows a marked leucocytosis, which in conjunction with clinical symptoms, may be indicative for pertussis in this age group.
- The differential blood count shows a relative and absolute lymphocytosis in infants and children without having sufficient diagnostic specificity.
- Measuring acute-phase proteins, such as CRP and the ESR, has no diagnostic relevance in pertussis.
- In outbreak situations and after household contacts, a positive PCR may also be found in patients with very little or no symptoms.
- PCR has highest sensitivity in the first 2 weeks:
  - The sensitivity of PCR decreases with the duration of cough, and it also depends on age and vaccination status; however, due to its higher sensitivity, it may be a useful tool for diagnosis up to 4–6 weeks of coughing.
  - Nasopharyngeal aspirates are the most suitable specimens for infants and young children.
  - Nasopharyngeal swabs taken from older children, adolescents and adults by trained personnel are adequate specimens in these age groups and are much better than throat swabs.
  - Nasopharyngeal swabs should be taken by gently inserting the swab into the nasopharynx under the inferior nasal choana, and the nose of the patient should be slightly bent upwards.
  - If possible, two nasopharyngeal swabs should be taken, one from each nostril. Small Dacron or rayon swabs, as well as flocked nylon swabs that are more convenient for the patient, may be used for *B. pertussis* PCR.
  - Sputum samples or throat washes are less suitable.
- Culture
  - Bacterial culture is not routinely done in hospital laboratories but remains important for following the evolution of the bacteria, for possible changes in antigens that are part of acellular vaccines and for monitoring antibiotic susceptibility, especially to macrolides.
- Serology
  - Pertussis in older vaccinated children, in adolescents and in adults is mostly diagnosed by serological tests as they tend to present in a later phase where PCR is less sensitive.
  - ELISAs or bead-based assays to quantify anti-pertussis toxin (PT) IgG antibody levels are recommended diagnostic techniques, whereas other techniques, such as agglutination, indirect fluorescence, immunoblotting or complement fixation, are discouraged.
  - Measuring IgM antibodies is not recommended.
  - Serology can be performed with paired (acute and convalescent phase) or single-serum samples.
  - Paired sample serology is an optimal method of diagnosis, but single-sample serology also provides good sensitivity and specificity to determine cases.

- Serology is unable to detect infection with *B. parapertussis*, and it cannot distinguish between vaccine- and infection-induced immunological responses (symptomatic or asymptomatic infection).
- Pertussis serology cannot be reliably interpreted for 1 year after vaccination with acellular vaccines.
- Antibodies are detectable after 3 weeks.

CLINICAL PEARL

In infants, PCR is most sensitive, while serology is the method of choice for adolescents and adults with longer-lasting coughs (PCR is most sensitive in the early period where pertussis is clinically not suspected, and patients are less likely to present to the GP).

DIFFERENTIAL DIAGNOSIS

- Adenoviruses, respiratory syncytial virus (RSV), human parainfluenza viruses, influenza viruses, *Mycoplasma pneumoniae*
- Shorter duration of symptoms (days opposed to weeks as seen in pertussis)

TREATMENT AND POST-EXPOSURE PROPHYLAXIS

- Treatment of choice is a macrolide.
- Most individuals appear to clear pertussis infection without antibiotic treatment within 6 weeks.
- Antibiotic treatment given during the early (catarrhal) phase may decrease the duration and severity of cough.
- The diagnosis is rarely established during this phase among adolescents and adults, except in situations of known outbreaks or contact with a person with pertussis infection.
- Antibiotic treatment later in the course of disease probably does not affect the course of symptoms, but it may be useful in reducing the spread of the infection to others.
- Household and other close contacts should be prescribed a macrolide as well.

CLINICAL PEARL

Possible causes for resurgence of cases of pertussis:

- Asymptomatic transmission of *B. pertussis* in those vaccinated with these vaccines, preventing herd protection
- Small genetic changes in *B. pertussis* leading to antigenic divergence from vaccine strains
- Faster waning of protection with the acellular vaccines
- Older adults who are susceptible to infection, owing to use of imperfect vaccines
- Increased awareness and reporting of pertussis cases
- Increase in the sensitivity of assays, resulting in more confirmed cases

PREVENTION

Pertussis vaccine is combined with vaccination against diphtheria and tetanus. The whole-cell pertussis vaccine (DTwP) was the vaccine type used before 1997.

DTwP was effective in preventing childhood pertussis but suffers from waning immunity 5–10 years after completing childhood vaccination. DTwP is also plagued by a high rate of adverse events including local reactions such as pain and redness and systemic reactions including fever and anorexia.

The acellular vaccine (DTaP) was introduced after 1997 and contains up to five purified antigens: pertussis toxin (PT), filamentous haemagglutinin (FHA), pertactin (PRN) and fimbria proteins 2 and 3. The upside of DTaP is a similar efficacy as DTwP, but lower rate of sideeffects. The downside is a shorter-term protection compared to DTwP.

Although DTaP prevents development of clinical symptoms, asymptomatic infection may still occur, and therefore, DTaP is ineffective at preventing transmission. Because of the short-term immunity, booster vaccines (Tdap) are recommended in later age groups. The use of DTaP also led to an epidemiological shift with increasing cases seen in adults compared to the pre-vaccine era, when pertussis was mostly seen in infants. Immunity from Tdap wanes even faster than that from DTaP.

CLINICAL APPROACH

INTERPRETATION SEROLOGY

- For single-sample serology, IgG-anti-PT antibodies below 40 IU/mL are not indicative of recent contact, whereas levels above 100 IU/mL can be used as indicators of recent contact with the bacteria.
- IgA-anti-PT may serve as an additional test for equivocal results (>40 and <100 IU/mL).

TREATMENT

- Antibiotic therapy may improve symptoms for patients who present within 3 weeks of cough onset.
- For individuals with persistent cough for 3–6 weeks, antibiotic treatment may not reduce cough duration or severity but may reduce the likelihood of pertussis transmission to others.
- For pregnant women, healthcare workers and individuals working with infants, antibiotic therapy is appropriate for those presenting with persistent cough for up to 6 weeks.
- Azithromycin and clarithromycin are the preferred options.
- Oral azithromycin for 5 days (500 mg day 1, followed by 250 mg days 2 through 5) or clarithromycin (500 mg twice daily for 7 days).
- Trimethoprim-sulfamethoxazole (TMP-SMX; one double-strength tablet twice daily for 14 days) is an acceptable alternative.
- *In vitro* susceptibility to amoxicillin has also been shown, but it does not effectively eradicate *B. pertussis* from the nasopharynx.

POST-EXPOSURE PROPHYLAXIS

- Prior booster should not be considered sufficiently protective to eliminate the need for antibiotic prophylaxis.
- Close contact is defined as face-to-face exposure within 3 feet of a symptomatic patient. Individuals with direct contact with respiratory, nasal or oral secretions may also be considered close contacts. Household contacts are considered close contacts.
- Post-exposure antibiotics should be offered to close contacts within 21 days of onset of cough in the index patient to prevent symptomatic infection. Antibiotic choice and dose are similar to treatment options.
- Post-exposure immunization, either passive with immunoglobulin or active with pertussis vaccine, does not protect contacts from infection.

INFECTION CONTROL

- Hospitalized patients with *B. pertussis* should be placed on droplet precautions (in addition to standard precautions).
- Patients with pertussis should avoid contact with young children and infants, particularly those who are unimmunized or incompletely immunized, until they have completed at least 5 days of appropriate antibiotic therapy.
- In addition, patients with pertussis working in schools, day-care centres, or healthcare facilities should not return to work until completing at least 5 days of appropriate antibiotic therapy.

BIBLIOGRAPHY

Guiso N. Pertussis vaccination and whooping cough: And now what? *Expert Rev Vaccines.* 2014 October;13(10):1163–1165.

Martinón-Torres F, Heininger U, Thomson A, Wirsing von König CH. Controlling pertussis: How can we do it? A focus on immunization. *Expert Rev Vaccines.* 2018 April;17(4):289–297.

Tiwari T, Murphy TV, Moran J. Recommended antimicrobial agents for the treatment and postexposure prophylaxis of pertussis: 2005 CDC Guidelines. *Morb Mortal Wkly Rep: RecommendRep.* 2005;54(14):1–16.

Wirsing von König CH. Pertussis diagnostics: Overview and impact of immunization. *Expert Rev Vaccines.* 2014 October;13(10):1167–1174.

4.8 Breast Abscess

Jennifer Tomlins and Simon Tiberi

CLINICAL CONSIDERATIONS

ESTABLISH THE LIKELY DIAGNOSIS

A breast abscess is a walled-off collection of inflammatory exudate (pus). It most commonly occurs as a complication of mastitis but may also be a primary presentation of breast infection. It is seen frequently in women aged 15–45 years and may be secondary to lactational mastitis or non-lactational causes such as duct ectasia (Table 4.8.1). Other causes including neonatal mastitis and systemic infection such as tuberculosis are rare. Mastitis during breastfeeding is common, with recent estimated prevalence reaching as high as 33%, and may lead to abscess in 3%–11% of these women. Duct ectasia occurs in older women, is associated with squamous metaplasia resulting in duct obstruction and has a prevalence of 5%–9%.

Clinical features include pain, swelling, a fluctuant mass and systemic signs of infection, such as a fever. An abscess typically presents 5–28 days after mastitis and diagnosis is easily established with an ultrasound demonstrating a fluid-filled collection. Lactational abscesses tend to be peripheral in location while non-lactational abscesses are more common in the subareolar region. Rupture of an abscess may result in a draining sinus that leads to fistula formation.

CONSIDER THE DIFFERENTIAL DIAGNOSIS

Differentials include:

- *Blocked duct*: Painful lump, overlying erythema, no fever
- *Galactocele*: Smooth, round, painless lump
- *Inflammatory breast cancer*: Oedema, erythema, peau d'orange skin
- *Granulomatous disease of the breast*: TB, actinomycosis, histoplasmosis, brucellosis, bartonellosis, syphilis, blastomycosis, *Corynebacterium*, giant cell arteritis, sarcoidosis, fat necrosis, foreign body reaction, filariasis, idiopathic granulomatous

CONSIDER THE MICROBIOLOGY

Staphylococcus aureus is by far (approximately half of all infections) the most common pathogen found in lactational abscesses. MRSA is increasingly common in some healthcare settings. Non-lactational and recurrent abscesses are more likely to be polymicrobial with isolation of other aerobes such as *Streptococcus* spp., *Enterobacterales* spp. and *Pseudomonas aeruginosa*. Anaerobes are commonly isolated in smokers, typically *Bacteroides* and anaerobic *Streptococcus* spp. Unusual causes include *Mycobacterium*, *Actinomyces*, *Brucella*, fungi and *Salmonella typhi*. Rare and emerging causes of breast infection are now easily detected by MALDI-TOF MS.

CLINICAL APPROACH

SIMPLE MEASURES

For lactational mastitis, the approach includes pain relief with non-steroidal anti-inflammatory drugs, warm compresses, continuation of breastfeeding or extraction (if breastfeeding, sudden cessation may precipitate abscess formation) and prompt antibiotic therapy.

TABLE 4.8.1

Risk Factors for Lactational versus Non-Lactational Mastitis

Lactational mastitis:

- Milk stasis—Poor infant attachment, reduction in the frequency of feeds, pressure on the breast
- Age

Non-lactational mastitis:

- Smoking is the most prominent risk factor (esp. for periductal)—nicotine accumulates in the breast tissue and causes damage to the ducts
- Nipple skin damage/piercing and trauma to the breast
- Ductal abnormality, cyst or tumour altering drainage of the breast
- Foreign body—e.g. silicone used in augmentation
- Immunosuppression—e.g. diabetes, HIV

Source: World Health Organization (WHO) Guideline Mastitis. *Causes and Management.* WHO, 2000.

ASPIRATION OR DRAINAGE OF THE ABSCESS

Antibiotics alone are mostly ineffective once an abscess is established. Rapid referral to a breast surgeon or interventional radiology may be required. Needle aspiration (18–21 gauge) with local anaesthetic is used for most simple abscesses; multiple aspirations may be required but this/these may be curative. If the overlying skin is compromised or necrotic, a mini-incision and drainage (I&D) may be performed (often in the outpatient setting). All necrotic skin must be removed. Large I&D is required for large abscess (>5 cm) or if other procedures fail. Biopsy is recommended in non-lactational or recurrent cases to exclude underlying malignancy.

HANDLING OF MICROBIOLOGICAL SAMPLES

Breast milk can be cultured, but may indicate colonization rather than infection, and is not routinely recommended (only recommended for mastitis failing to respond to antibiotics). Ideally, pus should be sent and specimens should be plated on several media including polysorbate (lipophilic bacteria) and incubated for 5–7 days. Recurrent breast abscesses should also be cultured for fungi and acid-fast bacilli and be sent for histopathology (to identify granulomatous disorders and malignancy).

ANTIMICROBIAL CHOICE AND OTHER ADVICE

For lactational abscesses, empirical choice should cover MSSA (flucloxacillin or clarithromycin/ clindamycin if penicillin allergic). Cover MRSA if known colonization or highly probable.

For non-lactational abscesses, empirical choice may include anaerobic cover (co-amoxiclav or clarithromycin and metronidazole if penicillin allergic).

Other antibiotics include trimethoprim/sulfamethoxazole (not during breastfeeding), doxycycline (debate on whether breastfeeding is safe or not) and intravenous vancomycin. The duration is 10–14 days post-aspiration; shorter courses have been associated with a higher rate of relapse. Staphylococcal carriage is associated with recurrence, so decolonization can be considered. Other advice includes smoking cessation, strict hand hygiene, frequent dressing changes and removal of any offending items, e.g. nipple rings.

CLINICAL VIGNETTES

A 47-year-old female is seen in the breast clinic with a recurrence of abscess beneath her left nipple. She has a history of obesity and diabetes mellitus and smokes 20 cigarettes a day. On examination, she has a tender, fluctuant swelling in the left subareolar region as well as a sinus tract in the peri-areolar region. The abscess was aspirated, and pus grew a combination of Proteus and Bacteroides spp. She responded to treatment with co-amoxiclav, and a plan was made for total ductal excision following recovery.

- Ninety percent of non-lactational abscesses are subareolar and are associated with periductal mastitis. Damage to the ducts (often caused by smoking) leads to infection, duct rupture, abscess and fistula formation.
- They are more common in women in the perimenopausal years.
- They have a chronic cause, with frequent relapse due to duct obstruction. Total duct excision may be required for resolution.
- They are more likely to be polymicrobial and caused by Gram-negative and anaerobic organisms.

A 38-year-old female is seen in the breast clinic complaining of chronic pain and swelling of her right breast. She has two children and takes the oral contraceptive pill but is otherwise fit and well. On examination, there is a tender, irregular lesion in the lower outer quadrant of her right breast. A biopsy shows perilobular granulomatous inflammation and suppurative lipogranulomas and is culture positive for Corynebacterium kroppenstedtii.

- Idiopathic granulomatous mastitis is a rare inflammatory condition of unknown aetiology.
- It is often found in young, parous women a few years after pregnancy on the oral contraceptive pill. Clinical features are similar to those of a malignancy, which needs to be excluded.
- Other causes of granulomas, e.g. TB, sarcoidosis, fungal infection and Wegener's granulomatosis, must be excluded.
- An association with *Corynebacterium* species, particularly *Corynebacterium kroppenstedtii*, has been found. It is essential that deep tissue samples be sent for culture and the lab is alerted to clinical concern for *Corynebacterium* spp.
- Treatment requires an multidisciplinary team (MDT) approach and may involve a combination of surgery, antibiotics and steroids.

BIBLIOGRAPHY

Boakes E, Woods A, Johnson N, Kadoglou N. Breast Infection: A Review of Diagnosis and Management Practices. *Eur J Breast Health.* 2018;14(3):136–143.
Dixon J, Khan L. Treatment of breast infection. *BMJ.* 2011;342:d396.
Taylor GB, Paviour SD, Musaad S, Jones WO, Holland DJ. A clinicopathological review of 34 cases of inflammatory breast disease showing an association between corynebacteria infection and granulomatous mastitis. *Pathology.* 2003;35(2):109–119.
UK Drugs in Lactation Advisory Service (UKDILAS). https://www.sps.nhs.uk/articles/ukdilas/.
World Health Organization (WHO) Guideline Mastitis. *Causes and Management.* WHO, 2000.

4.9 Bronchiectasis

Patrick Lillie

CLINICAL CONSIDERATIONS

Bronchiectasis is an increasingly common cause of respiratory illness and, from an infection perspective, can be associated with difficult-to-treat biofilm-forming organisms. Table 4.9.1 shows some of the common, and problematic, pathogens that are found in patients' sputum. *Pseudomonas aeruginosa* colonization of the sputum has been associated with worsening of the disease.

Cystic fibrosis (CF) bronchiectasis and non-CF bronchiectasis have overlapping microbiological profiles, with most evidence coming from the CF population. The inflammation induced in the airways is related to bacterial burden and is a driver of exacerbation frequency and disease progression.

CLINICAL APPROACH

ANTIBIOTICS

Antibiotics in patients with bronchiectasis play a key role in management. They are used in three main ways: (1) to attempt to eradicate certain bacteria, in particular *P. aeruginosa* and MRSA; (2) as suppressive therapy to reduce the extent of bacterial colonization; and (3) to treat infective exacerbations. All of these areas are guided by sputum culture and sensitivity results.

ERADICATION OF CERTAIN ORGANISMS

British Thoracic Society guidelines recommend attempting to eradicate *P. aeruginosa* and MRSA when they are identified in sputum for the first time. European guidelines also recommend attempting to eradicate newly isolated *P. aeruginosa* infection. The regime used should be guided by culture and sensitivity results, but for *P. aeruginosa* isolates sensitive to fluoroquinolones, a long course of high-dose ciprofloxacin, possibly supplemented with nebulized colistin or an aminoglycoside, has been recommended. In those patients with fluoroquinolone resistance, IV therapy with an anti-pseudomonal β-lactam with or without an aminoglycoside is needed. MRSA should be treated with either linezolid, a glycopeptide, or dual treatment with agents that are active such as trimethoprim/sulfamethoxazole or doxycycline.

SUPPRESSIVE ANTIBIOTICS

Suppressive therapy is intended to reduce exacerbations and improve symptoms in patients who have not had successful eradication treatment. Bacterial burden correlates with the degree of airway inflammation and nebulized antibiotics; commonly tobramycin, gentamicin or colistin are used to reduce the bacterial density over the longer term. The major advantage of nebulized antibiotics is in reducing systemic side effects and targeting the airways only. For some other pathogens such as *Staphylococcus aureus*, particularly in cystic fibrosis, long-term oral antibiotics may be of use in reducing symptoms and exacerbations from these organisms.

EXACERBATION TREATMENT

Exacerbations should be treated according to up-to-date sputum culture results. If no previous cultures are available, broad-spectrum cover, which should include *P. aeruginosa*, should be started prior to the results from the current exacerbation being available. In cases of resistance, combination

TABLE 4.9.1

Common Pathogens in Patients with Bronchiectasis

Early Disease	Established Disease	Problematic Organisms
Haemophilus influenzae	*Pseudomonas aeruginosa*	Non-tuberculous mycobacteria
Moraxella catarrhalis	*Stenotrophomonas maltophilia*	*Burkholderia cepacia*
Staphylococcus aureus		*Achromobacter xylosoxidans*

therapy may be needed to ensure adequate cover and this may necessitate the use of outpatient parenteral antibiotic services. Most patients will need 14 or more days of treatment for exacerbations.

LONG-TERM MACROLIDE TREATMENT

Long-term macrolide use has been studied in several studies and guidelines now recommend that patients with frequent exacerbations should be considered for long-term use of azithromycin or erythromycin as these agents reduce the frequency of exacerbations. The rate of macrolide resistance in oral streptococci in patients on daily azithromycin was high at 88%, and gastrointestinal disturbance was high in the azithromycin group as well.

CLINICAL VIGNETTES

A 29-year-old man with bronchiectasis secondary to congenital agammaglobulinaemia presents with an exacerbation. He has been treated extensively in the past and is on nebulized tobramycin and oral azithromycin. A pan-resistant Burkholderia multivorans *is isolated from sputum. Empirically, treatment is commenced with ceftazidime/avibactam together with aztreonam, whilst awaiting synergy testing results from a reference laboratory.*

In patients with extensive resistance profiles, combining antibiotics with β-lactamase inhibitors may be of use in an attempt to overwhelm the resistance mechanisms. In selected patients, possibly including those in whom surgical intervention or transplant is being considered, synergy testing may be of use, but its use in routine care is not recommended.

A 53-year-old woman with recently diagnosed bronchiectasis was having frequent exacerbations despite inhaled colistin. She was considered for azithromycin treatment but was found to have Mycobacterium avium *in her sputum on several isolates. She was commenced on clarithromycin, rifampicin and ethambutol, and her symptoms began to improve on this regime.*

Although macrolide therapy is now commonly used to reduce exacerbation frequency, it is important to exclude non-tuberculous mycobacterial disease before commencing macrolide monotherapy given the important role these agents play in treating these pathogens.

BIBLIOGRAPHY

Altenburg J, de Graaff CS, Stienstra Y et al. Effect of azithromycin maintenance treatment on infectious exacerbations among patients with non-cystic fibrosis bronchiectasis: The BAT randomized controlled trial. *JAMA*. 2013;309:1251–1259.

Chalmers JD, Smith MP, McHugh BJ, Doherty C, Govan JR, Hill AT. Short- and long-term antibiotic treatment reduces airway and systemic inflammation in non-cystic fibrosis bronchiectasis. *Am J Respir Crit Care Med*. 2012;186(7):657–665.

King PT, Holdsworth SR, Freezer NJ, Villanueva E, Holmes PW. Microbiologic follow-up study in adult bronchiectasis. *Respir Med*. 2007;101(8):1633–1638.

Pasteur MC, Bilton D, Hill AT; British Thoracic Society Bronchiectasis non-CF Guideline Group. British Thoracic Society guideline for non-CF bronchiectasis. *Thorax*. 2010;65 (Suppl 1):i1–i58.

Polverino E, Goeminne PC, McDonnell MJ et al. European Respiratory Society guidelines for the management of adult bronchiectasis. *Eur Respir J*. 2017;50(3):1700629.

4.10 Bronchitis

Patrick Lillie

CLINICAL CONSIDERATIONS

Bronchitis is a common problem, with estimates of up to 5% of adults suffering from an episode each year. It can be usefully characterized as acute with no existing lung disease, or acute on chronic in patients with chronic lung disease, especially COPD. Viral infection is commonly suspected, and the commonest microbial causes are shown in Table 4.10.1, although in most cases a cause is not found.

CLINICAL APPROACH

DIAGNOSTICS

In previously well, community-dwelling adults, bronchitis is a self-limiting (although the cough may persist for several weeks) illness and no investigations are indicated. For patients with pre-existing respiratory disease being seen in secondary care, it is sensible to perform a chest X-ray to exclude pneumonia, together with sputum cultures. As most episodes are due to respiratory virus infection, molecular testing of nasopharyngeal swabs should be performed as this may guide treatment (cessation of antibiotics or starting influenza treatment) and inform infection control practices and isolation.

TREATMENT

For acute episodes in previously well adults, no antibiotic treatment is required and supportive care alone is adequate. For patients with an exacerbation of COPD who have increased cough and worsening sputum purulence, an antibiotic active against *Streptococcus pneumoniae*, *Haemophilus influenzae* and *Moraxella catarrhalis* should be used. For mild-to-moderate exacerbations, doxycycline, amoxicillin or co-trimoxazole are possible options, with broader-spectrum agents such as co-amoxiclav or respiratory fluroquinolones being used for severe exacerbations. Consideration should be given to treatment of influenza during periods of transmission, and treating for this pending the results of investigations is recommended. In addition to antimicrobial therapy, oral corticosteroids and inhaled or nebulized bronchodilators are the mainstay of treatment. Steroid use and influenza are recognized risk factors for pulmonary aspergillosis.

CLINICAL VIGNETTES

A 32-year-old woman presented with a 12-day history of cough, which she described as causing her to vomit after prolonged episodes of coughing. A rapid molecular test on throat swab was positive for Bordetella pertussis, *and the patient was commenced on oral azithromycin.*

The major exception to the general rule of acute bronchitis not requiring antibiotics is for those with pertussis. Although if started beyond 3 weeks of symptoms, benefit is negligible, the diagnosis is often not considered until after this time. Diagnosis is by PCR of nasopharyngeal swab or culture (special media and swabs are needed and PCR is likely to be of more use). Serological testing can also confirm the diagnosis in those not recently vaccinated; however, the result may not be available in a clinically useful timeframe. Azithromycin is the preferred treatment.

TABLE 4.10.1
Aetiology of Infectious Bronchitis

	Acute	Acute or Chronic
Viral	Rhinovirus, RSV, influenza, human metapneumovirus	Rhinovirus, RSV, influenza, human metapneumovirus
Bacterial	*Mycoplasma pneumoniae, Chlamydophila pneumoniae, Streptococcus pneumoniae*	*Streptococcus pneumoniae, Haemophilus influenzae, Moraxella catarrhalis*

A 72-year-old man was admitted with an exacerbation of his severe COPD. He had been unwell for 6 days, had not responded to oral doxycycline and steroids, and was productive of purulent sputum. A CXR showed chronic changes only, and a rapid molecular test on a throat swab was positive for influenza B virus. He was commenced on oral oseltamivir and co-amoxiclav and made a slow recovery.

Viral infections are a very common cause of exacerbations of COPD and have limited treatment options. Although neuraminidase inhibitor treatment for uncomplicated influenza should be commenced within 48 hours of onset of symptoms, in those with severe potentially life-threatening disease, they are recommended irrespective of the duration of illness. Influenza vaccination is indicated in all patients with chronic lung disease, as well as in older patients and those with other comorbidity.

BIBLIOGRAPHY

Brendish NJ, Malachira AK, Armstrong L et al. Routine molecular point-of-care testing for respiratory viruses in adults presenting to hospital with acute respiratory illness (ResPOC): A pragmatic, open-label, randomised controlled trial. *Lancet Respir Med.* 2017;5(5):401–411.

Clark TW, Medina MJ, Batham S, Curran MD, Parmar S, Nicholson KG. Adults hospitalised with acute respiratory illness rarely have detectable bacteria in the absence of COPD or pneumonia; viral infection predominates in a large prospective UK sample. *J Infect.* 2014;69(5):507–515.

Public Health England. PHE guidance on use of antiviral agents for the treatment and prophylaxis of seasonal influenza Version 10.0, September 2019. https://assets.publishing.service.gov.uk/government/uploads/system/uploads/attachment_data/file/833572/PHE_guidance_antivirals_influenza_201920.pdf.

Wenzel RP, Fowler AA 3rd. Clinical practice. Acute bronchitis. *N Engl J Med.* 2006;355(20):2125–2130.

4.11 Brucellosis

Firza Alexander Gronthoud

CLINICAL CONSIDERATIONS

Brucellosis is the most common zoonotic infection in the world and diagnosis can be delayed or missed because the disease primarily presents as fever of unknown origin with nonspecific clinical signs and symptoms. Once infected, brucellosis is associated with high clinical morbidity and causes significant loss of productivity in animal husbandry in the developing world. Furthermore, *Brucella* spp. are hazard group 3 organisms, and laboratory personnel need to use special precautions to avoid laboratory transmission. With increased foreign travel and international tourism, brucellosis may be encountered more frequently in developed countries. It is therefore worthwhile to consider the following.

MICROBIOLOGY

Brucella species are small, oxidase- and urease-positive intracellular Gram-negative coccobacilli. Colonies resemble fine grains of sand. *Brucella* species belong to the same α2 subdivision of the proteobacteria as *Ochrobactrum, Rhizobium, Rhodobacter, Agrobacterium, Bartonella* and *Rickettsia.* Like other Gram-negative rods, *Brucella* spp. have a lipopolysaccharide (LPS) layer, which can be rough or smooth. Depending on the species, rough or smooth LPS increases or decreases its virulence. The medically most important species are *Brucella melitensis, Brucella abortus* and *Brucella suis.*

EPIDEMIOLOGY

Brucellosis is endemic in many parts of the world, including the Mediterranean basin, the Middle East, India, Mexico and Central and South America. High incidence has been reported in Iran, Algeria and Syria.

RESERVOIR

The animal reservoir of *B. melitensis* is goats, sheep and camels, whilst *B. abortus* is found in cows, camels, yaks and buffalo. *Brucella suis* has been reported in pigs, wild hares, caribou and reindeer.

TRANSMISSION

Transmission of brucellosis to humans occurs through consumption of infected, unpasteurized animal-milk products, through direct contact with infected animal parts (such as the placenta by inoculation through ruptures of skin and mucous membranes) and through inhalation of infected aerosolized particles (as occurs in laboratory-transmitted cases).

Hard cheese, yoghurt and sour milk carry a lower risk since both propionic and lactic fermentation takes place. Bacterial load in animal muscle tissues is low, but consumption of undercooked traditional delicacies such as liver and spleen has been linked to human infection.

OCCUPATIONAL RISK

Brucellosis is an occupational disease in shepherds, abattoir workers, veterinarians, dairy industry professionals and personnel in microbiologic laboratories.

PATHOGENESIS

After exposure, *Brucella* spp. are ingested by macrophages. About 15%–30% survive phagocytosis and are transported to the reticuloendothelial system, where they replicate. Mucous membranes are reservoir sites for *Brucella* spp. and could act as a reservoir for chronic infection.

Th1 cell-mediated immune response is important in protection against *Brucella* spp., and IFN-γ plays an essential role.

IgM against lipopolysaccharide can be detected during the first week of infection, followed by IgG as early as the second week. Antibody titres peak during the fourth week. The IgM titre may be higher than IgG for 6 months. IgM and IgG titres decline after antibiotic treatment but may remain elevated for a prolonged time (months-years).

INCUBATION PERIOD

The period of incubation usually ranges from 2–4 weeks but may be up to 6 months and, in rare cases, a year.

SIGNS AND SYMPTOMS

Almost all patients present with fever; up to a third of patients have malaise, weight loss and arthralgias; and in a minority of cases, hepatomegaly, splenomegaly and lymphadenopathy are seen. Fever is invariable and can be spiking and accompanied by rigors, if bacteraemia is present, or may be relapsing, mild or protracted. Malodorous perspiration is almost pathognomonic.

COMPLICATIONS OF BRUCELLOSIS

Osteoarticular disease is the most common complication of brucellosis, and manifests as peripheral arthritis, sacroiliitis and spondylitis. Peripheral arthritis is the most common and is nonerosive, since it usually involves the knees, hips, ankles and wrists in the context of acute infection. Prosthetic joint infection has also been reported. Spondylitis, predominantly involving the lumbar spine, is difficult to treat, and residual damage following treatment occurs frequently. Other important complications are neurobrucellosis and endocarditis.

CNS complications occur in 5%–7% of cases and manifest as meningitis, encephalitis, meningoencephalitis, meningovascular disease, brain abscesses or demyelinating syndromes.

Endocarditis remains the principal cause of mortality in the course of brucellosis. It usually involves the aortic valve and typically requires immediate surgical valve replacement.

Brucellosis can present as epididymo-orchitis in men. Brucellosis in pregnancy poses a substantial risk of spontaneous abortion. Hepatitis is common, usually manifesting as mild transaminitis. Granulomas can be present in liver biopsy specimens. Liver abscess and jaundice are rare. *Brucella* can cause peritonitis.

CLINICAL PEARL

Pedro Pons' sign, or anterior superior end erosion, occurs together with rounding of the vertebral end and level deformity and is a characteristic radiologic finding of spondylitis in brucellosis.

LABORATORY TESTING

Blood cultures have a reported sensitivity of 15%–70%, but it is generally low. Blood cultures which have remained negative after 7 days should be sub-cultured on agar plates for at least 4 weeks.

Bone marrow cultures are the gold standard for the diagnosis of brucellosis because of a high bacterial load but are difficult to obtain.

The main serology test used is an agglutination test where titres of 1:160 or higher in combination with clinical symptoms are compatible with brucellosis. In areas with higher prevalence, a higher cut-off of 1:130 is used. The test can cross-react with *Francisella tularensis*, *Escherichia coli* O157, *Salmonella urbana*, *Yersinia enterocolitica* O:9, *Vibrio cholerae* and *Stenotrophomonas maltophilia* owing to similarities in O antigen in the LPS.

Serology can be false negative if performed in the window period or due to a prozone effect (excess antibodies preventing agglutination), and not all patients seroconvert. ELISA tests exist which offer higher sensitivity and specificity. Rheumatoid factor cross-reacts with IgM.

Finally, molecular techniques such as PCR have been developed which can detect *Brucella* spp. as soon as 10 days after exposure; obviously, obtaining an adequate sample such as a bone marrow aspirate is not always feasible.

CLINICAL APPROACH

Important triggers for suspecting brucellosis are (1) fever, pancytopaenia and hepatosplenomegaly and (2) history of consumption of unpasteurized dairy products or culture-negative endocarditis.

BIOCHEMISTRY

The blood count is often characterized by mild leucopenia and relative lymphocytosis, along with mild anaemia and thrombocytopaenia. Pancytopaenia in brucellosis is multifactorial and is attributed to hypersplenism and bone marrow involvement.

MICROBIOLOGY TESTING

Specimens from patients suspected to have brucellosis should be handled in biosafety level 3 (BSL-3) conditions. It is therefore important that clinicians notify the microbiology laboratory if there is a clinical suspicion of brucellosis.

If a blood culture has remained negative for 7 days, the laboratory should sub-culture for 2–4 weeks. Meanwhile, a clotted blood sample should be collected for *Brucella* serology; if possible, a bone marrow aspirate for culture or PCR if available. Bacteraemia occurs in the early stages of infection and blood culture sensitivity is highest in the first 2 weeks.

Brucella spp. grow on most standard media, for example, blood agar and chocolate agar. Colonies can be identified using MALDI-TOF MS or agglutination tests. It must be noted that MALDI-TOF MS, API 20NE and VITEK 2 tests can misidentify *Brucella* species as *Ochrobactrum anthropi*. *Brucella* species do not grow on MacConkey agar, whereas *Ochrobactrum anthropi* does.

USING SEROLOGY FOR MONITORING TREATMENT RESPONSE

A rapid fall of IgG antibody titre is a prognostic indicator for a successful therapy, whereas persisting high IgG titre does not necessarily indicate treatment failure. Antibody titres decrease more slowly in patients with deep-seated infections, and a relapse is characterized by a second peak of anti-*Brucella* IgG and IgA, but not IgM.

CLINICAL PEARL

The Rose Bengal test is a rapid card agglutination test with high sensitivity and specificity, but with a low performance in patients who were exposed repeatedly to *Brucella* spp. or had a history of brucellosis and a low pre-test probability.

TREATMENT

The optimum treatment with the lowest relapse rate is oral doxycycline 100 mg twice daily for 6 weeks + streptomycin 15 mg/kg IV intramuscularly for 2–3 weeks.

Alternative regimen is oral doxycycline 100 mg twice daily + oral rifampicin 15 mg/kg (maximum 1200 mg/day) twice daily for 6 weeks.

Streptomycin is not available in some countries, in which case gentamicin 5 mg/kg IV for 5–7 days can be used.

Some people have used triple therapy with doxycycline + rifampicin + an aminoglycoside or any other triple combination containing trimethoprim/sulfamethoxazole 960 mg twice daily.

Other regimens used for brucellosis are oral ofloxacin 400 mg twice daily + oral rifampicin 600 mg twice daily.

For deep-seated infections such as spondylitis or CNS infection, treatment duration may need to be extended to 3 months and triple therapy could be considered.

Doxycycline + streptomycin has an efficacy of 90%–95%, compared to doxycycline + rifampicin, which has an efficacy of 75%–85%.

RELAPSE

Mild relapses are seen in 10% of the cases, usually in the first year after infection, and are treated with the same antibiotic regimen as used for the initial infection.

PREVENTION

Live, attenuated vaccines are used in animals to control the disease, but safe and effective vaccines for humans are not available yet.

BIBLIOGRAPHY

Al Dahouk S, Nöckler K. Implications of laboratory diagnosis on brucellosis therapy. *Expert Rev Anti Infect Ther.* 2011 July;9(7):833–845.

Hashemi SH, Gachkar L, Keramat F, Mamani M, Hajilooi M, Janbakhsh A, Majzoobi MM, Mahjub H. Comparison of doxycycline-streptomycin, doxycycline-rifampin, and ofloxacin-rifampin in the treatment of brucellosis: A randomized clinical trial. *Int J Infect Dis.* 2012 April;16(4):e247–e251.

Pappas G, Akritidis N, Bosilkovski M, Tsianos E. Brucellosis. *N Engl J Med.* 2005 June 2;352(22):2325–2336.

Poonawala H, Marrs Conner T, Peaper DR. The brief case misidentification of *Brucella melitensis* as *Ochrobactrum anthropi. J Clin Microbiol.* 2018 May 25;56(6).

Ruiz-Mesa JD, Sánchez-Gonzalez J, Reguera JM, Martín L, Lopez-Palmero S, Colmenero JD. Rose Bengal test: Diagnostic yield and use for the rapid diagnosis of human brucellosis in emergency departments in endemic areas. *Clin Microbiol Infect.* 2005 March;11(3):221–225.

Yousefi-Nooraie R, Mortaz-Hejri S, Mehrani M, Sadeghipour P. Antibiotics for treating human brucellosis. *Cochrane Database Syst Rev.* 2012 October 17;10:CD007179.

4.12 Candiduria

Firza Alexander Gronthoud

CLINICAL CONSIDERATIONS

- Candiduria often represents colonization not requiring treatment.
- In candiduria, colonization of indwelling urinary catheters is common.
- Previous antibiotic treatment promotes *Candida* growth in the genitourinary tract.
- The risk of *Candida* urinary tract infection (UTI) is highest in the presence of a bladder catheter or in critically ill patients, immunocompromised individuals and neonates.
- Neither pyuria nor quantitative cultures distinguish colonization from infection; hence, findings such as unexplained fever, leucocytosis and coexisting risk factors for invasive candidiasis should be investigated.
- Imaging of the urinary tract (ultrasound or CT scan) might reveal renal abscesses, hydronephrosis, urinary tract obstruction or fungus balls (more common in infants).
- The most common *Candida* species are *Candida albicans* followed by *Candida glabrata*.
- Clinical symptoms of a *Candida* UTI are indistinguishable from bacterial UTI.
- During candidaemia, *Candida* spp. may be found in the urine. However, the other way around whereby a Candida UTI progresses to a urosepsis with translocation into the bloodstream is rare.
- Pyelonephritis due to *Candida* spp. is often complicated by pyonephrosis or abscess and fungal ball formation.

CLINICAL PEARL

Candida in the urine most commonly represents contamination, genitourinary colonization or asymptomatic candiduria. In rarer cases, it represents a lower and upper urinary tract infection. Renal candidiasis is more likely caused by haematogenous spread as can occur in invasive candidiasis. Candiduria may also be an indicator of vaginal thrush.

CLINICAL APPROACH

GENERAL POINTS

- Asymptomatic candiduria treatment is not indicated unless low-birth-weight infant OR neutropaenic patient OR patient will be undergoing urological intervention.
- If symptomatic candiduria, send a repeat urine sample to rule out contamination. If an indwelling catheter is present, remove/change catheter first before taking a urine sample.
- Culture of urine in women with heavy colonization of vulvovaginal area may yield heavy growth of *Candida* spp. and may falsely indicate candiduria.
- Removal of an indwelling catheter usually resolves candiduria.
- Unlike bacterial UTI, the quantification of growth cannot be used to distinguish between colonization and infection.
- *C. glabrata* grows slower compared to *Candida albicans* and detection may take 72 hours.

TREATMENT OPTIONS

- 1st line: Cystitis: Fluconazole 200 mg once daily for 14 days. Pyelonephritis: Fluconazole 400 mg once daily for 14 days.
- 2nd line: IV Amphotericin B deoxycholate 0.3–0.6 mg/kg daily.
- Notes
  - Although flucytosine reaches high concentrations in the urine, resistance may develop quickly. Approximately 25% of *Candida albicans* isolates are resistant to flucytosine, but most *C. glabrata* isolates are susceptible.
  - Successful eradication of *Candida* bladder infections with flucytosine may occur in 70% of symptomatic individuals.
  - Flucytosine dose of 25 mg/kg every 6 hours for 7–10 days may be used if there are no other alternatives.
  - For fluconazole intermediate sensitive *C. glabrata*, fluconazole 800 mg once daily may be effective (the MIC range between sensitive and resistant is quite broad).
  - Colonized indwelling catheters should be removed.
  - Neither liposomal amphotericin B nor echinocandins nor azoles other than fluconazole reach therapeutic concentrations in the urine.
  - Voriconazole has excellent activity in renal parenchyma and is the preferred option for treatment of pyelonephritis.
  - Liposomal amphotericin B is not recommended for treating renal candidiasis because of poor penetration in the renal parenchyma.
  - Candiduria seldom leads to candidaemia or *Candida* pyelonephritis.
  - Removal of fungus balls and replacement of stents or nephrostomy tubes is recommended.

In candiduria, high urinary and tissue concentrations make fluconazole the first-line drug for prophylaxis in high-risk groups (e.g. patients with neutropaenia or post-urinary tract instrumentation) and for treatment of urinary tract infections caused by susceptible strains.

Amphotericin B deoxycholate bladder irrigation (50 mg/L sterile water daily for 5–7 days) may be considered for treatment of fluconazole-resistant species in patients with renal failure. However, relapse rate after local bladder irrigation is high. Although echinocandins have low urinary concentrations, treatment success has occasionally been reported.

BIBLIOGRAPHY

Alfouzan WA, Dhar R. Candiduria: Evidence-based approach to management, are we there yet? *J Mycol Med.* 2017 September;27(3):293–302.
Fisher JF, Sobel JD, Kauffman CA, Newman CA. *Candida* urinary tract infections—treatment. *Clin Infect Dis.* 2011 May;52(Suppl 6):S457–S466.
Malani AN, Kauffman CA. *Candida* urinary tract infections: Treatment options. *Expert Rev Anti Infect Ther.* 2007 April;5(2):277–284.
Pappas PG, Kauffman CA, Andes DR et al. Clinical practice guideline for the management of candidiasis: 2016 update by the Infectious Diseases Society of America. *Clin Infect Dis.* 2016 February 15;62(4):e1–50.

4.13 Cardiac Implantable Device Infections

Julian Anthony Rycroft and Simon Tiberi

CLINICAL CONSIDERATIONS

GRADE THE INVOLVEMENT OF THE DEVICE

Infection of cardiac implantable devices occurs at a rate of 5–20 per 1000 device-years—and infection is associated with increases in 30-day mortality observed, compared to patients with uninfected devices.

Infection of an implantable system occurs primarily on the intracardiac portion of the leads, which follows bacteria tracking down the leads from the subcutaneous pocket, or by haematogenous seeding during a bacteraemia from another focus. The former is to some extent protected against from 1 week following insertion, when leads contiguous with the intimal layer of the vein become partially covered in vascular endothelium.

CLINICAL PEARL

Risk factors for infection of cardiac implantable devices:

- *Patient factors*: Age, immunosuppression
- *Chronic comorbidities*: Diabetes mellitus, COPD, malignancy, heart failure
- *Drugs*: Corticosteroids, anticoagulants
- *Device factors*: Previous infection, epicardial leads, ICD (versus PPM), abdominal pocket
- *Procedural elements*: User inexperience, duration of insertion, haematoma post-procedure, re-intervention

---

Clinical infection can be divided into three presentations:

- *Superficial infection*: Stitch abscess or overlying erythema only, occurring within 30 days of insertion. May be confused with post-implantation inflammation seen in up to 30% of cases and is characterized by erythema but with an absence of exudate, fluctuance and dehiscence.
- *Pocket infection*: Marked by pain, erythema and swelling around the pocket. Erosion or purulent discharge may be present.
- *Systemic infection*: Pocket infection may not always be clinically apparent. As the infection tracks along the venous leads into the cardiac chambers, the patient will become febrile, and complications may occur resulting from haematogenous spread.

CONFIRM THE DIAGNOSIS AND ASSESS FOR COMPLICATIONS

The initial diagnosis should be made based on the clinical findings previously mentioned. If the patient is febrile or otherwise meets the criteria for sepsis, further investigations should include blood for culture (2–3 sets), a chest radiograph and an echocardiogram (transoesophageal if no evidence of valvular or lead involvement on transthoracic echocardiogram). In the case of the febrile patient with a cardiac device and no alternative proof for a septic focus, a CT/PET can confirm infection of the pocket and/or leads. White cell scintigraphy is an alternative to CT/PET. Percutaneous aspiration is not recommended.

CLINICAL PEARL

Complications of implant device-associated infections:

- Infective endocarditis following spread to valves contiguous to leads, particularly if the valve is abnormal or prosthetic.
- Embolic complications; pulmonary infiltrates seen in 20%–45%, with progression to pneumonia
- Metastatic spread following bacteraemia
- Direct spread from epicardial leads (pericarditis or mediastinitis)
- Septic shock, multiorgan failure and death

CLINICAL APPROACH

ANTIMICROBIAL CHOICE

Up to 90% of infections are caused by Gram-positive organisms—two-thirds of which are coagulase-negative staphylococci, with the majority of the remainder being *Staphylococcus aureus*. The most common Gram-negative organisms are *Enterobacterales* spp. and *P. aeruginosa*. Mycobacterial and fungal causes account for less than 1%. Infection is polymicrobial in around 11% of cases.

In reflection, empirical antimicrobials should be anti-staphylococcal—vancomycin (or daptomycin) should be used until the sensitivities are known for any isolated organisms. For methicillin-sensitive strains, antibiotics can later be rationalized to anti-staphylococcal penicillin or cefazolin. Gram-negative cover should be included empirically until the organism is identified—piperacillin/tazobactam or an aminoglycoside.

CONSIDER WHETHER OR NOT THE DEVICE SHOULD BE REMOVED

Superficial infections can be treated with oral antibiotics for 2 weeks and followed up on an outpatient basis. The device should not be removed.

Besides superficial infection, retention should be attempted only if any bacteraemia confirmed is a single episode, the organism is neither *S. aureus* nor *Candida* and there are no complications. After a 2-week course of antibiotics, the patient should be followed up with and surveillance blood cultures taken—and the device removed in the event of relapse.

Pocket infections should always prompt device removal if caused by *S. aureus* or *Candida* species, or if pocket infection is associated with persistent bacteraemia caused by any organism. In the absence of complications, pocket infections can be treated for 2 weeks following explantation and washout of the pocket.

If vegetations are seen on echocardiography, the entire device should be removed and antimicrobial management should then be as for infective endocarditis. If removal is indicated, the device should be removed as soon as possible. Device removal usually occurs transvenously, although open surgery may be required in the case of large vegetations. Assuming the local infection has resolved, a new device should not be implanted until 72 hours after the last negative blood culture (14 days if valvular vegetations on echocardiography).

Even though device removal in definite device infections is mandatory, device retention with chronic antibiotic suppression may be reasonable in patients who are not eligible for complete device extraction owing to multiple comorbidities.

CLINICAL PEARL

Indications for device removal:

- Lead or valvular vegetations seen on echocardiography
- *Staphylococcus aureus* identified as the cause (even in absence of bacteraemia)
- *Candida* species identified as the cause (even in absence of bacteraemia)
- Multiple positive blood cultures for the same organism
- Failure of retention attempt

CLINICAL VIGNETTES

The emergency medicine fellow calls you because 30 minutes after receiving piperacillin/ tazobactam, the patient experiences facial flushing, pruritus and chest pains. He would like to change the β-lactam.

Although a rash reaction to the penicillin would be in the differential diagnosis, the description is more typical of red man syndrome resulting from glycopeptide infusion. The condition is not benign, as haemodynamic instability and cardiac arrest may rarely occur, but the reaction does not contraindicate continuing vancomycin, and it does not contraindicate continued β-lactam therapy. The response is a rate-related infusion reaction, and opioids, radiocontrast and some anaesthetics increase the risk of developing it. On diagnosis, the infusion should be stopped and ranitidine given. If mild/moderate (no haemodynamic instability or chest pains), the infusion can be restarted at half the original rate; if severe (i.e. chest pain or hypotension), the infusion should not restart for 4 hours.

On day 2 of admission, Staphylococcus epidermidis *is identified in two of two blood culture bottles sent from the emergency department. The time to positivity was 14 hours for the aerobic bottle and 16 hours for the anaerobic bottle. A further set sent by the on-call SHO during the night contained Gram-positive cocci in clusters, again in both bottles.*

This organism is most likely the cause of the PPM infection, and the persistent bacteraemia should prompt removal of the device. The device and its leads, as well as pus and tissue from the pocket, should be sent for culture to the microbiology laboratory. In the absence of a microbiological diagnosis from culture, molecular testing can be used to identify the organism from sterile samples including pus. When the sensitivities are known, the antimicrobial prescription can be rationalized. Flucloxacillin can be used for methicillin-sensitive staphylococci; vancomycin may be used for methicillin-resistant organisms (as many coagulase-negative subspecies are)—daptomycin and linezolid are alternatives. Rifampicin should be added for synergy and anti-biofilm activity. Once the device is removed, the pocket washed out and patient is improving, other oral options that could be considered, depending on the sensitivities, might include ciprofloxacin or co-trimoxazole. Provided infective endocarditis is excluded, this patient would require 14 days of treatment after the first negative blood culture (not all of which would need to be intravenous).

After the microbiological diagnosis is made, a transthoracic echocardiogram is arranged, which confirms vegetations on the tricuspid valve.

This patient now has a diagnosis of infective endocarditis. The device should be removed, and antibiotics will be required for a minimum of 4–6 weeks depending on the organism and whether or not the valve is native. A permanent device should not be re-implanted until at least 2 weeks after the first negative blood culture—ideally longer. This may require a temporary system depending upon the ongoing indication for a cardiac device.

REFERENCES

Arber N, Pras E, Copperman Y et al. Pacemaker endocarditis: Report of 44 cases and review of the literature. *Medicine (Baltimore)*. 1994;73(6):299–305.

Baddour LM, Epstein AE, Erickson CC et al. Update on cardiovascular implantable electronic device infections and their management: A scientific statement from the American Heart Association. *Circulation*. 2010;121(3):458–477.

Peacock JE, Stafford JM, Le K et al. Attempted salvage of infected cardiovascular implantable electronic devices: Are there clinical factors that predict success? *Pacing Clin Electrophysiol*. 2018;41:524–531.

Sandoe JA, Barlow G, Chambers JB et al. Guidelines for the diagnosis, prevention and management of implantable cardiac electronic device infection. Report of a joint Working Party project on behalf of the British Society for Antimicrobial Chemotherapy (BSAC, host organization), British Heart Rhythm Society (BHRS), British Cardiovascular Society (BCS), British Heart Valve Society (BHVS) and British Society for Echocardiography (BSE). *J Antimicrob Chemother*. 2015;70(2):325–359.

Tan EM, DeSimone DC, Sohail MR et al. Outcomes in patients with cardiovascular implantable electronic device infection managed with chronic antibiotic suppression. *Clin Infect Dis*. 2017;64(11):1516–1521.

4.14 *Chlamydia trachomatis*

Anda Samson

CLINICAL CONSIDERATIONS

Chlamydia is an ancient infection that has adapted to life in various species; various *Chlamydia* strains exist. *Chlamydia trachomatis* is the strain most commonly infecting humans. Different serotypes of *Chlamydia trachomatis* are prone to causing infection at different body sites; serotypes A to C most commonly cause ocular trachoma, and serotypes D to K most commonly cause genital infection, although these are not exclusive to the genital tract. Lymphogranuloma venereum (LGV) is a more systemic manifestation of *Chlamydia trachomatis* caused by *Chlamydia* serovars L1, L2 and L3. Most infections take place in the young (16–24 year olds), but people with a new partner or men having sex with men are also at a higher risk.

INFECTION

Ocular infection occurs most in areas of crowding and with lack of access to hygienic washing facilities; once living environments improve, there is usually a spontaneous decrease in infection rates. Most active trachoma infections occur in children under 5; they often get reinfected due to lack of face cleaning facilities.

Genital *Chlamydia trachomatis* in women is usually asymptomatic. Co-infection with *Mycoplasma genitalium* or *Neisseria gonorrhoeae* is common. However, it may, like other STDs, lead to increased vaginal discharge, post-coital bleeds and dyspareunia, dysuria and abdominal pain. A significant number of women also have asymptomatic rectal infection irrespective of history of anal intercourse. In men, *Chlamydia* causes urethritis as well; in only around 1 in 8 cases, it becomes symptomatic. In practice, it is not possible to reliably distinguish clinically between gonococcal urethritis and that caused by *Chlamydia trachomatis*.

LGV may manifest as fever, malaise and arthritis as well as perihepatitis, pneumonitis, painful or painless ulceration in the mouth or haemorrhagic proctitis, and as lymphadenopathy in draining lymph node sites. In advanced stages, it can mimic inflammatory bowel disease with proctitis, proctocolitis and fistulation.

COMPLICATIONS OF *CHLAMYDIA* INFECTIONS

In children and young adults, reinfection of the eyes over prolonged periods of time may lead to scarring of the cornea and other ocular anatomy, ultimately leading to blindness.

In women, genital *Chlamydia* infections can lead to endometritis, salpingitis and pelvic inflammatory disease. This can, in turn, lead to infertility or ectopic pregnancy. In men, the infection can lead to epididymitis and prostatitis. Rectal or vaginal LGV infection can lead to fistulae and scarring of the surrounding tissue, and long-term damage to the lymphatic system can lead to elephantiasis of the draining tissue.

Genital *Chlamydia* infection is known to cause reactive arthritis in 1% of patients. Usually, reactive arthritis will settle after treatment of the primary cause, but incidentally, short-lived anti-inflammatory therapy is needed.

CLINICAL APPROACH

DIAGNOSIS

Chlamydia trachomatis is an intracellular Gram-negative organism. It is one of the smallest microorganisms that uses the host cell machinery to replicate effectively. Because it is intracellular, it cannot be readily identified on a Gram stain. Only trachoma can be diagnosed on clinical grounds; infections at other sites may occur silently before they lead to complications and are clinically not distinguishable from other venereal diseases.

NAAT

The most effective way to diagnose *Chlamydia* is a nucleic acid amplification test (NAAT) assay (PCR). A self-obtained vulvo-vaginal swab in women or a first-catch urine sample in men and women is an acceptable sample for a NAAT test. They are very sensitive and specific, although not all NAAT assays can automatically distinguish between LGV and other strains of *Chlamydia trachomatis*. It is therefore important to flag the possibility of LGV to the laboratory.

Because NAATs detect DNA or RNA and not live organisms, they can remain positive for up to 3 weeks post-treatment. It is therefore not recommended to use them as a test of cure, except in pregnant women and in rectal infections.

CLINICAL PEARL

Repeat NAAT as test of cure is only recommended in pregnancy and in rectal infections.

TREATMENT OF *CHLAMYDIA* INFECTION

Doxycycline 100 mg 12-hourly for 7 days is now recommended as first-line treatment for uncomplicated urogenital, pharyngeal and rectal *Chlamydia* infections. Because of increasing evidence for co-infection with *M. genitalium*, which is often resistant to azithromycin, azithromycin is no longer recommended as first-line treatment for *Chlamydia*. Additionally, doxycycline is superior to azithromycin in curing rectal infections.

TREATMENT IN PREGNANCY AND DURING LACTATION

Because doxycycline is potentially teratogenic, it is contraindicated in pregnancy and during lactation. Recommended treatment regimens are: erythromycin 500 mg four times a day for 7 days, azithromycin 1 g on day 1 followed by 500 mg on days 2 and 3, or amoxicillin 500 mg three times a day for 7 days. Test of cure with repeat NAAT is recommended.

LGV should be treated with doxycycline 100 mg 12-hourly for 3 weeks. Azithromycin 1 g stat and 1 g weekly for 3 weeks or erythromycin 500 mg four times daily for 21 days are alternative regimens. Fluctuating lymph nodes (buboes) can be aspirated through healthy skin, not through surgical incision. Again, test of cure with repeat NAAT is recommended.

Pelvic inflammatory disease treatment should always include antibiotics that cover *N. gonorrhoeae* and anaerobes; a good option would be one dose ceftriaxone 250 mg intramuscularly or 2 g intravenously PLUS doxycycline 100 mg 12-hourly and metronidazole 400 mg 8-hourly for 14 days (see Chapter 4.46 for more treatment options).

PREVENTION OF *CHLAMYDIA TRACHOMATIS*

Unfortunately, there is no vaccine available for primary prophylaxis. The effort of prevention is therefore aimed at primary prevention strategies.

In order to prevent trachoma infections, overall improvement of sanitation and access to clean water and latrines are paramount. Mass treatment programmes with azithromycin have been shown to be effective, but the effect only lasts around 6 months to a year. A combination of improvement of living standards and repeat mass treatment programmes is therefore likely to have the biggest impact.

Universal screening and treating of pregnant women have been widely recognized to prevent mother-to-child transmission, and *Chlamydia* infections, when treated in pregnancy, do not appear to have an effect on rates of stillborn or premature babies or birth weight.

Lastly, universal screening programmes for genital *Chlamydia* are not proven to be cost-effective so far, but systematic screening of higher-risk groups seems effective in preventing further dissemination of the infection.

CLINICAL PEARL

Universal screening of pregnant women for *Chlamydia* infections is recommended.

CLINICAL PEARL

Improvement in sanitation and access to clean water are paramount in halting ocular trachoma epidemics.

CLINICAL VIGNETTES

A 12-week pregnant, 25-year-old woman is checked in for her first routine pregnancy check. Along with the booking bloods, a Chlamydia *screen is performed on a urine sample, which comes back positive. This comes as a complete surprise to the patient because she had absolutely no symptoms. She is treated with erythromycin and her partner is tested and subsequently treated as well.*

A 35-year-old man is referred to the gastroenterology clinic because of rectal bleeding and abdominal pain. A colonoscopy is performed, which shows inflammation of the ileo-coecal area. Cultures show no growth, but NAAT for Chlamydia *spp. is positive; a subsequent test shows that there is indeed infection with serovar L1. He is treated with doxycycline and recovers swiftly. A full STI screen is negative.*

BIBLIOGRAPHY

2015 BASHH guideline for Chlamydia (2018 update), 2019 BASHH guideline for PID, 2013 BASHH guideline for LGV. In: Bennett JE, Dolin R, Blaser MJ (eds). *Mandell, Douglas, and Bennett's Principles and Practice of Infectious Diseases*. Philadelphia, PA: Elsevier/Saunders, 2015.

Dukers-Muijrers NHTM, Wolffs PFG, De Vries H et al. Treatment effectiveness of azithromycin and doxycycline in uncomplicated rectal and vaginal *Chlamydia trachomatis* infections in women: A Multicenter Observational Study (FemCure). *Clin Infect Dis*. 2019;69(11):1946–1954.

Reekie J, Roberts C, Preen D et al. *Chlamydia trachomatis* and the risk of spontaneous preterm birth, babies who are born small for gestational age, and stillbirth: A population-based cohort study. *Lancet Infect Dis*. 2018;18:452–460.

Taylor HR, Burton MJ, Haddad D, West S, Wright H. Trachoma. *The Lancet*. 2014;384(9960):2142–2152.

4.15 Cholangitis

Firza Alexander Gronthoud

CLINICAL CONSIDERATIONS

Cholangitis is an acute infection that may not always respond to antibiotic therapy. It is then worthwhile to review the source of infection and consider the following.

DIAGNOSING CHOLANGITISS

Classical symptoms such as fever, jaundice and pain in the right upper quadrant (Charcot's triad) may be absent in 30% of patients.

Reynolds' pentad, consisting of Charcot's triad, altered mental status and hypotension, indicates severe cholangitis.

Biochemistry often shows a cholestatic picture with increased liver function tests, but the increased bilirubin, Gamma-glutamyl transferase (GGT) and alkaline phosphatase should raise suspicion. An ultrasound may show dilated biliary ducts, aerobilia, stricture and stones. The most frequent cause of cholangitis is biliary stones.

BILIARY OBSTRUCTION

Cholangitis is inflammation and infection in the biliary duct associated with obstruction of the biliary duct caused by gall stones, stricture or compression due to a malignancy. The presence of parasites in the bile duct such as *Fasciola hepatica*, *Clonorchis sinensis*, *Opisthorchis* spp. or *Ascaris lumbricoides* can cause significant obstruction and can be overlooked if no travel history is taken.

BILIARY INFECTION AND TRANSLOCATION

Progressive obstruction causes an increased pressure which leads to stasis and inflammation of bile. Biliary obstruction causes local immune dysfunction and subsequently increases small bowel bacterial colonization. It is believed that bacteria gain access to the biliary tree by retrograde ascent from the duodenum or from portal venous blood. Progressive biliary obstruction results in cholangiovenous and cholangiolymphatic reflux, with translocation of bacteria into the bloodstream resulting in septicaemia.

BACTERIAL AETIOLOGY

The most frequent organisms isolated are *Escherichia coli*, *Klebsiella pneumoniae* and *Klebsiella oxytoca*. *Aeromonas hydrophila* has also been found in a minority of cases. In immunocompromised individuals with multiple courses of antibiotics, cholangitis *Pseudomonas aeruginosa*, *Enterococcus faecium* and *Candida* spp. may be involved.

CLINICAL PEARL

Interventions to relieve biliary obstruction, such as ERCP and stent placing, are risk factors themselves for cholangitis. Sepsis post-ERCP increases the likelihood of cholangitis.

CLINICAL APPROACH

DRAINAGE

- *When*: Moderate-to-severe cholangitis.
- *How*: Drainage via ERCP, percutaneously or, less common, surgically. Alternatively, a stent may be placed in the biliary duct.
- *Rationale*: A stent restores biliary flow via internal drainage, which is often performed in the case of duct compression by a malignancy.

MICROBIOLOGICAL INVESTIGATION

- Blood cultures
- Bile culture

MEDICAL MANAGEMENT

The severity of acute cholangitis can be classified into three grades (see Table 4.15.1). Grade I cholangitis can be managed with antimicrobial therapy. Empirical therapy should be based on expected associated pathogenic bacteria, the presence of comorbidities such as hepatic or renal failure, patient allergies, local susceptibility patterns, previous culture results and recent history of antibiotic usage. Blood cultures can be used to guide antimicrobial therapy. Other important components are intravenous fluids and analgesia. It is important to frequently monitor the patient as acute cholangitis may rapidly progress to a severe form, particularly in elderly patients.

ANTIBIOTIC CHOICE

Empirical treatment commonly consists of amoxicillin/clavulanic acid, cefuroxime or ceftriaxone with or without gentamicin. Anaerobes are rarely involved, and metronidazole is generally not indicated. Antibiotic therapy should be rationalized based on blood culture and/or biliary cultures.

DURATION OF TREATMENT

For grade I cholangitis, a treatment duration of 7–10 days is indicated. For grade II cholangitis, after successful biliary drainage, a short course of antibiotics can be discontinued after as early as 3 days provided the patient has clinically and biochemically improved. Grade III cholangitis may require a longer course up to 7 days. The presence of a concomitant bacteraemia does not influence the antibiotic course length.

TABLE 4.15.1
Grading and Corresponding Treatment

Grade I	Grade II	Grade III
Observation + antimicrobial therapy	Antimicrobial therapy + early biliary drainage	Antimicrobial therapy + organ support + urgent biliary drainage

CLINICAL VIGNETTE

You receive a phone call from the night SHO regarding a 68-year-old male with pancreatic cancer with a biliary stent in situ. He was treated for a cholangitis 12 days ago and re-admitted with a recurrent septic episode on day 7 of piperacillin/tazobactam and vancomycin for a presumed relapsed cholangitis. Blood cultures were negative. Patient had a spiking temperature but was clinically stable. The night SHO calls asking you if piperacillin/tazobactam should be changed to meropenem. You advise to continue current antibiotics but to request a CT abdomen to look for any persistent source of infection. The following day, the CT scan shows two small abscesses amenable to drainage. A successful drainage is attempted after which the fever settled.

Antibiotic therapy is supportive. The mainstay is source control. If a patient is clinically stable but keeps spiking temperature, that indicates a persistent source of infection in need of source control. Escalation of antibiotic therapy won't be beneficial. Liver abscess is a complication of cholangitis and requires drainage, and 4–6 weeks of antibiotics is often needed.

BIBLIOGRAPHY

Doi A, Morimoto T, Iwata K. Shorter duration of antibiotic treatment for acute bacteraemic cholangitis with successful biliary drainage: A retrospective cohort study. *Clin Microbiol Infect.* 2018 November;24(11):1184–1189.

Gomi H, Takada T, Hwang TL et al. Updated comprehensive epidemiology, microbiology, and outcomes among patients with acute cholangitis. *J Hepatobiliary Pancreat Sci.* 2017;24(6):310–318.

Mayumi T, Okamoto K, Takada T et al. Tokyo Guidelines 2018: management bundles for acute cholangitis and cholecystitis. *J Hepatobiliary Pancreat Sci.* 2018;25(1):96–100.

Park TY, Choi JS, Song TJ, Do JH, Choi SH, Oh HC. Early oral antibiotic switch compared with conventional intravenous antibiotic therapy for acute cholangitis with bacteremia. *Dig Dis Sci.* 2014 November;59(11):2790–2796.

Uno S, Hase R, Kobayashi M et al. Short-course antimicrobial treatment for acute cholangitis with Gram-negative bacillary bacteremia. *Int J Infect Dis.* 2017;55:81–85.

van Lent AU, Bartelsman JF, Tytgat GN, Speelman P, Prins JM. Duration of antibiotic therapy for cholangitis after successful endoscopic drainage of the biliary tract. *Gastrointest Endosc.* 2002 April;55(4):518–522.

4.16 Deep Neck Space Infection

Firza Alexander Gronthoud

CLINICAL CONSIDERATIONS

Deep neck space infections (DNSIs) are a challenging problem because of the complex anatomy and potentially fatal complications that may occur. The spaces of the neck communicate with one another, forming avenues by which infections may spread over large areas. It may therefore be worthwhile to consider the following.

AETIOLOGY

The most common cause of deep neck space infections is odontogenic infection, and unsurprisingly, the submandibular space is the area most involved. Other spaces that can be involved are the masticatory space, sublingual space, parotid space and pharyngeal space. The infection can present as a cellulitis and/or abscess.

SYMPTOMS

Symptoms consist of neck swelling, dysphagia, trismus, dyspnoea, dysphonia and fever.

RISK FACTORS

Pharyngitis, peritonsillar abscess, sialadenitis, parotitis, lymphadenitis, trauma, surgery or diabetes mellitus.

CLASSIFICATION

Cellulitis versus abscess, monolateral or bilateral, involved spaces: lateral pharyngeal space, retropharyngeal space, prevertebral space, parotid space, masticatory space, visceral vascular space and anterior visceral space.

MICROBIOLOGY

The microbiological pattern of DNSIs is generally polymicrobial, including aerobes and anaerobes. The predominant anaerobic organisms are *Prevotella* spp., *Porphyromonas* spp., *Fusobacterium* spp., and *Peptostreptococcus* spp.; aerobic organisms are group A *Streptococcus*, viridans streptococci, *Staphylococcus aureus* and *Haemophilus influenzae*. More than two-thirds of deep neck infections contain β-lactamase-producing bacteria.

COMPLICATIONS

The rate of complications is associated with the presence of diabetes mellitus, age older than 65 years, secondary submandibular infection, bilateral submandibular infection, multiple space involvement and visceral space involvement. It is important to maintain a safe and secure airway in submandibular space infections.

In patients with bilateral submandibular swelling, an airway obstruction can be the result of the tongue pushing against the roof of the mouth and the posterior pharyngeal wall, or a consequence of anterior visceral space involvement with laryngeal oedema.

Both the submandibular and lateral pharyngeal space communicate with the anterior visceral space, which in turn extends from the hyoid bone down to the superior mediastinum, posing a potential route for descending mediastinitis. The anterior visceral space contains the larynx, thyroid gland, trachea and cervical oesophagus, and this space may play a key role in determining airway obstruction as well as the spread of infection to the anterior mediastinum. Other complications could be pleural empyema, pericarditis, jugular vein thrombosis and septic shock.

CLINICAL PEARL

Ludwig's angina is a potentially life-threatening bilateral diffuse gangrenous cellulitis of the submandibular and sublingual spaces.

CLINICAL APPROACH

DIAGNOSIS

An initial CT with contrast can show which structures are involved, presence of abscesses and the extent of infection, e.g. mediastinal involvement. An area of low attenuation with a complete circumferential rim of enhancement is considered the hallmark of abscess. Early CT findings may not differentiate between cellulitis and abscess formation.

TREATMENT

The mainstay of treatment of DNSIs consists of airway control, antibiotic treatment and, if necessary, surgical drainage. Airway control can be achieved with (fibreoptic-guided) endotracheal intubation.

Indications for immediate drainage: descending infection, anterior visceral space involvement with the abscess involving more than two deep neck spaces and patients with abscesses larger than 3.0 cm. In other cases, a decision on drainage can wait 48 hours for the effect of antibiotics. A repeat CT can be done to evaluate response to therapy.

Empiric antibiotic therapy should be targeted at aerobic and anaerobic pathogens.

Initial antibiotic therapy can consist of amoxicillin/clavulanic acid 1.2 g 8-hourly or 6-hourly or ceftriaxone 2 g IV once daily plus metronidazole 500 mg 8-hourly IV. Alternative options are intravenous vancomycin or teicoplanin plus metronidazole or clindamycin IV. Oral stepdown can consist of co-amoxiclav 625 mg 8-hourly PO, clindamycin 600 mg 8-hourly PO or doxycycline 100 mg 12-hourly plus metronidazole 500 mg 8-hourly PO. Duration of antibiotic treatment should be at least 5 days after source control has been achieved and, if necessary, extended. This should be decided on a case-by-case basis.

Other interventions that may be necessary are tracheostomy or thoracotomy.

BIBLIOGRAPHY

Bakir S, Tanriverdi MH, Gün R, Yorgancilar AE, Yildirim M, Tekbaş G, Palanci Y, Meriç K, Topçu I. Deep neck space infections: A retrospective review of 173 cases. *Am J Otolaryngol*. 2012 January–February;33(1):56–63.

Boscolo-Rizzo P, Da Mosto MC. Submandibular space infection: A potentially lethal infection. *Int J Infect Dis*. 2009 May;13(3):327–333.

Boscolo-Rizzo P, Marchiori C, Montolli F, Vaglia A, Da Mosto MC. Deep neck infections: A constant challenge. *ORL J Otorhinolaryngol Relat Spec*. 2006;68(5):259–265. Epub 2006 May 4.

Huang TT, Liu TC, Chen PR, Tseng FY, Yeh TH, Chen YS. Deep neck infection: Analysis of 185 cases. *Head Neck*. 2004 October;26(10):854–860.

4.17 Empyema

Patrick Lillie

CLINICAL CONSIDERATIONS

Pleural infection is a serious and not uncommon complication of pneumonia and can also occur after thoracotomy and trauma. Infection of the pleural space leads to an exudative effusion with a low pH and can be frankly purulent. Fibrin deposition and loculation of the effusion can impair drainage and may require formal surgical intervention. Light's criteria for differentiating between a transudate and an exudate are of use and Table 4.17.1 shows some of the fluid differences between complicated and uncomplicated empyema.

Microbiological studies on the pleural fluid should include standard bacterial culture (including fluid that has been directly inoculated into blood culture bottles), mycobacterial cultures, Gram staining and molecular testing for 16S rRNA, as molecular testing identifies pathogens in a greater number of cases than standard culture-based techniques alone. Streptococci and *S. aureus* are the commonest organisms isolated, with Gram-negative bacteria being more common in post-operative empyema and hospital-acquired cases. Anaerobes may be involved as well.

CLINICAL APPROACH

IMAGING STUDIES

Standard chest radiographs will show the presence of reasonably large volumes of pleural fluid and while it is the first-line imaging modality, both CT scanning and pleural ultrasound have the advantage of showing the presence or absence of loculation and may be of use in guiding drainage of the effusion.

DRAINAGE/SURGICAL INTERVENTION

All patients with empyema will require pleural drainage with a chest drain. Parapneumonic effusions that have a pH of >7.2, are not cloudy/purulent and have no positive cultures can be managed with antibiotics alone initially, with a low threshold for chest drain placement if not improving. Debate about the size of the chest drain has been long ongoing, with little evidence that size is important in free-flowing effusions. Fibrinolytic treatments are of little use on their own and need to be combined with DNase to improve outcomes. In those patients who do not respond to standard pleural drainage, early referral for surgical drainage is warranted.

ANTIBIOTIC THERAPY

Antibiotic therapy should include coverage against streptococci, *S. aureus* and anaerobes and should penetrate the pleural space well. For hospital-acquired cases, post-traumatic cases, and those who have had multiple courses of antibiotics, then coverage should also include Gram-negative *Enterobacterales*. In most cases, a broad spectrum β-lactam would be a reasonable initial treatment, possibly with metronidazole or clindamycin as extra cover against anaerobes. Intrapleural administration is not recommended. In areas of high MRSA prevalence, including vancomycin

TABLE 4.17.1
Biochemical Analysis of Pleural Fluid in Patients with Suspected Empyema

Feature	Transudate	Simple Parapneumonic Effusion	Empyema
Volume of fluid/viscosity	Minimal	Moderate, free flowing	Moderate to large, viscous
Appearance	Straw coloured	Cloudy	Purulent
LDH	<200 U/L	>200 U/L	>>200 U/L
Protein	<3 g/dL	>3 g/dL	>>3 g/dL
pH	>7.2	<7.2	N/A

or linezolid in the initial regime is prudent. Antibiotics should be modified in the light of culture results and can be switched from IV to oral when the patient is improving. Oral antibiotics with good bioavailability and penetration in the pleural space should be used, with clindamycin, fluroquinolones and linezolid all being useful in this situation. Duration of therapy is dependent on clinical response and, for standard organisms, is generally at least 3 weeks from source control.

CLINICAL VIGNETTES

A 44-year-old woman presents with a 1-day history of severe left-sided chest pain after a bout of vomiting. A CXR shows a left-sided pleural effusion, which on aspiration is cloudy, and Gram stain shows Gram-positive cocci and yeasts. A CT scan shows a rupture of the lower oesophagus.

Polymicrobial, and especially fungal, empyema should prompt consideration of oesophageal rupture or contamination from a sub-diaphragmatic source. Drainage and broad-spectrum antibiotic and antifungal cover are required.

A 38-year-old Somalian woman presents with a 4-week history of fever, weight loss and chest pain. A CXR shows a large left-sided pleural effusion which, on aspiration, is serous in nature but has a raised LDH and protein. Gram and AFB staining are negative, but on thoracoscopy, the pleura is covered in nodules which, on biopsy, show acid-fast bacilli.

Worldwide, tuberculosis remains a common cause of pleural infection and should be considered in the differential diagnosis of pleural effusion. Pleural fluid is rarely smear positive and biopsy of the pleura allows for both microbiological and histological confirmation of the diagnosis. Treatment is with the same regimen as for pulmonary disease. Other causes of chronic pleural infection include *Nocardia* and *Actinomyces* infections, both of which would require prolonged antibiotic treatment.

BIBLIOGRAPHY

Birkenkamp K, O'Horo JC, Kashyap R et al. Empyema management: A cohort study evaluating antimicrobial therapy. *J Infect.* 2016;72(5):537–543.
Davies HE, Davies RJ, Davies CW; BTS Pleural Disease Guideline Group. Management of pleural infection in adults: British Thoracic Society Pleural Disease Guideline 2010. *Thorax.* 2010;65(Suppl 2):ii41–ii53.
Light RW. Pleural effusion. *N Engl J Med.* 2002;346:1971–1977.
Maskell NA, Batt S, Hedley EL, Davies CW, Gillespie SH, Davies RJ. The bacteriology of pleural infection by genetic and standard methods and its mortality significance. *Am J Respir Crit Care Med.* 2006;174(7):817–823.
Rahman NM, Maskell NA, West A et al. Intrapleural use of tissue plasminogen activator and DNase in pleural infection. *N Engl J Med.* 2011;365(6):518–526.

4.18 Encephalitis

Firza Alexander Gronthoud

CLINICAL CONSIDERATIONS

Encephalitis is an inflammation of the brain parenchyma which can result from a direct infection of the central nervous system (CNS) or as a post-infectious, immune-mediated complication. Non-infectious causes are outside the scope of this book. Although encephalitis can be caused by many pathogens, clinical presentation may be similar and specific tests need to be requested in order to find the cause. It is therefore worthwhile to consider the following.

CLINICAL PRESENTATION

The main presenting symptom of encephalitis is altered mental status and it can be accompanied by current or recent fever, seizures and focal neurological signs such as ataxia. Altered mental status can include lethargy, drowsiness, confusion, disorientation and coma. Other features of encephalitis can include severe headache, nausea and vomiting, disorientation, speech disturbances and behavioural changes. These symptoms can also be seen in individuals with systemic sepsis without encephalitis. Encephalitis can have an acute onset or run an indolent course.

PATHOGENESIS

In contrast to herpes simplex virus (HSV), varicella zoster virus (VZV) infects vascular endothelial cells of large and small cerebral vessels, at times followed by spread of the infection into brain parenchyma. In this process, VZV may involve large or small vessels to produce focal or multifocal ischemic injury or may cause vessel wall necrosis with arterial dissection, aneurysm formation, or haemorrhage within the subarachnoid space or brain parenchyma. Human herpes virus (HHV)-6 DNA has also been found in normal brain tissue and CSF, raising questions about the specificity of this finding. HHV-6 reactivation frequently occurs during acute infections with other viruses and also in the setting of other neurologic conditions, including multiple sclerosis.

ENCEPHALITIS IN IMMUNOCOMPETENT INDIVIDUALS

Viral: Herpes simplex virus (HSV) encephalitis is the most commonly diagnosed viral encephalitis. Most HSV encephalitis is due to HSV-1, but about 10% is caused by HSV-2.

The latter typically occurs in immunocompromised individuals and neonates, in whom it can cause a disseminated infection. Varicella zoster virus (VZV) is also a relatively common cause of viral encephalitis, especially in the immunocompromised. Encephalitis caused by VZV at the time of primary infection (chickenpox) may follow the rash at an interval of days or weeks, though it occasionally occurs before the rash, or even in patients with no rash. Enteroviruses most often cause aseptic meningitis but can also be an important cause of encephalitis. Measles can cause encephalitis (see Chapter 4.37).

Other less common infectious causes of encephalitis are:

Bacterial: *Listeria monocytogenes*, syphilis, *Mycoplasma pneumoniae*, *Borrelia burgdorferi*, leptospirosis.

Parasites: *Naegleria fowleri*, *Balamuthia mandrillaris* (amoebic encephalitis), cysticercosis, trichinosis.

CLINICAL PEARL

Adults over 20 years old, the immunocompromised, or those with cranial dermatome involvement, disseminated skin disease or immune compromise are at increased risk of encephalitis following chickenpox. The presentation may be acute or subacute with fever, headache, altered consciousness, ataxia and seizures. An acute cerebellar ataxia is also seen in association with chickenpox; typically this is seen in children, but adults are occasionally affected. Reactivation of VZV may also lead to encephalitis, especially in the elderly or the immunocompromised. The onset is typically insidious, and there may be no zoster rash, fever or CSF pleocytosis; sometimes there is a brainstem encephalitis associated with Ramsay Hunt syndrome. The primary cause is thought to be immune-mediated reaction to the virus replicating at low levels, rather than viral cytopathology itself. A small-vessel vasculitic or large-vessel stroke syndrome may also be seen.

ENCEPHALITIS IN RETURNING TRAVELLERS

Trypanosoma brucei gambiense and *Trypanosoma brucei rhodesiense* (African sleeping sickness), *Angiostrongylus cantonensis* (rat lungworm), malaria, encephalitis due to flaviviruses: West Nile, dengue, Japanese encephalitis, Zika virus and tick-borne encephalitis should be considered in a traveller presenting with encephalitis. Less common is rabies encephalitis and *Rickettsia*. It is important to consider geographical differences, as West Nile virus may be the most common cause of encephalitis in the United States whilst Japanese encephalitis may be the most common cause of encephalitis worldwide. Tick-borne encephalitis virus (TBE) is a quite prevalent cause of encephalomyelitis in Europe and Russia.

ENCEPHALITIS IN IMMUNOCOMPROMISED PATIENTS

Viral: Cytomegalovirus (CMV) is seen almost exclusively in the immunocompromised. Varicella zoster and herpes simplex type 2 are other frequent causes of viral encephalitis in immunocompromised individuals. Reactivation of JC virus can cause progressive multifocal leukoencephalopathy (PML). Other herpes viruses reported to cause encephalitis are HHV-6 and -7.

Parasites: Reactivation of *Toxoplasma gondii* in individuals with HIV with a CD4 count of ≤100 can lead to toxoplasmosis, characterized by fever, headaches and seizures. In contrast to toxoplasmosis, headache and seizures are unusual with PML.

Fungi: *Cryptococcus* in HIV with CD4 <100 is an important cause of meningoencephalitis.

POST-INFECTIOUS

Acute disseminated encephalomyelitis is an immune-mediated inflammatory demyelinating condition that can be triggered by an infection. It has an acute onset and is associated with polyfocal neurologic deficits and typically is self-limiting. Corticosteroids are often given.

NON-INFECTIOUS

Antibody-associated encephalitis, which may or may not be paraneoplastic: encephalitis associated with antibodies to the voltage-gated potassium channel complex, or N-methyl-D-aspartate antibody (NMDA) receptors are increasingly recognized.

IMAGING FINDINGS

Early CT scan has two clear roles: suggesting the diagnosis of viral encephalitis and indicating an alternative diagnosis. An initial CT scan soon after admission will show a suggestive abnormality in about ≥25% of patients with herpes simplex virus (HSV) encephalitis, though it is not, on its own, diagnostic. Almost all those with proven HSV encephalitis and a negative initial scan will have abnormalities on a second scan.

A CT can rule out shift of brain compartments, due to mass lesions and/or oedema, which might make a subsequent lumbar puncture (LP) dangerous. Reduction of the CSF pressure below the lesion following an LP could precipitate herniation of the brainstem or cerebellar tonsils. This may occur in patients with brain abscess, subdural empyema, tumour or a necrotic swollen lobe in encephalitis. Thus, in selected patients, with appropriate clinical features, a scan is performed to see if there is significant brain swelling and shift, or whether there is space around the basal cisterns.

Ring-enhanced lesions: Neurotoxoplasmosis is characterized by single or multiple hypodense or hypointense lesions in white matter and basal ganglia with mass effects. Lesions may enhance in a homogeneous or ring pattern with contrast.

Demyelinization: JC virus causing progressive multifocal leukoencephalopathy (PML), measles, multiple sclerosis, African trypanosomiasis (slow onset: West African or *Trypanosoma brucei gambiense*, rapid onset is East African trypanosomiasis caused by *Trypanosoma brucei rhodesiense*).

DIAGNOSTIC TESTS

Diagnosis is confirmed with a positive CSF or blood sample. If there is a possibility of raised intracranial pressure, it is recommended to perform an urgent CT or MRI first. In anticoagulated patients, adequate reversal (with protamine for those on heparin and vitamin K, prothrombin complex concentrate or fresh frozen plasma for those on warfarin) is mandatory before LP. Patients on warfarin should be treated with heparin instead, and this should be stopped before lumbar puncture. Consider imaging before lumbar puncture in patients with known severe immunocompromise (e.g. advanced HIV). A lumbar puncture may still be possible if the platelet count is 50×10^9/L; seek haematological advice. LP may also be harmful in patients with coagulopathy because of the chance that the needle may induce a subarachnoid haemorrhage or the development of spinal subdural and epidural haematomas. A rapidly falling platelet count is also a contraindication.

An acellular CSF is also described in encephalitis caused by other viruses, including VZV, EBV and CMV; it occurs more frequently in the immunocompromised. Although a lymphocytic CSF pleocytosis is typical of viral CNS infections, bacterial infection can give a similar picture, particularly in tuberculosis, listeriosis, brucellosis and partially treated acute bacterial meningitis. CSF lactate may be helpful in distinguishing bacterial meningitis from viral CNS infections; in particular, a CSF lactate of <2 mmol/L is said to rule out bacterial disease.

CLINICAL PEARL

Most viral encephalitis is acute, but subacute and chronic presentations are characteristic of particular pathogens, especially in the immunocompromised.

CLINICAL APPROACH

- Assess ABCD and glucose
- Take two sets of blood cultures
- Send EDTA blood and clotted blood for storage

- Is there a contraindication to LP without neuroimaging?
  - Glasgow Coma Scale <13, focal neurological signs (excluding cranial neuropathies), papilloedema, seizures, immunocompromised, systemic shock, respiratory insufficiency, platelets < 100×10^9/L, relative bradycardia with hypertension
- Perform lumbar puncture and assess (see Chapter 2.8 for interpretation of CSF)
  - Opening pressure
  - White cell count and differentiation
  - Red blood cell count
  - Protein
  - Glucose CSF:blood ratio
  - Lactate
- Is the patient immunocompetent: Request PCR for HSV (1 and 2), *Enterovirus*, VZV, *Cryptococcus* if CD4 <100
- CSF antibody testing for VZV has a higher sensitivity than PCR
- Is the patient immunocompromised: Add PCR for toxoplasma, CMV, EBV, VZV, JC virus, consider HHV-6/-7
- Consider meningococcus if a purpuric rash is present: If a vesicular rash is present, consider hand foot and mouth disease, varicella zoster and rickettsial disease.
- Water contact: naegleria fowleri, Balamuthia mandrillaris
- Exposure to mice or hamster: request PCR for lymphocytic choriomeningitis virus (LCMV)
- Recent travel to an area where these pathogens are endemic: Zikavirus, dengue, west-nile, St. Louis encephalitis, Japanese encephalitis
- Animal contact: Rabies encephalitis
- Recent vaccination: consider ADEM
- A sub-acute presentation, orofacial dyskinesia, choreoathetosis, faciobrachial dystonia, intractable seizures or hyponatraemia, may suggest an antibody-mediated encephalitis

TREATMENT

The most common cause of viral encephalitis is HSV. If there is a delay of >6 hours for performing the LP, start acyclovir 10 mg/kg 8-hourly IV immediately.

BIBLIOGRAPHY

Bookstaver PB, Mohorn PL, Shah A, Tesh LD, Quidley AM, Kothari R, Bland CM, Weissman S. Management of viral central nervous system infections: A primer for clinicians. *J Cent Nerv Syst Dis.* 2017 May 1;9:1179573517703342.
Cunha BA. The clinical and laboratory diagnosis of acute meningitis and acute encephalitis. *Expert Opin Med Diagn.* 2013 July;7(4):343–364.
Levin SN, Lyons JL. Infections of the nervous system. *Am J Med.* 2018 January;131(1):25–32.
Studahl M, Lindquist L, Eriksson BM, Günther G, Bengner M, Franzen-Röhl E, Fohlman J, Bergström T, Aurelius E. Acute viral infections of the central nervous system in immunocompetent adults: Diagnosis and management. *Drugs.* 2013 February;73(2):131–158.
Venkatesan A, Michael BD, Probasco JC, Geocadin RG, Solomon T. Acute encephalitis in immunocompetent adults. *Lancet.* 2019 February 16;393(10172):702–716.

4.19 Endocarditis

Anda Samson

CLINICAL CONSIDERATIONS

Patients with infective endocarditis may not improve or may even deteriorate despite appropriate antimicrobial therapy. It is then worthwhile to revisit the source of infection and consider the following.

PERSISTENT FOCUS OF INFECTION

Infective endocarditis is a deep-seated infection which is prone to metastasize to other places in the body. In left-sided endocarditis, aortic root abscess, stroke, splenic abscesses and splinter haemorrhages are a few frequently occurring complications. The emboli from right-sided endocarditis are usually filtered by the lungs, leading to septic pulmonary emboli or lung abscesses. Any of these complications may cause a less-than-ideal response to therapy. If there are any abscesses, these are preferably drained as soon as possible.

INSUFFICIENT ANTIMICROBIAL DRUG ACTIVITY

Patients with septic cerebral emboli may develop cerebral abscesses. When choosing your antibiotic, it is necessary to consider whether or not the antibiotic will cross the blood–brain barrier for it to work. Similarly, some antibiotics may work less in abscesses or may not penetrate in certain tissues.

> **CLINICAL PEARL**
>
> If a patient is clinically not improving or even deteriorating despite targeted antimicrobial therapy, assess whether there are metastatic foci of infection that need draining, or whether the infected valve needs operating on sooner.

CLINICAL APPROACH

THE ROAD TO VALVE SURGERY

- *Who*: Patients with ongoing infection despite adequate antibiotic therapy and patients with substantive destruction of cardiac valves leading to haemodynamic compromise. Patients with a vegetation >10–15 mm have a relative indication for surgery.
- *When*: Early operation within the first 3 weeks of hospitalization in patients with native valve endocarditis (NVE) reduces long-term mortality by 40%–50%. In patients with prosthetic valve endocarditis, this difference is not as pronounced.
- *What to resect*: All infected material.
- *Rationale*: Complete removal of the source of infection.

> **CLINICAL PEARL**
>
> Early surgery in native valve endocarditis reduces mortality significantly.

DURATION OF ANTIMICROBIAL THERAPY

- The duration of antimicrobial therapy in infective endocarditis varies per organism, as shown in the ESC and IDSA guidelines on infective endocarditis, but is generally 4–6 weeks.
- For selected patients with right-sided endocarditis, oral antibiotics may be a feasible option; all others would need to be treated with IV antibiotics.
- Antibiotics can generally be stopped 2 weeks after removal of the infected valve assuming pre-operative cultures are negative AND there are no further sources of infection/abscesses.
- If the pre-operative cultures are positive, the duration of therapy starts the day of surgery.

CLINICAL PEARL

Consider whether any seeding infection needs longer treatment than the infective endocarditis itself (e.g. multi-level discitis, abscesses).

CLINICAL PEARL

Suppressive oral therapy should be considered in patients with prosthetic valve endocarditis (PVE) who do not undergo surgery since prosthetic devices can maintain an infection or significantly increase the risk of recurrence.

The following clinical vignettes illustrate how differently patients with infective endocarditis can present.

CLINICAL VIGNETTES

The medical team is treating a 54-year-old woman for a Streptococcus gallolyticus *bacteraemia. She remains febrile and unstable despite treatment with benzylpenicillin according to the hospital guidelines. They phone you to ask whether or not they should broaden the antibiotic therapy. You notice that she had three blood cultures with the same microorganism. The MIC for penicillin is 0.25, which makes the* Streptococcus *intermediate sensitive to penicillin. You change the antibiotic to ceftriaxone because you suspect infective endocarditis. Additionally, you advise an urgent echocardiogram.*

The penicillin MIC dictates the duration and the dose of benzylpenicillin or switch to alternative agent in endocarditis caused by streptococci.

The transthoracic echocardiogram does not show any vegetation. The cardiology team does not believe that there is endocarditis and refers back to the medical team. Because of ongoing fevers, you persist in your diagnosis. You also note several splinter haemorrhages and haematuria without clear signs of a urinary tract infection, as well as a splenic abscess on ultrasound, making the patient a case of definite endocarditis according to the Modified DUKE criteria (See Table 4.19.1). A transoesophageal echocardiogram is then made, which shows a vegetation on the aortic valve. The splenic abscess is drained. Because there is no haemodynamic complication or valve destruction, the patient is treated with 4 weeks of ceftriaxone.

TABLE 4.19.1
Modified Duke Criteria for Infective Endocarditis

Major Criteria	Minor Criteria

• Microorganisms demonstrated by culture or histologic examination of a vegetation, a vegetation that has embolized or an intracardiac abscess specimen; or
• Pathologic lesions; vegetation or intracardiac abscess confirmed by histologic examination showing active endocarditis
• Typical microorganisms consistent with infective endocarditis (IE) from 2 separate blood cultures: viridans streptococci, *Streptococcus bovis,* HACEK group, *Staphylococcus aureus*; community-acquired enterococci, in the absence of a primary focus; or
• Microorganisms consistent with IE from persistently positive blood cultures, defined as follows:
  • At least 2 positive cultures of blood samples drawn 12 h apart; or
  • All of 3 or a majority of >4 separate cultures of blood (with first and last sample drawn at least 1 h apart)
  • Single positive blood culture for *Coxiella burnetii* or antiphase I IgG antibody titre 1:800
• Echocardiogram positive for IE, defined as oscillating intracardiac mass on valve or supporting structures, in the path of regurgitant jets or on implanted material in the absence of an alternative anatomic explanation; or abscess; or new partial dehiscence of prosthetic valve
• New valvular regurgitation (worsening or changing of pre-existing murmur not sufficient)
	• Predisposing heart condition or injection drug use
	• Temperature >38.5°C
	• Vascular phenomena, major arterial emboli, septic pulmonary infarcts, mycotic aneurysm, intracranial haemorrhage, conjunctival haemorrhages and Janeway's lesions
	• Immunologic phenomena: Glomerulonephritis, Osler's nodes, Roth's spots and rheumatoid factor
	• Positive blood culture but does not meet a major criterion as noted or serological evidence of active infection with organism consistent with IE

Source: Baddour LM et al. *Circulation.* 2015;132:1435–1486.

A vegetation seen on echocardiogram is a *possible* but **not** a *necessary* part of the diagnosis of infective endocarditis. Endocarditis is clinically diagnosed if either 2 Major criteria OR 1 Major criteria and 3 Minor criteria OR 5 Minor criteria are met. The sensitivity of the modified Duke Criteria can be further increased with additional imaging studies including MRI, CT and PET/CT. Although a negative Duke core reduces the likelihood of endocarditis, it does not completely rule out endocarditis.

A 64-year-old male is transferred from a neighbouring hospital with aortic regurgitation but no vegetation on his prosthetic aortic valve. He has a history of a stroke 4 months ago. His blood results show a CRP of 40 and a normal white cell count. He says he feels quite ok except for the breathing problems. When prompted, he does remember drenching night sweats since the time of the stroke. Given the clinical picture, infective endocarditis is suspected and you advise to take 3 blood cultures at least 2 hours apart and to await the outcome. You advise not to start antibiotics yet.

Patients with a prosthetic valve, in particular bioprosthetic valves, have a vastly increased risk of infective endocarditis.

All three blood cultures flag up with a coagulase-negative Staphylococcus. *You start your patient on vancomycin, rifampicin and gentamicin. Because of interactions, you change his warfarin to heparin. Transoesophageal echocardiogram again does not show a vegetation, only the already recognized aortic regurgitation. Subsequently, a cardiac CT is made, which shows a beginning aortic root abscess. The patient undergoes aortic valve replacement and recovers well.*

BIBLIOGRAPHY

Baddour LM, Wilson WR, Bayer AS et al. Infective endocarditis in adults: Diagnosis, antimicrobial therapy, and management of complications: A scientific statement for healthcare professionals from the American Heart Association. *Circulation*. 2015;132:1435–1486.

Habib G, Lancellotti P. 2015 ESC Guidelines for the management of infective endocarditis: The Task Force for the Management of Infective Endocarditis of the European Society of Cardiology (ESC) Endorsed by: European Association for Cardio-Thoracic Surgery (EACTS), the European Association of Nuclear Medicine (EANM). *Eur Heart J*. 2015;36(44):3075–3128.

Li JS, Sexton DJ, Mick N et al. Proposed modifications to the Duke criteria for the diagnosis of infective endocarditis. *Clin Infect Dis*. 2000;30(4):633–638.

Liang F, Song B, Liu R, Yang L, Tang H, Li Y. Optimal timing for early surgery in infective endocarditis: A meta-analysis. *Interact Cardiovasc Thorac Surg*. 2016;22:336–345.

4.20 *Neisseria gonorrhoeae*

Anda Samson

CLINICAL CONSIDERATIONS

Gonorrhoea has been around for a long time. In many countries, the incidence is unknown; in the Western world, infections soared up to as many as 468/100,000 people in the early 1970s in the United States, which has come down to around 120–130/100,000 since then. In the UK, the incidence is around 75/100,000 but this number is increasing. Transmission can occur via oral, vaginal or anal sex, with the risks greatest for receptive vaginal or anal sex partners. Because the infection can be symptomless and drug resistance is an emerging concern, it is therefore worthwhile to consider the following.

CLINICAL DIAGNOSIS

There is an incubation period of about 40 hours after infection in men; in men, infection usually causes an acute inflammatory reaction which expresses as acute urethritis. Untreated gonorrhoea usually resolves spontaneously within a few weeks. However, in one-half to three-quarters of women, the infection is symptomless. Those who do develop symptoms usually do so within 1–2 weeks.

CLINICAL PEARL

Infection in women is often asymptomatic but can nevertheless lead to severe complications.

DISSEMINATED INFECTION

Infection can disseminate locally. In men, this can lead to epididymo-orchitis or, less frequently, lymphangitis or prostatitis. In about half of infected women, the infection ascends into the female genital tract, and 10%–20% can contract pelvic inflammatory disease (PID) or perihepatitis (Fitz-Hugh–Curtis syndrome).

Systemic dissemination can also occur and can lead to arthritis-dermatitis syndrome. Patients are often bacteraemic during this phase and have asymptomatic arthralgia in mostly the knees, elbows and ankles. The skin may show various bullae, pustules and papules. After a few days, the skin lesions may disappear and an overt arthritis may appear in one or two joints. Other manifestations of disseminated gonococcal infection, such as endocarditis, pericarditis and conjunctivitis, are increasingly rare. Although gonococcal arthritis is rare in the UK, with a rate of 1:1,000,000, in patients without a clear cause or a response to treatment, it should be considered (see Chapter 4.57).

LABORATORY DIAGNOSIS

Neisseria gonorrhoeae (gonococci) are intracellular Gram-negative diplococci. Although they grow well when the right cultures are set up with 95% sensitivity, they only grow under specific circumstances and need to be transported in a transport media to prevent drying out as they rapidly perish outside the mucosal environment; therefore, if the diagnosis is not considered, it can be easily missed. The genital and oropharyngeal tract can be colonized with *Neisseria meningitidis*,

TABLE 4.20.1
Summary of BASHH Treatment Guidelines 2019

	Men	2nd Line
Uncomplicated urethritis/pharyngitis/ cervicitis/rectal infections	Ceftriaxone 1 gram IM one-off dose	Ciprofloxacin 500 mg PO once-off dose if sensitivity known Gentamicin 240 mg IM PLUS azithromycin 2 g orally Cefixime 400 mg orally AND azithromycin 2 g orally
Meningitis	Ceftriaxone 2 g IV OD 14 days PLUS azithromycin 2 g PO one-off	Depending on culture results
Endocarditis	Ceftriaxone 2 g IV OD for 4 weeks PLUS azithromycin 2 g PO one-off	Depending on culture results
Ophthalmia neonatorum	Ceftriaxone 25–50 mg/kg IV or IM, not exceeding 125 mg	
Arthritis	Ceftriaxone 2 g IV OD 14 days PLUS azithromycin 2 g PO one-off	Depending on culture results

which is easier to grow and can be mistaken for gonococci. Identifying the exact species is therefore recommended.

Many genitourinary physicians reply on direct Gram stains as a diagnostic aid when assessing urethritis in men; diplococci in association with neutrophils are pathognomonic. Microscopy is about 95% sensitive for diagnosing gonococcal urethritis; for other sites, the technique is very unreliable and much more dependent on experience. More recently, various nucleic acid amplification tests (NAAT or PCR) have become available. They are all about as sensitive as appropriately set up cultures, but are very specific and retain specificity even in samples that would in normal culture settings be vulnerable to contamination, such as self-obtained vaginal swabs and urine samples. PCR becomes negative 1–2 weeks after treatment. The caveat is that some commercially available PCR platforms cross-react with other *Neisseria* species.

CLINICAL PEARL

PCR is very sensitive and specific in making a diagnosis of gonorrhoea.

CLINICAL PEARL

Neisseria meningitidis is a common colonizer of the oropharyngeal and genital tract; specific identification of species is therefore important.

CLINICAL APPROACH

LOCAL TREATMENT GUIDELINES

Treatment guidelines may differ per country depending on local susceptibility patterns; it is recommended to review national guidelines when treating patients because of changes in susceptibility that may occur rapidly (see Table 4.20.1, for the 2019 UK guideline).

In most countries these days, *Gonorrhoeae* infections are usually treated with ceftriaxone intramuscularly. Azithromycin is often the go-to second-line drug with 2 g as an oral (single) dose, and in some countries, dual therapy is recommended. Other drugs such as ciprofloxacin and tetracycline have been used in the past, but their use is currently contraindicated without culture confirmation of a sensitive organism because of a high risk of resistance and thus treatment failure.

Worryingly, there is also an increase even in the number of isolates that are relatively or completely resistant to ceftriaxone and azithromycin. A patient with multidrug-resistant *Gonorrhoeae* was treated successfully in the UK in 2018 with ertapenem.

SPECIAL GROUPS

HIV-positive individuals can be treated with the same regime as non-HIV-positive individuals. For pregnant women, treatment regimens containing ceftriaxone and azithromycin are generally safe. Tetracyclines and quinolones are not recommended because of risk of foetal complications.

CLINICAL PEARL

Antimicrobial resistance in *N. gonorrhoeae* is rapidly emerging. Erring on side of caution with a higher drug dose and/or dual therapy is advisable.

CLINICAL PEARL

HIV-positive individuals can be treated the same way as HIV-negative individuals.

BIBLIOGRAPHY

Bennett JE, Dolin R, Blaser MJ. *Mandell, Douglas, and Bennett's Principles and Practice of Infectious Diseases*. Philadelphia, PA: Elsevier/Saunders, 2015.

Curry A, Williams T, Penny ML. Pelvic inflammatory disease: Diagnosis, management, and prevention. *Am Fam Physician*. 2019 September 15;100(6):357–364.

Fifer H, Saunders J, Soni S, Sadiq ST, FitzGerald M. *British Association for Sexual Health and HIV national guideline for the management of infection with* Neisseria gonorrhoeae *(2019)*. London: British Association for Sexual Health and HIV, 2019.

Rutherford AI, Subesinghe S, Bharucha T, Ibrahim F, Kleymann A, Galloway JBA. Population study of the reported incidence of native joint septic arthritis in the United Kingdom between 1998 and 2013. *Rheumatology (Oxf)*. 2016 December;55(12):2176–2180.

4.21 Hepatitis A

Anda Samson

CLINICAL APPROACH

Hepatitis A is transmitted via the fecal-oral route. Consequently, it is endemic in places where access to hygienic cooking facilities, clean drinking water and sewage systems are poor. It is therefore worthwhile to consider the following.

INFECTION IN ADULTHOOD AND CHILDHOOD

Children are often asymptomatic or become mildly jaundiced. Adults are more likely to develop symptomatic hepatitis, and those over 40 are at most risk of serious complications, rarely even leading to liver transplants. Symptoms of hepatitis include fatigue, flu-like symptoms, dark urine, pale stool, abdominal pain, loss of appetite and signs of jaundice, including yellow skin and eyes.

OUTBREAKS

Although most outbreaks take place in developing countries, occasionally in developed countries, outbreaks occur, usually in nurseries, care homes or other places where many people live tightly together.

RELAPSE

One in 5–10 patients develops a relapse within 6 months, during which they are infectious. This relapse is also self-limiting. Other causes should be ruled out, including drug toxicity and other infectious including hepatitis E, B and C, and an ultrasound of the liver to exclude a problem in the biliary tree would be appropriate.

CLINICAL APPROACH

TREATMENT

The vast majority of patients improve without medical contact. There is no specific treatment available for hepatitis A. A small number of patients will develop severe hepatitis for which supportive treatment or, ultimately, liver transplant is the only option.

PREVENTION

There are several effective vaccines on the market. In some countries like the United States that have adopted childhood vaccination, outbreaks of hepatitis A have plummeted.

Despite a low case fatality rate, hepatitis A remains one of the leading causes of vaccine-preventable illnesses worldwide.

CLINICAL PEARL

The vast majority of patients get better without any medical contact. Supportive treatment is the only treatment available for hepatitis A.

CLINICAL VIGNETTE

You are phoned by the director of a nursery. One of the children attending had diarrhoea and was diagnosed with hepatitis A yesterday, and he phones you in your public health role. Two other children have diarrhoea, but no other people have been affected. You advise to vaccinate all employees who have worked with the child in the last 14 days as well as the children attending the nursery and the household contacts of the affected child.

- Aggressive vaccination is sometimes required to stop an emerging epidemic.
- Close contacts (household contacts, sexual partners) are usually the only ones vaccinated.
- Children under 12 months, immunocompromised patients and patients with severe liver disease are eligible for immunoglobulins.

BIBLIOGRAPHY

Bennett JE, Dolin R, Blaser MJ, Mandell GL, Douglas RG. *Mandell, Douglas, and Bennett's Principles and Practice of Infectious Diseases.* 2015.
Matheny SC, Kingery JE. Hepatitis A. *Am Fam Physician.* 2012 December 1;86(11):1027–1034; quiz 1010-2.
Willner IR, Uhl MD, Howard SC et al. Serious hepatitis A: An analysis of patients hospitalized during an urban epidemic in the United States. *Ann Intern Med.* 1998 January 15;128(2):111–114.

4.22 Hepatitis B

Anda Samson

CLINICAL CONSIDERATIONS

There are around 250 million people worldwide that are hepatitis B surface-antigen positive. Around 600,000 people die each year; a large proportion may potentially be prevented by early diagnosis and treatment where needed. Hepatitis B is a DNA virus that infects only hepatocytes and can be incorporated into human DNA, which makes complete eradication impossible at the moment. Some people are able to generate an accurate immune response that will stop the virus from replicating and become 'naturally immune' to hepatitis B.

CLINICAL PEARL

Patients infected with hepatitis B virus need to be tested for all other blood-borne viruses including hepatitis A, C, D, as well as Human Immunodeficiency Virus (HIV).

CHRONIC INFECTION VERSUS ACUTE INFECTION VERSUS IMMUNIZED PATIENT

Serology combined with hepatitis B DNA levels can easily distinguish between acute infection, chronic infection (that may or may not need treatment) and vaccinated persons.

- *Vaccinated*: HBsAg negative, HBsAb positive, Anti-HBc negative (IgM and IgG), HBeAg/Ab negative
- *Acute infection*: HBsAg positive, HBsAb negative, Anti-HBc IgM positive, IgG negative, HBeAg positive or negative, HBeAb negative
- *Chronic infection*: HBsAg positive, HBsAb negative, Anti-HBc IgM negative, IgG positive, HBeAg positive or negative, HBeAb positive or negative

DECIDING WHO NEEDS TREATMENT

The goal of therapy is to prevent cirrhosis and hepatocellular carcinoma (HCC). The majority of patients with a chronic hepatitis B infection do not need treatment. Patients with hepatitis B infection who do need treatment are those that have a high viral replication rate or those with an inflammatory response to hepatitis B that may lead to liver fibrosis and ultimately cirrhosis. The EASL Guidelines provide detailed guidance on treating hepatitis B.

DECIDING WHOM TO SCREEN FOR HEPATOCELLULAR CARCINOMA

Patients with cirrhosis, as well as patients with a high risk of developing HCC (see Table 4.22.1.), need to be screened for hepatocellular carcinoma on a 6-monthly basis via ultrasound with or without AFP measurements. There is no clear-cut guidance on how often to screen patients outside this risk group; an initial ultrasound at the start of monitoring and then every 3–5 years may be a practical guide.

TABLE 4.22.1
Risk Factors for Hepatocellular Carcinoma

Cirrhotic Patients	All
Patients with increased risk of cirrhosis	African patients >20 years old
	Asian men >40 years old
	Asian women >50 years old
Patients with high HBV DNA or persistent inflammatory activity	Co-infected patients (HCV, HIV, HDV)
	HBV DNA >2000 IU
	Core mutant virus

CLINICAL APPROACH

TREATING WITH NUCLEOSIDE ANALOGUES

The nucleoside analogues (NAs) that are recommended are entecavir (ETV) 0.5 mg/day, tenofovir disoproxil fumarate (TDF) 245 mg/day and tenofovir alafenamide (TAF) 25 mg/day. The choice depends on renal and bone health; these should be monitored whilst on treatment. Older nucleoside analogues such as lamivudine, adefovir and telbivudine are no longer recommended because of resistance development in the longer term.

Nucleoside analogues should be taken long-term if treatment is indicated, and in many cases lifelong treatment is necessary. Full viral suppression can take up to 12–18 months; HCC screen should not be stopped after achieving viral suppression. Failure due to resistance has been described in (pre-treated) patients on ETV, but not in patients on TDF or TAF. Compliance should be thoroughly monitored and a resistance test sent off in case of treatment failure.

Treatment should never be stopped in cirrhotic patients. Patients in whom stopping therapy may be *considered* are those at increasing risk of a flare-up of the hepatitis B:

- Those with HBsAg loss (regardless of antibody development)
- Those with HBeAg seroconversion to HBeAb AND a suppressed viral load for a minimum of 12 months
- HBeAg-negative patients who have been virologically suppressed for >3 years

TREATMENT WITH PEGINTERFERON

The treatment aim of this 48-week subcutaneous treatment is a hepatitis B viral load of <2000 and ideally hepatitis BeAg to antibody conversion. Peginterferon is also the only available therapy for patients infected with hepatitis delta virus (HDV).

Some patients may achieve a period of >5 years off daily NA therapy this way. The success rate is, depending on genotype and fibrosis stage, between 10% and 50%. However, treatment-limiting psychiatric, neurological and endocrinological side effects are common. Treatment by an experienced team is highly recommended.

IMMUNOCOMPROMISED PATIENTS

Hepatitis B reactivation occurs mostly in HBsAg-positive patients but may even occur in the case of anti-HBs carriers. Patients undergoing immunosuppressive therapy should therefore always receive a full serological screen before start of their therapy, especially if this therapy involves rituximab or other cytotoxic forms of chemotherapy. These patients need chemoprophylaxis in the form of

TDF, TAF or entecavir. A riskier option in patients with a very high anti-HBs titre who do not wish immediate treatment is monitoring anti-HBs levels and starting only when there is a significant decline.

PREGNANT WOMEN

Treatment of pregnant women has two aims: prevention of transmission to the child and monitoring and sometimes treating a flare of the hepatitis B. This flare can occur up to a few weeks postpartum, so closer monitoring is encouraged. Breastfeeding is not contraindicated in HBsAg-positive, untreated women or those on TDF-based treatment or prophylaxis. Entecavir is not used in pregnancy.

CLINICAL PEARL

Pregnant women should be started on tenofovir at week 24–28 of gestation when:

- There is advanced fibrosis or cirrhosis
- The HBV DNA is >200,000 IU/mL or HbsAg is >4 $\log_{10}$ IU/mL at that point

---

HEALTHCARE WORKERS

Hepatitis B infection alone is never a reason to deter people from working in the healthcare profession. Healthcare workers performing exposure-prone procedures with serum HBV DNA >200 IU/mL may be treated with NAs to reduce transmission risk and be followed up on a 3–6-monthly basis.

CLINICAL PEARL

Healthcare workers in a procedure-prone environment (e.g. surgery, dentistry, etc.) can be offered treatment with a nucleoside analogue if their HBV DNA is >200 IU.

LIVER TRANSPLANT PATIENTS

Patients undergoing liver transplant with an undetectable viral load have a significantly reduced risk of 5% for reinfecting the transplant with hepatitis B.

CHILDREN

Most children do not need treatment; liaison with a paediatric infectious disease physician or hepatologist is advised when considering treatment.

CLINICAL VIGNETTES

A 23-year-old female is admitted for analysis of jaundice. Hepatitis serology shows that hepatitis B surface antigen is positive, hepatitis B anti-core IgM positive, hepatitis B anti-core IgM is negative, and her anti-hepatitis B surface antibody is negative. Her ALT is around 5000 and PT is normal. They want to know if they should treat the infection. You tell them to hold off treatment but to repeat tests tomorrow.

Acute hepatitis B infection can cause extremely high ALT levels, but treatment is only needed in 5% of patients.

The SHO phones you 5 days later: The ALT is 5500 but the PT has climbed up to 16 and the bilirubin is rising too. You advise to start tenofovir 245 mg OD and contact a liver transplant centre, from which the staff advise to start adjunctive prednisolone.

- The hallmark of disease severity is a rise in PT.
- Prednisolone use has been shown effective in trials with older medication; however, use with the newer agents (tenofovir, entecavir and TAF) has never been tested.
- In case of liver function deterioration, always contact a liver transplant centre early.

The patient is accepted by the transplant centre; however, the patient starts to improve within the next week. Three months later, her liver enzymes have almost normalized.

A 36-year-old police officer is presenting to the emergency room on Friday night after a human bite incident involving a lot of blood 2 hours ago. One of the persons involved told him he was recently tested for HIV, hepatitis B and C and that he is hepatitis B positive. The police officer doesn't remember whether he has had any vaccinations. The A&E SHO asks you what to do. You advise to try to get some new samples from the source patient to confirm hepatitis B/C and HIV status, to give immunoglobulins against hepatitis B (HBIG) and to start vaccination prior to getting in touch with the occupational health team on Monday.

- Patients who have not been vaccinated, patients who are known non-responders to vaccination or patients who have become severely immunocompromised since vaccination need HBIG as well as vaccination; in others, vaccinations alone suffice.
- Treat with 500 units of HBIG IM (deltoid muscle) within 12–24 hours of the incident—maximum 1 week post-exposure—and start hepatitis B vaccination scheme at the same time.

BIBLIOGRAPHY

2017 EASL guidelines for the treatment of hepatitis B infection. *J Hepatol.* 2017;67:370–398.

Bruix J, Sherman M. Management of hepatocellular carcinoma. *Hepatology.* 2005 November;42(5):1208–1236.

Choi J, Lim YS. Characteristics, prevention, and management of hepatitis B virus (HBV) reactivation in HBV-infected patients who require immunosuppressive therapy. *J Infect Dis.* 2017 November 16;216(suppl_8):S778–S784.

Galle PR, Forner A, Llovet JM, Mazzaferro V, Piscaglia F, Raou J-L, Schirmacher P, Vilgrain V. European Association for the Study of the Liver. EASL Clinical Practice Guidelines: Management of hepatocellular carcinoma. *J Hepatol.* 2018;69(1):182–236.

Lok AS, Ward JW, Perrillo RP et al. Reactivation of hepatitis B during immunosuppressive therapy: Potentially fatal yet preventable. *Ann Intern Med.* 2012 May 15;156(10):743–745.

Terrault NA, Lok ASF, McMahon BJ et al. Update on prevention, diagnosis, and treatment of chronic hepatitis B: AASLD 2018 hepatitis B guidance. *Hepatology.* 2018;67(4).

4.23 Hepatitis C

Anda Samson

CLINICAL CONSIDERATIONS

Hepatitis C is a small RNA virus that only affects the liver. It is a chronic infection with a mostly indolent course, but it could lead to problems later in life. The aim of hepatitis C treatment is thus the prevention of those complications, in particular cirrhosis of the liver and hepatocellular carcinoma. About 20%–25% of patients infected will clear the virus spontaneously; the rest will convert to chronic hepatitis C. Infection can remain silent or can go with a prominent episode of clear liver inflammation. Those with a strong inflammatory response may be more likely to clear the virus spontaneously. It is therefore worthwhile to consider the following.

EVALUATION OF LIVER HEALTH

Before starting a patient on antivirals, it is important to evaluate their liver health. There needs to be a clinical assessment of the possibility of other causes for raised liver enzymes, particularly hepatis B or HIV co-infection, as well as non-infectious causes. An assessment of the amount of fibrosis or cirrhosis of the liver needs to occur as well. If there is cirrhosis of the liver, there is a small chance that the patient may decompensate whilst initiating treatment.

Where a liver biopsy was used previously, a non-invasive FibroScan is the current standard of care to assess whether there is likely fibrosis or cirrhosis. Although the scan is very sensitive and specific at the more severe end of the spectrum, it is not reliable in assessing whether or not a patient has F2–F3 fibrosis.

CLINICAL APPROACH

SELECTING A TREATMENT

The modern direct-acting antivirals (DAAs) are all highly effective, with a success rate of 95%–98%, although there is a slight variation amongst drugs in effectiveness depending on the genotype of hepatitis that is being treated.

Patients with cirrhosis should remain under the care of a hepatologist even after clearing the hepatitis C for ongoing hepatocellular carcinoma surveillance and further management of the cirrhosis. Patients who have a FibroScan score of F0 or F1 and have cleared the hepatitis can be discharged. The opinions are divided still on how to treat those who had a high FibroScan score but did not quite classify as cirrhotic. In some centres, a repeat FibroScan is made if the value has normalized.

TYPES OF TREATMENT

Current medication regimes consist of DAAs. The antivirals are directed against specific sites in the genome—there are protease inhibitors (also called NS3/NS4A inhibitors) glecaprevir and grazoprevir, NS5A inhibitors velpatasvir, elbasvir, pibrentasvir and ledipasvir, and NS5B inhibitor sofosbuvir. Treatment with DAAs is associated with significantly improved survival and overall improvement in morbidity in hepatitis C positive patients, whether or not they are cirrhotic. These new antivirals are generally very well tolerated and need to be taken for a duration of 8–16 weeks usually, depending on the treatment chosen.

Drug interactions, including any illicit substances, should be considered before starting treatment. Treatment with DAAs is dependent on genotype, as well as cirrhosis/fibrosis state. It is recommended to follow national or international guidelines such as the EASL's Clinical Practice Guidelines to ensure appropriate antiviral prescribing.

Prior to DAAS, treatment with peginterferon was the treatment of choice for hepatitis C. It is, however, associated with serious complications such as hypo- and hyperthyroidism, other autoimmune illnesses and, most widespread, depression. The addition of ribavirin to the treatment regime increased the success rate somewhat, but anaemia was a common complication. In some parts of the world, however, peginterferon with or without ribavirin is still the only available treatment for hepatitis C.

PEP AND PrEP

The risk of contracting hepatitis C after a needlestick incident is around 1.8%. Unfortunately, there are no drugs available as pre- or post-exposure prophylaxis. The first patients receiving organs from hepatitis C–positive donors have been successfully treated for 4 weeks.

REINFECTION RISK

Patients with hepatitis C are susceptible to reinfections. Proper patient education and needle-exchange programs, as well as exchange of all gear, may help prevent reinfection. Quite often, patients do not realize it is not just the needles, but also other paraphernalia used, including citric acid, which increases risk of transmission of hepatitis C.

CLINICAL PEARL

By treating a patient who is actively injecting drugs for hepatitis C, provided they are educated on transmission risks, treatment may work as prevention of further new hepatitis C infections in others.

CLINICAL PEARL

Hepatitis C treatment is now a lot easier and possible for most patients. The right timing and patient education are paramount, though.

The following clinical vignettes illustrate how hepatitis C treatment can be used in varying circumstances.

CLINICAL VIGNETTES

A young, otherwise healthy hepatitis C–positive person dies in a tragic car accident. Their family expresses the patient's strong wish to be an organ donor, although they are aware this is a controversial topic still. The doctors consult the donor coordinators in the hospital. They liaise with patients and doctors awaiting an organ and decide to accept the organs. Three people received a heart, liver and kidneys alongside a month of anti-hepatitis C drugs. Six months after the transplants, the organ recipients have remained hepatitis C negative.

Although there have not been definitive changes to transplant practice, early reports suggest that there may be a role for transplanting organs from hepatitis C–positive donors to hepatitis C–negative recipients.

A 50-year-old man is admitted to hospital with decompensated cirrhosis of the liver with a MELD score of 26. He previously drank alcohol excessively but stopped this 5 years ago. He tests positive for hepatitis C, and there is a discussion about whether or not to treat his hepatitis C. There is no hepatocellular carcinoma. It is decided to consult a liver transplant centre, and the patient is transferred straightaway. He is lucky enough to receive a donor organ almost instantly. His hepatitis C is treated after the transplant.

- Patients with decompensated cirrhosis should not receive protease inhibitors, but either sofosbuvir-ledipasvir with ribavirin, or sofosbuvir-velpatasvir.
- Patients with Child B or C cirrhosis should be treated in an expert centre.
- Patients with a MELD score of <18–20 should be treated before proceeding to liver transplant. Those with higher MELD scores should be transplanted before treatment of hepatitis C.

BIBLIOGRAPHY

Bennett JE, Dolin R, Blaser MJ. *Mandell, Douglas, and Bennett's Principles and Practice of Infectious Diseases*. Philadelphia, PA: Elsevier/Saunders, 2015.

European Association for the Study of the Liver. EASL recommendations on treatment of hepatitis C 2018. *J Hepatol*. 2018 August;69(2):461–511.

4.24 Hepatitis E

Anda Samson

CLINICAL CONSIDERATIONS

After the discovery of the hepatitis E virus as a separate entity, it has become clear that it is a significant cause of endemic hepatitis in developing countries. Because genotypes 1 and 2 of hepatitis E are transmitted via the fecal-oral route, it is endemic in places where access to hygienic cooking facilities, clean drinking water and sewage systems is poor. Depending on the location, it may comprise 25%–70% of acute hepatitis cases. More recently, however, it has become clear that in developed countries, genotypes 3 and 4 cause hepatitis through consumption of pig and wild boar meat. Possibly, other animals are a reservoir for hepatitis E too, though it is as yet unclear how many transmissions to man occur through these other animals. Screening of blood donors in Europe showed that 5%–30% are seropositive for hepatitis E IgG and that 1:600 to 1:7000 patients are viraemic. Some countries have introduced screening of blood donors for hepatitis E because of documented transmission through blood transfusion; however, screening of donated blood is not universal yet.

INFECTION IN ADULTHOOD AND CHILDHOOD

Contrary to hepatitis A, the highest incidence in hepatitis E infections appears to be in early adulthood in endemic areas. It does not appear to be due to decreasing infection in childhood because the findings in age groups have remained stable for over a decade now.

GENERAL CHARACTERISTICS OF HEPATITIS E INFECTION

- Incubation period is 15–60 days following exposure, with an average of 40 days.
- Increase in ALT occurs 4–5 weeks after exposure and persists for 3–13 weeks.
- Symptoms occur when liver enzymes are elevated.
- Viraemia starts from 3 weeks following exposure (or a week prior to onset of symptoms) and lasts for 2 weeks.
- Excretion of HEV in stool usually from 1 week before symptoms occur until 1 week after, but can be longer, especially in immunocompromised individuals.
- Both HEV IgM and IgG are detectable 3–4 weeks after exposure. HEV IgM is usually negative after 13 weeks; HEV IgG persists lifelong.
- Chronic HEV infection in immunocompetent individuals is rare.
- More and more cases of hepatitis E with progression to chronic hepatitis and chronic liver disease are being reported among HEV genotype 3 cases acquired in the developed countries. These chronic cases are exclusively among persons who are on immunosuppressive treatment for solid organ transplant.

MORTALITY OF HEPATITIS E

In outbreaks of hepatitis E in refugee camps, mortality was between 1%–2%.
    For unclear reasons, pregnant patients are extra vulnerable when it comes to hepatitis E infection. There is a staggering 25% mortality in pregnant patients, owing to fulminant liver disease. In patients

with acute or chronic liver disease, case fatality may be equally high or even higher than in pregnancy, but in patients with a normal liver function and immune system, the infection usually is self-limiting.

CLINICAL PEARL

Mortality of hepatitis E infection in pregnant women and patients with chronic liver disease can be as high as 25%.

ACUTE AND CHRONIC INFECTIONS

Acute hepatitis E is indistinguishable from other types of hepatitis and often comes with general malaise, myalgia and icterus. It can pass unnoticed, but in severe cases, ALT can rise to 40× the upper limit or normal. Bilirubin and other markers of cholestasis are often slower to recover.

In severely immunocompromised patients, hepatitis E can become a chronic infection. ALT is usually less pronounced than in immunocompetent patients, and serum RNA levels may vary. Early detection and treatment are important though, since RNA levels and progression to fibrosis or cirrhosis seem to be independent.

CLINICAL PEARL

Progression to fibrosis or cirrhosis in a transplant patient is independent of hepatitis E RNA levels.

EXTRAHEPATIC MANIFESTATIONS

Although the virus itself has not been found outside the liver and digestive tract, like other forms of hepatitis, hepatitis E can cause extrahepatic manifestations. The most common extrahepatic manifestations are neurological: Guillain–Barré–syndrome, mononeuritis simplex and myositis are examples. Glomerulonephritis and acute kidney injury are also described.

CLINICAL APPROACH

DIAGNOSIS OF HEPATITIS E

Although serology is widely available, the specificity of the IgM assays is variable, making it an unreliable test in non-endemic countries. The gold standard for diagnosing acute Hepatitis E infection is currently done by PCR on blood or stool. In patients living in or travelling from endemic countries who present with acute hepatitis, hepatitis E should be tested as first-line testing. In countries with a lower endemicity, it can be used as a second-line test after the more prevalent other types of hepatitis have been excluded.

TREATMENT OF HEPATITIS E INFECTION

The vast majority of patients improve without medical contact; some may need supportive measures.

MANAGEMENT OF HEPATITIS E IN THE IMMUNOCOMPROMISED PATIENT

In immunocompromised patients, lowering the dose of immunosuppressive agents, if feasible, will contribute to clearing the infection in about half of the patients. Those patients who remain viraemic can be considered for an initial 3-month course of ribavirin; if either stool or blood PCR is still positive after the 3 months, a second but longer (6 months) course of ribavirin can be tried.

In liver transplant patients, after failure of ribavirin monotherapy, peginterferon could be considered, but in kidney transplant patients, this has led to increased numbers of graft rejection. More recently, a combination of ribavirin and sofosbuvir has been suggested; however, although some successes have been claimed with this combination, there are multiple failures described in the literature.

PREVENTION OF HEPATITIS E INFECTION

The most effective way to prevent hepatitis E infection is access to sanitation and clean drinking water, as well as avoidance of consumption of undercooked meat.

Vaccines are not yet commercially available but there are promising options in the development pipeline.

CLINICAL PEARL

The vast majority of patients get better without any medical contact.

CLINICAL PEARL

Although some antiviral agents can be used to clear hepatitis E, the hallmark of cure seems to be, first and foremost, the lowering of immunosuppressive agents.

CLINICAL VIGNETTES

A 57-year-old woman with a renal transplant who was transplanted 4 years ago is admitted with acute hepatitis. Serology suggests hepatitis E infection, which is confirmed by RNA testing. Her immunosuppressive agents consist of prednisolone, tacrolimus and mycophenolate mofetil. Her prednisolone dose is significantly reduced, and her target tacrolimus levels are lowered, but hepatitis E RNA is still present 3 months later and there is still a rise in ALT levels. Further reduction of her immunosuppressive agents is deemed unsafe for her transplant kidney. She is then treated with ribavirin for 3 months, and the hepatitis E is cleared.

A 35-year-old pregnant refugee who has just arrived in the UK is admitted with nausea, vomiting and general malaise. A few days into her admission, her ALT levels start to rise and reach 2000 U/L; at this point, her albumin is dropping and her clotting is deranged. She is transferred to a liver transplant centre and worked up for a possible liver transplant. Although ribavirin is known to be teratogenic, treatment with ribavirin is considered; however, unfortunately, the patient dies of fulminant liver disease a few days after transfer to the transplant centre.

BIBLIOGRAPHY

Bennett JE, Dolin R, Blaser MJ. *Mandell, Douglas, and Bennett's Principles and Practice of Infectious Diseases*. Philadelphia, PA: Elsevier/Saunders, 2015.

Denner J, Pischke S, Steinmann E et al. Why all blood donations should be tested for hepatitis E virus (HEV). *BMC Infect Dis*. 2019;19:541.

European Association for the Study of the Liver. EASL clinical practice guidelines on hepatitis E virus infection. *J Hepatol*. 2018;68:1256–1271.

Zhang J, Zhang XF, Huang SJ et al. Long-term efficacy of a hepatitis E vaccine. [published correction appears in *N Engl J Med*. 2015 Apr 9;372(15):1478]. *N Engl J Med*. 2015;372(10):914–922.

4.25 Histoplasmosis

Firza Alexander Gronthoud

CLINICAL CONSIDERATIONS

Histoplasmosis is caused by *Histoplasma capsulatum* and is the most endemic mycosis worldwide. It can cause a self-limiting, mild pneumonia or an invasive disease with multiorgan failure. It is therefore worthwhile to consider the following.

GLOBAL DISTRIBUTION

Histoplasmosis has a global distribution and is endemic in areas in North America (Ohio and Mississippi River valleys), Central and South America, Africa, Australia, India and Malaysia.

CLINICAL MANIFESTATIONS

After a primary infection, a mild and transient pneumonia develops with symptoms similar to a community-acquired pneumonia (CAP). In immunocompromised patients, it can then progress to severe pneumonia with acute respiratory distress syndrome (ARDS). Pulmonary manifestations are broad and can resemble a bacterial pneumonia, malignancy, sarcoidosis, tuberculosis, *Nocardia* or aspergillosis. Pulmonary manifestations with arthritis or arthralgia plus erythema nodosum may also occur. In immunocompromised individuals, histoplasmosis may also progress to disseminated disease characterized by fever, malaise, weight loss, pancytopaenia, hepatosplenomegaly, deranged liver function tests, necrosis of the adrenal glands and mucosal lesions (seen in >60% of patients). Disseminated disease can further progress to septic shock with ARDS and multiorgan failure. A chronic complication is meningitis.

CLINICAL PEARL

Pulmonary manifestations in immunocompromised individuals: pneumonia with mediastinal or hilar lymphadenopathy, mediastinal or hilar masses, pulmonary nodule and cavitary lung disease.

CLINICAL APPROACH

DIAGNOSIS

Histoplasma can be diagnosed by detecting antigen in urine or serum. Urine has a higher sensitivity and may be easier to obtain. Microscopy and culture can be performed on blood cultures, bone marrow aspirates or biopsy of liver, skin and mucosal lesions or respiratory samples such as bronchoalveolar lavage, lung tissue and lymph nodes.

Due to a similarity in cell wall antigens, false-positive galactomannan results are seen in patients with histoplasmosis; conversely, a histoplasma antigen test will test negative in patients with aspergillosis.

MANAGEMENT

The choice and duration of antifungal treatment depend on the severity of disease as well as complications such as cavitation and dissemination (see Table 4.25.1).

Methylprednisolone (0.5–1.0 mg/kg daily intravenously) during the first 1–2 weeks of antifungal therapy is recommended for patients with respiratory complications, including hypoxaemia or significant respiratory distress.

TABLE 4.25.1
Treatment Options for Histoplasmosis

Mild-to-Moderate Acute Pulmonary Histoplasmosis	Chronic Cavitary Pulmonary Histoplasmosis	Disseminated Histoplasmosis
Treatment is usually unnecessary unless immunocompromised. If treatment, then: Itraconazole 200 mg 3 times daily for 3 days and then 200 mg once or twice daily for 6–12 weeks for patients with symptoms >1 month. *Moderate-to-severe disease*: Ambisome 3.0–5.0 mg/kg daily IV for 1–2 weeks followed by itraconazole 200 mg 3 times daily for 3 days and then 200 mg twice daily, for a total of 12 weeks.	Itraconazole 200 mg 3 times daily for 3 days and then once or twice daily for at least 1 year, but some prefer 18–24 months in view of the risk for relapse. Blood levels of itraconazole should be obtained after the patient has been receiving this agent for at least 2 weeks to ensure adequate drug exposure.	*Mild-to-moderate disease*: Itraconazole 200 mg 3 times daily for 3 days and then twice daily for at least 12 months. Lifelong suppressive therapy with itraconazole 200 mg daily may be required in immunosuppressed patients if immunosuppression cannot be reversed and in patients who relapse despite receipt of appropriate therapy. Blood levels of itraconazole should be obtained to ensure adequate drug exposure. *Moderate-to-severe disease*: Ambisome 3.0 mg/kg daily for 1–2 weeks, followed by oral itraconazole 200 mg 3 times daily for 3 days and then 200 mg twice daily for a total of at least 12 months. *Progressive disease*: 1st-line amphotericin B deoxycholate 1.0 mg/kg daily for 4–6 weeks. 2nd-line amphotericin B deoxycholate 1.0 mg/kg daily for 2–4 weeks followed by itraconazole 5.0–10.0 mg/kg daily in 2 divided doses to complete 3 months of therapy. Longer therapy may be needed for patients with severe disease, immunosuppression or primary immunodeficiency syndromes. Lifelong suppressive therapy with itraconazole 5.0 mg/kg daily, up to 200 mg daily may be required in immunosuppressed patients if immunosuppression cannot be reversed and in patients who experience relapse despite receipt of appropriate therapy. Blood levels of itraconazole should be obtained to ensure adequate drug exposure.

MONITORING TREATMENT

Antigen levels should be measured during therapy and for 12 months after therapy has ended to monitor for relapse. If antigen levels have not decreased significantly after 3 months, then treatment should be changed to a different agent. Persistent low-level antigenuria may not be a reason to prolong treatment in patients who have completed appropriate therapy and have no evidence of active infection.

BIBLIOGRAPHY

Kauffman CA. Histoplasmosis: A clinical and laboratory update. *Clin Microbiol Rev.* 2007 January;20(1):115–132.
Wheat LJ, Freifeld AG, Kleiman MB, Baddley JW, McKinsey DS, Loyd JE, Kauffman CA; Infectious Diseases Society of America. Clinical practice guidelines for the management of patients with histoplasmosis: 2007 update by the Infectious Diseases Society of America. *Clin Infect Dis.* 2007 October 1;45(7):807–825.

4.26 Human Immunodeficiency Virus and Opportunistic Infections

Anda Samson

CLINICAL CONSIDERATIONS

After more than three decades of development, there is no such thing as the typical HIV epidemic. There are regional differences where access to medication, stigma and prosecution dictate which group is most at risk. Despite advances in the treatment and prevention, every year 1.7 million people are newly infected with HIV and around 1 million people died from HIV in 2017. You may note prejudice and fear even within the healthcare system. It is our collective task as infection professionals to stand up to this stigma and educate our colleagues where appropriate.

CLINICAL CONSIDERATIONS

DIAGNOSIS

Fourth-generation HIV1/2 antibody/antigen ELISA tests are recommended as a first-line screening method. They have a 4-week window period, which means that they can reliably exclude HIV four weeks post-exposure. Rapid tests, or bedside tests, are available too, but specificity is much lower than the ELISA tests, meaning there are more false-positive results. The consent rules for HIV testing are the exact same as 'normal' good medical practice prescribes.

CLINICAL PEARL

Patients should know about and consent to ALL tests they undergo, including HIV testing, but there is no special status.

FIRST CLINICAL ASSESSMENT

When assessing your patient, you'll need to do a full physical exam and establish whether or not there is a risk the patient has an opportunistic infection. You will need a CD4 (lymphocyte subset) count. The lower the CD4 count, the higher the risk of opportunistic infections, although there are no absolute cut-offs for the counts; see Table 4.26.1 for reference of frequently diagnosed infections.

CLINICAL PEARL

The height of the CD4 count is a good indicator of the overall risk of opportunistic infections.

TABLE 4.26.1

Relationship between CD4 Count and Risk of Opportunistic Infections

CD4 Count	Infection/Syndrome	Whom	Prophylaxis
500	Guillain–Barré		No prophylaxis
	Chronic demyelinating neuropathy		
	Idiopathic thrombocytopaenia		
	Reiter's syndrome		
	Polymyositis		
	Sjögren's syndrome		
	Bell's palsy		
200–500	Tinea, onychomycosis	If active TB excluded and	No prophylaxis
	Gingivitis	positive screen	Rifampicin/INH 3–4 months, OR
	Seborrhoeic dermatitis		INH 9 months, OR rifabutin/INH 1
	Molluscum contagiosum		month
	Herpes zoster		
	Tuberculosis		
	Kaposi's sarcoma		
	Sinusitis		
	Non-Hodgkin's lymphoma		
	Cervical intraepithelial neoplasia		
<200	Oral candidiasis	CD4 <200	No prophylaxis
	Hairy leukoplakia	CD4 <200 AND AB +ve	No prophylaxis
	Pneumocystis jirovecii pneumonia	CD4 <50	Co-trimoxazole 480–960 mg OD
	(PCP)	CD4 >50	No prophylaxis
	Herpes simplex		Co-trimoxazole 480–960 OD OR
	Toxoplasmosis		Dapsone PLUS pyrimethamine
	Cryptococcosis		No prophylaxis
	Cytomegalovirus		3-monthly retinal screen
	Mycobacterium avium complex		Azithromycin 1250 mg once weekly

TREATMENT OF HIV

There is no curative treatment available for HIV, but combination antiretroviral therapy (cART), (previously called highly active antiretroviral therapy, HAART) is highly effective, and life expectancy of a treated HIV patient is now close to normal. Once a patient is established on therapy and has an undetectable viral load, they are not cured, but the virus cannot be passed on to others. Most treatment-naïve patients start on a combination of two nucleoside reverse transcriptase inhibitors (NRTIs)—usually a fixed-dose combination of abacavir/lamivudine or tenofovir/emtricitabine—plus an integrase inhibitor or non-NNRTI (NNRTI) (see Table 4.26.2). Patients on treatment need to be adherent to their medication every day; some are restricted to taking with or without food. If changing medication whilst the viral load is not suppressed, or unreliable timing of tablets, HIV resistance to medication can occur.

- Patients with low CD4 count will need prophylaxis for opportunistic infections.
- The current advice is to start a patient on antiretroviral therapy regardless of CD4 count.
- All protease inhibitors in current use are boosted with either low-dose ritonavir or cobicistat. This boosting effect can lead to significant drug-drug interactions.
- Expert advice is recommended when changing or stopping antiretroviral drugs.
- Not all mainstay antiretrovirals are suitable for HIV-2 treatment.

TABLE 4.26.2
Current Antiretroviral Agents Used for HIV Treatment

Integrase inhibitors	**Dolutegravir**
	Raltegravir
	Elvitegravir (boosted)
	Bictegravir*
Protease inhibitors	**Darunavir**
	Atazanavir
	Fosamprenavir
	Lopinavir
	Nelfinavir, indinavir
	Ritonavir (usually as a booster only)
Nucleoside reverse transcriptase inhibitors (NRTIs)	**Abacavir**
	Emtricitabine
	Lamivudine
	Tenofovir (DF/AF)
	Zidovudine
	Stavudine
	Didanosine
Non-nucleoside reverse transcriptase inhibitors (NNRTIs)	**Efavirenz**
	Etravirine
	Nevirapine
	Rilpivirine
	Doravirine*
Fusion and entry inhibitors	Maraviroc
	Enfuvirtide
	Albuvirtide*
	Fostemsavir*
Post-attachment inhibitors	Ibalizumab*

Note: Bold text indicates currently widely used.
* Not yet approved for use in all countries.

CLINICAL PEARL

Consider drug-drug interactions when starting or changing medication, using, for example, https://www.hiv-druginteractions.org/.

CLINICAL PEARL

Patients with an undetectable viral load cannot pass their HIV on to others in ANY way.

NON-HIV-RELATED TREATMENT FOR HIV PATIENTS

HIV patients need various vaccinations because of a higher risk of acquiring infections or a higher risk of a severe course of disease when contracting the illness; a summary of the recommended vaccines can be found in the most recent BHIVA guideline for vaccinations. Keep in mind that live vaccines in patients with a low CD4 count are generally not safe.

Bone health and cardiovascular health in HIV patients are again areas of concern; incidents occur more frequently and at an earlier age than the general population, either due to medication, inflammation, the HIV itself or lifestyle factors, so active screening via tools such as the FRAX score or QRISK are imperative.

POST-EXPOSURE PROPHYLAXIS

Post-exposure prophylaxis should be given to individuals who have been at a higher risk (>1:1000) or moderate risk (1:1000–1:10,000) as soon as possible after exposure. The BHIVA PEP guideline has a good overview of the risks per particular exposure. Overall, if the prevalence in the area is low, the risk of transmission—(the risk that the source is positive, which varies per area) × (risk per exposure)—will automatically also be low.

PRE-EXPOSURE PROPHYLAXIS

The fixed-dose combinations of tenofovir/emtricitabine or tenofovir/lamivudine have now been approved as effective prevention of HIV when taken according to instructions.

CLINICAL VIGNETTES

A 56-year-old man is brought into hospital with shortness of breath and a dry cough. He is able to speak in full sentences but unable to get up the stairs without getting out of breath. A chest X-ray shows a bilateral fine interstitial pattern which was missed initially. You advise to do a BAL and treat for Pneumocystis jirovecii pneumonia (PJP) empirically until the results come back.

- Patients with PJP can often look entirely normal, but with minimal exertion their SpO_2 levels drop dramatically.
- If the PO_2 is under 8, addition of steroids is advised according to EACS and BHIVA guidelines.

The HIV test comes back positive, and the patient has a CD4 count of 34. BAL indeed shows pneumocystis. His pneumonia is static despite treatment but he is now also complaining of headaches. Toxoplasma antibody is negative but cryptococcal antigen is positive in his blood. You decide to do a CT scan of his brain, and if there are no mass lesions, do a lumbar puncture.

- Patients with a low CD4 count and a positive cryptococcal antigen on blood should always have a lumbar puncture performed; CSF should be sent for culture, antigen testing and staining.
- Opening pressure should always be measured when performing an LP and suspecting cryptococcal meningitis.

A 40-year-old woman is admitted with shortness of breath and very quickly needs intubation and ventilation. She has a history of cervical lymphadenopathy without any clear cause and has visited her GP several times for bacterial pneumonia over the past 2 years. CT thorax/abdomen shows several large lymph nodes in her abdomen, axilla and mediastinum. There is a reasonable amount of pleural fluid as well. A lymphoma is diagnosed, and as part of her work-up, an HIV test is performed which is positive. The patient unfortunately dies due to respiratory failure and disseminated lymphoma.

- In cases of lymphadenopathy that is not understood, HIV should always be part of the work-up.
- Many patients who are 'late presenters' might have been diagnosed earlier if signs had been picked up earlier. Multiple courses of antibiotics in an otherwise healthy person should trigger HIV testing.

BIBLIOGRAPHY

2015 Joint BHIVA/BASHH guideline for PEP/PEPSE.

BHIVA treatment guidelines https://www.bhiva.org/guidelines.

EACS guidelines http://www.eacsociety.org/guidelines/eacs-guidelines/eacs-guidelines.html.

https://www.bashh.org/documents/PEPSE%202015%20guideline%20final_NICE.pdf.

Bennett JE, Dolin R, Blaser MJ.*Mandell, Douglas, And Bennett's Principles and Practice of Infectious Diseases*, Philadelphia, PA: Elsevier/Saunders, 2015.

UNAIDS unaids.org.

4.27 Infections in Haematopoietic Stem Cell Transplants

Patrick Lillie

CLINICAL CONSIDERATIONS

Stem cell transplantation is a method of rescuing the patient's haematopoietic function after high-dose chemotherapy or disease has damaged the recipient's bone marrow beyond recovery. Stem cell transplants are broadly split into autografts (using the patient's own stem cells) or allografts (using donor stem cells). Whilst both procedures have a risk of procedure-related mortality and morbidity, of which infection is a significant cause, allografts have a higher risk and also have a risk of infection that continues after engraftment, with a changing spectrum of organisms as time passes (see Table 4.27.1).

Infections in the pre-engraftment period are often related to neutropaenia, and these will be covered in Chapter 4.40.

CLINICAL APPROACH

PROPHYLAXIS

Viral

Because of the very high risk of infection in the early post-transplant period, prophylaxis against several organisms is indicated. Herpes viruses reactivate post-transplant very frequently and aciclovir prophylaxis is routinely given to prevent HSV-1, HSV-2 and VZV reactivation. CMV reactivation/infection is dependent on many factors, with the serostatus of the donor and recipient of an allograft being the major determinant (R+/D− being highest risk for reactivation). CMV prophylaxis in the form of ganciclovir/valganciclovir is often used for a prolonged period of time after the transplant; however, some centres monitor CMV viral load using weekly PCR and will commence treatment based upon this.

Bacterial

Profound and prolonged neutropaenia in the peri-transplant period is almost ubiquitous. Prophylaxis directed against enteric Gram-negative bacilli is commonly given until neutrophil counts have recovered. This is usually in the form of fluroquinolones, with levofloxacin being commonly used. Longer-term prophylaxis is less commonly employed, with the exception of co-trimoxazole for pneumocystis prophylaxis and also in those patients who are functionally asplenic. Some patients may require IV immunoglobulin infusions in the longer term if they become hypogammaglobulinaemic.

Fungal

In the early post-transplant period, *Candida* and *Aspergillus* are the commonest fungal infections encountered. Mould-active azole prophylaxis is given to reduce the incidence of this and, in high-risk allograft patients, would be continued for a prolonged period of time, especially if there is ongoing graft-versus-host disease, with posaconazole being the preferred agent in most cases. For patients unable to receive azoles for any reason, both liposomal amphotericin and echinocandin infusions

TABLE 4.27.1

Spectrum of Infections Occurring during Pre- and Post-Engraftment in HSCT Recipients

	Pre-Engraftment	Early Post-Engraftment	Late Post-Engraftment
Bacterial	Gram-negative rods, oral streptococci, coagulase-negative staphylococci		Encapsulated bacteria, e.g. *Streptococcus pneumoniae*
Viral	Herpes simplex	CMV, VZV, adenovirus	Respiratory viruses, EBV-related post-transplant lymphoproliferative disease (PTLD)
Fungal	*Candida* spp., *Aspergillus* spp.	*Pneumocystis jirovecii*, *Aspergillus* spp.	

have been used as prophylaxis. *Pneumocystis* infection is another fungal infection that is common in the period after transplant, and prophylaxis with co-trimoxazole is usually given from the time of engraftment for at least 6 months.

CLINICAL PEARL

Prophylactic regimens need to take into account both the degree and duration of immune suppression, as well as patient comorbidities and exposures.

MONITORING FOR BREAKTHROUGH/NEW INFECTION

Most transplant centres will have protocols for monitoring allograft patients for the development of occult infections in the post-transplant period. This will generally include PCR on blood for viruses such as CMV, EBV, HHV-6 and adenovirus to allow for early pre-emptive treatment of these if detected before symptoms occur. Other serological/PCR-based monitoring could include fungal biomarkers (1,3-β-D-glucan and galactomannan), toxoplasmosis and South American trypanosomiasis dependent on recipient and donor serological profiles.

CLINICAL PEARL

A thorough history, including a travel history, should be taken ideally before transplant occurs so as to guide screening and prophylaxis for less-common infections that might complicate the treatment.

CLINICAL VIGNETTES

A 26-year-old man who received an allogenic stem cell transplant for aplastic anaemia 9 months earlier presented with fever, coryza and shortness of breath. A viral throat swab was positive for RSV at a high viral load and his CXR showed diffuse bilateral infiltrates. He was treated with ribavirin (given orally due to bronchospasm when initially nebulized) and pooled human normal immunoglobulin for 5 days and made an uneventful recovery.

Even several months after engraftment, patients with allogenic transplants have an ongoing high risk of certain infections, and patients should be advised about contact precautions for respiratory viruses. Household contacts should receive inactivated influenza vaccine to reduce the potential for transmission. Live, attenuated influenza vaccine should not be used, owing to the risk of disease from this. For viral pneumonitis in which there is a paucity of other therapeutic options, polyvalent immunoglobulin may be of use alongside antiviral medications such as ribavirin.

A 43-year-old man who received a matched, unrelated donor, allogenic transplant for high-risk myelodysplasia 5 months earlier presented with a fever, skin rash and diarrhoea. He was taking prophylactic co-trimoxazole and aciclovir, and his CMV PCR on blood was negative. A subsequent skin biopsy was consistent with graft-versus-host disease (GvHD), and his immunosuppression was increased to treat this.

In addition to infective complications, GvHD is a serious complication that can occur either in the early post-transplant period or as a longer-term chronic complication. The importance of GvHD for infection teams is that it can mimic infection (diarrhoea, rash and fever being common manifestations of both) but also that chronic GvHD is a significant risk factor for developing infective complications, both from the condition itself and the increased intensity immunosuppression used to treat it. During flares of GvHD it may be appropriate to re-commence prophylaxis against mould infections and possibly also viral disease as well.

BIBLIOGRAPHY

Mikulska M, Averbuch D, Tissot F et al. Fluoroquinolone prophylaxis in haematological cancer patients with neutropenia: ECIL critical appraisal of previous guidelines. *J Infect*. 2018;76(1):20–37.
Cornely OA, Maertens J, Winston DJ et al. Posaconazole vs. fluconazole or itraconazole prophylaxis in patients with neutropenia. *N Engl J Med*. 2007;356(4):348–359.
Tomblyn M, Chiller T, Einsele H et al. Guidelines for preventing infectious complications among hematopoietic cell transplantation recipients: A global perspective. [published correction appears in *Biol Blood Marrow Transplant*. 2010 Feb;16(2):294. Boeckh, Michael A [corrected to Boeckh, Michael J]]. *Biol Blood Marrow Transplant*. 2009;15(10):1143–1238.
Ullmann AJ, Lipton JH, Vesole DH et al. Posaconazole or fluconazole for prophylaxis in severe graft-versus-host disease. [published correction appears in *N Engl J Med*. 2007 Jul 26;357(4):428]. *N Engl J Med*. 2007;356(4):335–347.

4.28 Infections in the ICU

Firza Alexander Gronthoud

CLINICAL CONSIDERATIONS

Critically ill patients in the intensive care unit (ICU) are at increased risk of infections because of underlying morbidities, surgical interventions, presence of intravascular devices and mechanical ventilation. Viral and fungal infections are more common, and timely pathogen recognition and appropriate treatment are more challenging in the intensive care. It is therefore worthwhile to consider the following.

INCREASED RISK OF INFECTION

Increased risk of infection is multifactorial. Important factors are disruption of natural anatomical barriers because of invasive procedures and presence of catheters. Severe sepsis can lead to immune paralysis and ageing has been associated with impairments in both innate and adaptive immunity, a phenomenon called immunosenescence.

BACTERIAL INFECTIONS

Most infections in the ICU are bacterial infections. Central venous catheter (CVC) associated bloodstream infections are common and often occur without any surrounding soft tissue infection. Patients may be admitted to the ICU with respiratory failure due to a severe community-acquired pneumonia or develop a hospital-acquired pneumonia or ventilator-associated pneumonia during admission. One of the most common reasons for admission to the ICU is post-surgery and intra-abdominal infections such as secondary peritonitis after bowel surgery. Other post-operative infections are surgical site wound infections which may be complicated by cellulitis or rarely necrotizing fasciitis. Finally, patients may develop urosepsis due to a combination of dehydration, electrolyte disturbances and acute kidney injury further facilitated by the presence of an indwelling bladder catheter.

MAIN CAUSES OF ICU-ACQUIRED BACTERAEMIA

Most of the bacteraemias in the ICU are CVC associated; other sources are the lower respiratory tract and the gastrointestinal tract (see Chapters 2.2 and 4.6). The main pathogens encountered in blood cultures are coagulase-negative staphylococci, *Escherichia coli*, *Klebsiella* spp., *Pseudomonas aeruginosa* and enterococci. With regard to gastrointestinal sources, the main causes of bacteraemias are cholangitis and secondary peritonitis with intra-abdominal abscesses, and polymicrobial bacteraemias can occur.

HIGHER PREVALENCE OF MULTIDRUG RESISTANCE IN THE ICU

Antibiotic resistance is more common in the ICU. Critically ill patients are more likely to have frequent exposure to antibiotics, which increases risk of multidrug-resistant infections through selection pressure. Consequently, there is also a reduced gut colonization resistance and increased colonization pressure in the ICU (see Chapter 1.1, 'Pillars of Infection Management'). Other factors associated with resistance are duration of hospitalization, use of invasive devices and immunosuppression and foreign travel. Especially with increased medical tourism, patients are more likely to harbour multidrug-resistant organisms.

DRUG-RESISTANT ORGANISMS ENCOUNTERED IN THE ICU

Extended-spectrum β-lactamase-producing *Enterobacterales* (ESBL-E), multidrug-resistant (MDR) *Pseudomonas aeruginosa*, carbapenem-resistant *Acinetobacter baumannii* and carbapenemase-producing *Enterobacterales* (CPE), methicillin-resistant *Staphylococcus aureus* (MRSA) and vancomycin-resistant enterococci (VRE).

ANTIBIOTIC STEWARDSHIP ON THE ICU IS CHALLENGING

In contrast to clinically stable febrile patients on the wards where antibiotics may be held until culture results come back, in critically ill patients with sepsis, this is difficult owing to the severity of their clinical condition. It must be noted though that up to 50% of febrile episodes may not be infectious. Another challenging factor is the typical slow turnaround time of bacterial culture and the reduced sensitivity of culture as patients may have frequent antibiotic exposure.

The ICU would especially benefit from rapid point-of-care tests and more rapid sensitive methods in the laboratory, such as molecular techniques which can provide rapid identification and detection of common resistance mechanisms and whole genome sequencing. Another method to improve diagnostics is use of biomarkers to rule out infection; an example is procalcitonin. This would ensure that adequate antibiotic therapy is given, whilst reducing unnecessary antimicrobial consumption.

PHARMACOKINETIC (PK) CONSIDERATIONS

Critically ill patients have altered physiology which impacts antibiotic dosing strategies. Factors such as increased volume of distribution (Vd) and increased or augmented renal clearance can rapidly decrease antibiotic effectiveness of hydrophilic antibiotics such as β-lactams, aminoglycosides, glycopeptides or colistin. Hypoalbuminaemia further contributes to increased Vd of highly protein-bound antibiotics such as β-lactams. Renal impairment, on the other hand, increases toxicity of antibiotics and drugs such as aminoglycosides and colistin need to be used with caution.

PHARMACODYNAMIC CONSIDERATIONS

β-lactams are time-dependent antibiotics whereby effectiveness can be increased by the use of continuous or extended infusions (see Chapter 3.8). For concentration-dependent antimicrobials, such as aminoglycosides or colistin, increased doses should be used. Higher doses of antibiotics may be indicated in critically ill with albuminaemia, increased volume of distribution or augmented renal function.

THERAPEUTIC DRUG MONITORING

Therapeutic drug monitoring (TDM), therefore, is important in reducing risk of antimicrobial toxicity and maximizing antibiotic effectiveness. Antibiotics for which TDM is routinely performed are aminoglycosides, glycopeptides and some azoles, but TDM should perhaps also be used for other antimicrobials such as β-lactams.

EMPIRIC ANTIBACTERIAL TREATMENT

Empiric antibiotic regimens should be based on local resistance patterns and individual risk factors for multidrug resistance and should cover likely bacterial flora associated with suspected source of infection. Most infections are endogenous, and knowledge of commensal flora and association with infection is useful (see Chapter 2.1).

The choice of antibiotics is also influenced by previous antibiotics used and positive results. The use of combination therapy consisting of β-lactam with aminoglycoside remains controversial but is used in immunocompromised patients with septic shock with no clear source of infection and high local prevalence of MDR bacteria. If the source of infection is known, for example, a pneumonia, then monotherapy is reasonable. Broad-spectrum antibiotics should be rationalized based on clinical improvement and microbiology results. Course duration should be as short as possible to reduce risk of colonization and emergence of MDR bacteria (See Chapter 1.1). Source control is essential.

SOURCE CONTROL

The aim of source control is to physically remove the infection and it can be achieved by drainage, debridement, device removal and compartment decompression (see Chapter 3.9). Source control also facilitates short antibiotic courses and allows for taking clinical samples for microbiology from the site of infection. Central venous catheters and an indwelling bladder catheter should be changed or removed in patients with septic shock without an obvious other source of infection.

STOPPING ANTIBIOTICS

If the patient is clinically stable and immunocompetent, and if microbiology cultures are negative and there is no obvious source of infection, then antibiotics could be stopped, with close monitoring of the patient.

INFECTION CONTROL

Infection control is essential in preventing transmission of MDRO, and key components are hand hygiene, isolation measures, environmental cleaning and, depending on local background prevalence, also surveillance culture for MRO.

VIRAL INFECTIONS

Viral infections are also more common in the ICU. Influenza is a common reason for ICU admission, owing to respiratory failure, and requires organ support and treatment with oseltamivir or zanamivir. These agents are most effective if started within 48 hours of onset of symptoms. Zanamivir is usually reserved for immunocompromised individuals or if there is a high likelihood that the strain is resistant to oseltamivir.

Respiratory syncytial virus can cause life-threatening respiratory distress in premature children, children up to the age of 1 year and patients with chronic lung disease, congenital heart disease, neuromuscular disorders or immunodeficiency. Systemic ribavirin or aerosolized ribavirin have been used with success.

Herpes simplex can reactivate and has been linked to ventilator-associated pneumonia. Critically ill patients with haematopoietic stem cell transplants are at risk of reactivation with cytomegalovirus and adenovirus. Epstein–Barr virus is a major concern in transplant recipients, owing to risk of post-transplant lymphoproliferative disease.

FUNGAL INFECTIONS

Most fungal infections in the ICU are caused by *Candida* spp. and present mainly as candidaemia or intra-abdominal candidiasis; important risk factors are broad-spectrum antibiotics, increased colonization with *Candida* spp., intravascular devices and surgery (see Chapter 4.32).

Invasive pulmonary aspergillosis can complicate patients on high-dose steroids (for exacerbation of COPD), liver cirrhosis, profound neutropaenia (i.e. on treatment for haematological malignancies or HSCT recipients), mechanical ventilation, ECMO, influenza, and Child–Pugh C hepatic cirrhosis and sepsis-induced immunoparalysis (see Chapter 4.34).

CLINICAL APPROACH

EMPIRICAL ANTIBACTERIAL TREATMENT

Empirical treatment and choice of antibiotics should be informed by suspected location of infection, previous antibiotic exposure, previous positive cultures and immune-host factors. The choice of antibiotics should be based on local and national guidelines and informed by local antimicrobial susceptibilities.

EMPIRICAL ANTIFUNGAL TREATMENT

Empirical antifungal therapy should be considered in patients with sepsis and known risk factors for fungal infection (see 'Fungal Infections' section), patients in whom no clear source has been identified and those who are not responding to antibacterial treatment. The decision to start fungal treatment should be discussed with an infection specialist.

Empirical treatment for invasive candidiasis in the ICU is an echinocandin. A 1,3-β-D-glucan should be collected. If negative, then echinocandin should be stopped.

If aspergillosis is suspected, then first-line treatment is voriconazole, but care should be taken for risk of drug-drug interactions (see Chapter 3.7), and therapeutic drug monitoring should be undertaken.

Daily review of antimicrobial treatment:

- Clinical signs and symptoms of infection
- Suspected source of infection
- Microbiology results
- Dosing strategy
- Daily consideration of de-escalating to narrow-spectrum agents and shorter duration of treatment

When no clinical response to antibiotic therapy, consider:

- Empiric therapy that is not active against the infecting organism
- Lack of source control, i.e. inadequate drainage of collection, infected intravascular or indwelling catheters
- Altered volumes of distribution leading to subtherapeutic serum concentrations of antibiotics
- Development of secondary infections of hospital-acquired, MDR microbes, i.e. VAP due to MDR *Pseudomonas aeruginosa*

CLINICAL PEARL

Dosing of antimicrobials should be reviewed frequently because fluctuations in fluid status, organ function (i.e. renal function) and perfusion can affect antibiotic pharmacokinetics and therefore antibiotic efficacy at the site of infection.

- Consider post-operative complications

- Selection of *Candida*, enterococci or *Pseudomonas aeruginosa*
- Patient-specific factors such as immunosuppression may impair recovery of infection and increase risk of viral reactivation or opportunistic infections (i.e. aspergillosis, *Nocardia*, PJP, toxoplasma)

BIBLIOGRAPHY

Campion M, Scully G. Antibiotic use in the intensive care unit: Optimization and de-escalation. *J Intensive Care Med.* 2018 December;33(12):647–655.

Colombo AL, de Almeida Júnior JN, Slavin MA, Chen SC, Sorrell TC. Candida and invasive mould diseases in non-neutropenic critically ill patients and patients with haematological cancer. *Lancet Infect Dis.* 2017 November;17(11):e344–e356.

Monneret G, Venet F, Kullberg BJ, Netea MG. ICU-acquired immunosuppression and the risk for secondary fungal infections. *Med Mycol.* 2011 April;49(Suppl 1):S17–S23.

Timsit JF, Bassetti M, Cremer O et al. Rationalizing antimicrobial therapy in the ICU: A narrative review. *Intensive Care Med.* 2019 February;45(2):172–189.

Timsit JF, Soubirou JF, Voiriot G, Chemam S, Neuville M, Mourvillier B, Sonneville R, Mariotte E, Bouadma L, Wolff M. Treatment of bloodstream infections in ICUs. *BMC Infect Dis.* 2014 November 28;14:489.

Zafrani L, Azoulay E. How to treat severe infections in critically ill neutropenic patients? *BMC Infect Dis.* 2014 November 28;14:512.

4.29 Infectious Diarrhoea

Firza Alexander Gronthoud

CLINICAL CONSIDERATIONS

Infectious diarrhoea is one of the most common diseases in the world and one of the five most important causes of death. Aetiology and diagnostic tests for infective diarrhoea depend on duration of symptoms, if the diarrhoea is community or hospital acquired, whether the patient is immunocompromised and if there is a travel history. It is therefore worthwhile to consider the following.

Common causes of infectious diarrhoea overall:

- Community acquired: *Campylobacter* spp., *Salmonella* spp., norovirus and rotavirus
- Hospital acquired: *Clostridium difficile*, norovirus
- Children: Rotavirus, norovirus
- Immunocompromised: *Cryptosporidium parvum* and cytomegalovirus

INFECTIOUS CAUSES ACCORDING TO DURATION

Infectious acute diarrhoea lasts less than 14 days. Infectious diarrhoea lasting more than 14 days is called persistent diarrhoea. Diarrhoea lasting up to 14 days is almost always infectious. Infectious chronic diarrhoea persists more than 30 days and is more likely to be caused by parasites.

Infectious causes according to type of stool:

- *Watery diarrhoea*: This indicates secretory gastroenteritis of proximal small intestine caused by *Vibrio cholerae, Clostridium perfringens, Bacillus cereus, Staphylococcus aureus, Escherichia coli* (enterotoxigenic [ETEC], enteropathogenic [EPEC], enteroaggregative [EAEC], heat-labile toxin [LT], heat-stable toxin [ST]), *Giardia lamblia*, rotavirus, norovirus, *Cryptosporidium* spp., microsporidia (HIV and transplant recipients) and *Cyclospora cayetanensis*.
- *Dysentery*: This indicates colitis caused by *Shigella* spp., STEC, *Salmonella* spp. (not *Salmonella typhi/paratyphi*), *Vibrio parahaemolyticus, Clostridioides difficile, Campylobacter* spp., *E. coli* (enterohaemorrhagic [EHEC], enteroinvasive [EIEC]), *Salmonella enteritidis, Vibrio parahaemolyticus, Campylobacter jejuni* and *Entamoeba histolytica*.
- *Enteric fever*: Invasive disease caused by *Salmonella enterica* serotype Typhi and *S. enterica* serotype Paratyphi A, B and C.

CLINICAL PEARL

With increasing frequency, in high-income nations, the aetiology of diarrhoea is non-infectious. In these cases, diarrhoea is caused by food intolerances, reactions to medication, intestinal disorders such as irritable bowel syndrome or intestinal diseases, including Crohn's disease, ulcerative colitis and celiac disease.

COMMUNITY-ACQUIRED DIARRHOEA

Common Causes of Bacterial Gastroenteritis

Bacterial gastroenteritis typically has an acute onset with fever and watery diarrhoea. Enterohaemorrhagic *E. coli* O157:H7 is an important cause of bloody gastroenteritis.

Medically important *Salmonella* spp. causing diarrhoea are *S. choleraesuis*, *S. typhimurium* and *S. enteritidis*. Most infections are acquired by eating poultry, eggs or dairy products and are transmitted through the fecal-oral route. *Shigella* spp. cause dysentery, which is a clinical syndrome consisting of fever, bloody diarrhoea and abdominal pain. Shigellosis is primarily caused by *S. dysenteriae*, *S. flexneri*, *S. boydii* and *S. sonnei*. *Shigella* spp. are genetically very similar to *E. coli* and are now biogroups within the species *E. coli*. Humans are the only reservoir for *Shigella* spp., with more than half of all infections occurring in children younger than 10 years. Shigellosis is transmitted person-to-person by the fecal-oral route through contaminated hands and, less commonly, contaminated water or food. *Yersinia enterocolitica* can grow in cold temperature and can grow to high numbers in refrigerated food or blood products and is associated with transfusion-related sepsis. Enteric disease in children may manifest as enlarge mesenteric lymph nodes and mimic acute appendicitis. Yersinosis is a zoonotic infection, with humans as accidental hosts.

Viral Gastroenteritis

Norovirus is an important cause of diarrhoea in children and a major cause of hospital outbreaks of diarrhoea and vomiting. Enterovirus is another viral cause of community-acquired diarrhoea, and incidence is highest in the summer months. Adenovirus and rotavirus gastroenteritis are mainly seen in infants, children and immunocompromised individuals. From 2006 onwards, countries have been implementing rotavirus vaccination in infants as part of national immunization schedules which led to a dramatic reduction in cases of more than 70%.

In immunocompromised individuals presenting with bloody colitis, the most common viral causes are cytomegalovirus, adenovirus, Epstein–Barr virus and, less often, herpes simplex. Rotavirus can cause severe morbidity in immunocompromised individuals: prolonged diarrhoea, extraintestinal manifestations and associations with other gastrointestinal pathology such as graft-versus-host disease (GvHD), mucositis and colitis have been described. Other common viral causes of community-acquired diarrhoea are sapovirus and astrovirus.

CLINICAL PEARL

Rotavirus is a non-enveloped RNA virus and the most common cause of diarrhoea and vomiting in children and can lead to life-threatening dehydration and death. Rotavirus can be divided into serotypes A, B, C, D and E, with serotype A accounting for >90% of all human infections. It can also be divided into genotypes, with G1, G2, G3, G4 and G9 being the most common genotypes. The rotavirus vaccine efficacy is >80%–90%. The vaccine strain is also shed in the stool for at least 14 days; however, the risk of transmission and vaccine-derived disease is lower compared to the wild-type strain. The risk of intussusception is 1–2 cases per 100,000 first doses in some populations. To avoid this risk, the first dose is given at 6–15 weeks of age and the final dose at maximum age of 32 weeks.

Parasitic Gastroenteritis

The most common parasitic causes of diarrhoea in the developed world are *Giardia lamblia* and *Cryptosporidium* spp. Especially in the immunocompromised, *Cryptosporidium* spp. causes severe and potentially life-threatening diarrhoea. There is no proven treatment for crypotosporidiosis but nitazoxanide has been used with some success.

HOSPITAL-ACQUIRED DIARRHOEA

Hospital-acquired diarrhoea occurs after >72 hours in the hospital. The most common cause is *Clostrioides difficile*, an anaerobic Gram-positive, spore-forming rod. Diarrhoea is caused by toxins A and B and is elicited by broad-spectrum antibiotics including ciprofloxacin, clindamycin and has also been linked to third-generation cephalosporins. Proton-pump inhibitors are linked to *C. difficile* colonization. Clinical manifestations vary from asymptomatic, mild or severe colitis (see Chapter 5.9 for diagnosis, management and prevention). Norovirus is an important cause of outbreaks of diarrhoea and vomiting causes many wards to close in order to contain outbreaks.

Besides classifying gastroenteritis according to type of diarrhoea or community acquired versus hospital acquired, it is also helpful when taking a patient history to explore specific risk factors associated with infectious diarrhoea.

INFECTIOUS CAUSES ACCORDING TO SPECIFIC RISK FACTORS

Contaminated Water

Aeromonas spp. are ubiquitous in aquatic habitats, and risk of *Aeromonas* infection is highest during summer months when the temperature of the water peaks. *Aeromonas* spp. can be found in poultry, lamb, veal, pork and ground beef. Consumption of these food products or contact with water during, i.e. recreational sports, are the most common sources of infection. *Aeromonas* spp. can also be found in asymptomatic carriers. Parasitic infections occurring in untreated fresh or drinking water are *Giardia lamblia* and *Cryptosporidium* spp.

Sanitation

Cholera is caused by *Vibrio cholerae*, a Gram-negative rod. Typical diarrhoea has a rice-water appearance. Cholera is a disease of poverty and poor sanitary conditions. Complications of cholera are severe dehydration, metabolic acidosis and hypokalaemia. The key principle is aggressive rehydration. Ringer's lactate is preferred over saline. Antibiotic treatment consists of a tetracycline or quinolone and rehydration. Blood pressure should be monitored.

Food-Borne Gastroenteritis

- Unpasteurized dairy products: *Listeria monocytogenes*, *Brucella* spp.
- Shellfish: *Plesiomonas*, *Aeromonas*
- Raw or undercooked meat or poultry: *Campylobacter* spp., *Salmonella* spp., *Yersinia enterocolitica*, *E. coli*
- Consumption of undercooked eggs: *Salmonella* spp., *Shigella* spp.

Food Poisoning

Food poisoning is another form of gastroenteritis acquired in the community. It typically occurs within hours after consuming a contaminated meal. Clinical symptoms are nausea, vomiting and diarrhoea. It is most caused by toxins produced by *S. aureus*, *B. cereus* and *C. perfringens*.

CLINICAL APPROACH

Indications for sending stool sample to the laboratory:

- *Type of stool*: Severe, prolonged or bloody diarrhoea
- *Clinical symptoms*: Fever of ≥38.5°C, dehydration or systemic signs of infection
- *Medical history*: Significant comorbidities, immunocompromised, recent use of antibiotics

Clinical information on test request:

- Acute/outbreak case
- Immune status
- Healthcare or community acquired; if patient is hospitalized, then the date of admission and date of onset of symptoms should be on the request form
- Recent foreign travel (2–3 weeks) including location
- Exposure to recreational water facilities, fresh water sources and animal exposure
- Food intake (e.g. shellfish, chicken)
- Recent antibiotic use
- Other information (i.e. suspected food poisoning, viral gastroenteritis, contact with cases)
- Day-care centre visits

Test requests:

- Bacterial culture and sensitivity testing.
- If the patient develops diarrhoea after 48 hours of admission, then only *C. difficile* should be tested.
- Prolonged diarrhoea should prompt testing for parasitic causes.
- In children, stool should initially be investigated for rotavirus, adenovirus and norovirus. Several rapid tests and ELISA kits exist, but the most sensitive method is PCR.
- In immunocompromised individuals, the gold standard for diagnosing CMV colitis is a histology on a tissue sample showing nuclear inclusion bodies. A PCR can also be performed but cannot distinguish between latent infection and active infection. EDTA blood can also be sent for PCR, but a negative blood PCR does not rule out localized gut infection.

LABORATORY DIAGNOSIS

Modern laboratories nowadays detect common bacterial pathogens with multiplex PCR, which is highly sensitive and there is no added benefit of sending a repeat sample. Limitations of PCR is that it can only detect specific pathogens and cannot differentiate between colonization and infection. It is therefore important to ensure detailed clinical information is on the request form so the microbiology laboratory, if indicated, can perform extra tests for bacterial pathogens not included in their multiplex PCR.

Some laboratories still perform bacterial culture and it may be useful to send a second stool sample.

The laboratory diagnosis of *C. difficile* follows a two-tier or three-tier testing algorithm which is discussed in detail in Chapter 5.9. Stool samples sent within 7 days of the first sample are almost always negative. In addition, *C. difficile* can be detected in the stool for up to 28 days (or longer) after successful treatment, and a recurrent *C. difficile* infection within this interval is diagnosed based on clinical symptoms.

Tests for parasitic eggs and cysts should be performed in returning travellers with persistent gastrointestinal symptoms, or development of symptoms after exposure to outbreaks, or if immunocompromised such as HIV or bone marrow transplant. Similar to bacterial testing, PCR is becoming more mainstream and suffers from the same limitations.

TREATMENT

Rather, the primary goal for the patient with acute diarrhoea is symptomatic relief, rehydration (or prevention of dehydration) and preventing transmission of the infection. Treatment is indicated for severe cases of salmonellosis, shigellosis or *Campylobacter* spp., or in infections in the immunocompromised. *Campylobacter* infections are treated with a macrolide, quinolone or, alternatively, a tetracycline. *Salmonella* and *Shigella* infections are treated with ciprofloxacin or trimethoprim/sulfamethoxazole. Alternatively, azithromycin can be used. Treatment duration is 7 days. For immunocompromised individuals, a longer course may be necessary. *Salmonella* infections can be complicated by long-term carriage (see Chapter 4.56).

Treatment for CMV colitis consists of 3 weeks of (val)ganciclovir and two negative consecutive PCR results.

CLINICAL PEARL

Antibiotic therapy for gastroenteritis can have negative consequences. Antibiotics are associated with inducing HUS in STEC infection by stimulating toxin production. Antibiotics can also prolong carriage of *Salmonella* and can induce *C. difficile* disease in patients colonized with *C. difficile*. Finally, antibiotics increase risk of emergence of antibiotic drug resistance by disrupting the gut microbiota and reducing colonization resistance (see Chapter 1.1).

BIBLIOGRAPHY

Bruijning-Verhagen P, Nipshagen MD, de Graaf H, Bonten MJM. Rotavirus disease course among immunocompromised patients; 5-year observations from a tertiary care medical centre. *J Infect.* 2017 November;75(5):448–454.

Corcoran MS, van Well GT, van Loo IH. Diagnosis of viral gastroenteritis in children: Interpretation of real-time PCR results and relation to clinical symptoms. *Eur J Clin Microbiol Infect Dis.* 2014 October;33(10):1663–1673.

Humphries RM, Linscott AJ. Laboratory diagnosis of bacterial gastroenteritis. *Clin Microbiol Rev.* 2015 January;28(1):3–31.

Lübbert C. Antimicrobial therapy of acute diarrhoea: A clinical review. *Expert Rev Anti Infect Ther.* 2016;14(2):193–206.

Shane AL, Mody RK, Crump JA et al. . 2017 Infectious Diseases Society of America clinical practice guidelines for the diagnosis and management of infectious diarrhea. *Clin Infect Dis.* 2017 November 29;65(12):e45–e80.

4.30 Influenza

Firza Alexander Gronthoud

CLINICAL CONSIDERATIONS

Influenza is caused by influenza A and influenza B. Influenza can range from a mild, self-limiting illness to respiratory failure. Although the best method for preventing influenza is vaccination, the efficacy of the vaccine depends on how well it is matched with the circulating strain. Antiviral treatment is most effective if given within a couple of days after onset of symptoms and post-exposure prophylaxis may be indicated in some patients. It is therefore worthwhile to consider the following.

PATHOGENESIS

Viral proteins involved in the pathogenesis of influenza A are hemagglutinin (HA) and neuraminidase (NA). There are 16 HA subtypes and 9 NA subtypes. In contrast, there are only two antigenically distinct lineages of influenza B.

Gradual mutations in genes encoding for HA and NA result in antigenically different influenza strains, which are not recognized by circulating antibodies, offering influenza a way of evading the immune system, a process called antigenic drift.

The term antigenic shift is used when a novel influenza subtype is introduced in the population. This can be a result of exchange of genetic material between different influenza subtypes, a process called 're-assortment'. Consequently, novel HA and/or new HA and NA proteins emerge. This antigenic shift is clinically more significant than antigenic drift, not only because it provides influenza A the ability to escape the immune system, but also because an influenza virus previously only circulating in the animal reservoir now also can cross over to humans, such as in the case of the 2009 pandemic swine flu, H1N1. Antigenic drift and shift are the main reason why every year the influenza vaccines need to be updated in order to match the circulating influenza strains in that particular year.

INCUBATION PERIOD

The incubation period is between 1 and 4 days.

SYMPTOMS

Symptoms can range from fever, sore throat, myalgia, general malaise, diarrhoea to respiratory failure. Infection with influenza may also be asymptomatic, during which patients may still be shedding the virus in the oropharynx and are at risk of spreading it to others. Symptoms of influenza usually lasts between 3 and 7 days, although cough and malaise can persist for >2 weeks, especially in elderly people and those with chronic lung disease.

COMPLICATIONS

Complications include bacterial superinfections with *Streptococcus pneumoniae*, *Pseudomonas aeruginosa* and *Staphylococcus aureus*. Other complications are respiratory failure, multiorgan failure, encephalopathy and worsening of pre-existing medical conditions.

TRANSMISSION

Transmission occurs through droplets and contaminated hands, facilitating rapid transmission. The environment may also become contaminated. Aerosol generating procedures such as intubation cause aerosolization, which enables Influenza to spread through the airborne route.

PERIOD OF SHEDDING

The period of shedding is commonly between 5 and 7 days, but may be prolonged, i.e. in immunocompromised individuals. It is therefore highly advisable that even when the symptoms have resolved, patients continue to have good hand hygiene.

RISK FACTORS FOR COMPLICATED INFLUENZA

Risk factors for complications are patients with underlying chronic diseases, diabetes mellitus, elderly >65 years, pregnant women, infants <6 months, morbid obesity and severe immunosuppression (i.e. bone marrow and solid organ transplant recipients, primary immunodeficiencies, HIV with CD4 <200/µL and high dose corticosteroid use).

ANTIVIRAL TREATMENT

The two main antivirals, oseltamivir and zanamivir, inhibit the neuraminidase enzyme. Oseltamivir is only available by mouth whereas zanamivir is available intravenously and as a powder for inhalation. Zanamivir is usually reserved as a second line. Considerations for zanamivir are circulating strain is high-risk for development of oseltamivir resistance (i.e. pandemic 2009 H1N1 is high risk) in immunocompromised individuals or severe disease not responding to oseltamivir.

Both agents have a reduced effectiveness if administered beyond 48 hours from onset of symptoms. Oseltamivir has been shown to reduce influenza symptoms by one day, albeit with a reduction in influenza-related complications. Oseltamivir drug resistance is an emerging concern.

PREVENTION

Vaccination remains the cornerstone of prevention and control of seasonal epidemics. There are three types of influenza vaccines available: a live, attenuated influenza vaccine (LAIV), an inactivated influenza vaccine (IIV) and a recombinant HA vaccine. The main shortcoming of influenza vaccines is that annual updates are needed to retain effectiveness because of antigenic shift occurring. It takes about 14 days for the vaccine to become protective, with a vaccine effectiveness generally ranging between 40% and 70%. Furthermore, the vaccine is less effective in the elderly, requiring a vaccine adjuvant or a higher dose potentially. Recently, a vaccine for avian influenza H5N1 has been developed.

Inactivated influenza vaccines (IIVs) are the most used influenza vaccines.

Haemagglutinin is the most immunogenic viral protein and is the primary target of IIV-induced antibody response. The degree of antibody cross-reactivity with other influenza subtypes is dependent on antigenic similarities in HA between different subtypes. Inactivated vaccines do not provide immediate protection, and it may take up to 14 days before it is protective. The LAIV cannot be used in immunocompromised individuals. LAIV are grown in eggs which takes a considerate amount of time during which a new circulating influenza subtype can emerge, rendering the growing LAIV ineffective. There is also a risk of occurrence of mutations rendering LAIV ineffective.

CLINICAL APPROACH

CLINICAL DIAGNOSIS

The positive predictive value of any adult influenza case definition has ranged from 18%–87% compared with laboratory-confirmed influenza. During periods of influenza prevalence, clinical diagnosis (based on the acute onset of high fever and cough) can be highly predictive of influenza (PPV 79%–87%; NPV 39%–75%). The probability of a patient having confirmed influenza increases with increasing fever and acute presentation (within 36–48 hours of onset).

DIAGNOSIS

The best samples are nasopharyngeal aspirate, nasopharyngeal swab and deep respiratory samples. Alternatively a nose & throat swab can be taken. Many laboratories offer a highly sensitive multiplex PCR in which multiple respiratory viruses can be detected, including influenza. Rapid point-of-care tests are either antigen based or rapid commercial PCR.

ANTIGEN-BASED, RAPID POINT-OF-CARE TESTS

First generation antigen-based tests have a sensitivity which varies from 40% to 80%. Newer digital antigen tests have an improved sensitivity of 70%–80%.

Nasal aspirates, nasal washes, sputa and nasopharyngeal swabs, especially those specimens containing cellular material, are preferable to nasal swabs and throat swabs.

Rapid tests cannot distinguish amongst influenza A subtypes. Especially during peak influenza season, the negative predictive value is low and negative results should be confirmed with PCR.

During low influenza activity, the positive predictive value is low and negative predictive value high. Therefore, during low influenza activity, a positive test needs to be confirmed with PCR.

Rapid tests are recommended to be used only when they can influence timely patient management.

TREATMENT

First-line treatment is oseltamivir 75 mg 12-hourly for 5 days. If there is a high risk of development of oseltamivir in the circulating strain and the patient is immunocompromised, then first-line treatment is zanamivir by inhalation 10 mg twice daily for 5 days. If inhalation is not possible or in severe complicated illness, then the alternative is intravenous zanamivir 600 mg twice daily. It is reasonable to extend the course duration in immunosuppressed individuals based on clinical response. Dose adjustments for oseltamivir and zanamivir need to be made based on renal function.

ANTIBACTERIAL TREATMENT

Influenza may be complicated by a bacterial superinfection. It is reasonable to start antibacterial treatment pending culture results in severely unwell patients or in patients with a chest X-ray suggesting bacterial pneumonia, i.e. lobar infiltrate.

PREVENTION

Patients with influenza should be isolated in a single room. Infection control precautions may vary per institution. Some institutions recommend a surgical mask to be worn within 2 metres distance, and in the case of an aerosol-generating procedure such as intubation or suctioning, a FFP3 or N95 mask should be worn, whereas in other hospitals, it is recommended to always wear a respirator. It is therefore recommended to adhere to local infection control guidelines.

If a patient with influenza needs to go to radiology for an X-ray, it is recommended that the patient wears a surgical mask to avoid spreading influenza to the environment.

DURATION OF ISOLATION

Duration of shedding is usually similar to duration of symptoms. Risk of transmission is highest when patients are symptomatic. It is therefore reasonable to isolate patients until symptoms have resolved. In an immunocompromised individual, some institutions repeat a PCR to see if the virus has been cleared before the patient is de-isolated. However, a PCR may not distinguish between a viable ('live') and a nonviable ('dead') virus.

POST-EXPOSURE PROPHYLAXIS

Post-exposure prophylaxis (PEP) is needed for contacts of influenza who are at risk for complicated influenza. PEP consists of oseltamivir 75 mg once daily for 10 days and should be given within 48 hours after exposure. If oseltamivir cannot be used, then zanamivir by inhalation 10 mg once daily should be started within 36 hours after exposure. Contacts who have been vaccinated $\geq$14 days ago do not require PEP unless the vaccine is not well matched with the circulating strain or if the patient is severely immunosuppressed.

ASPERGILLUS AND INFLUENZA

In recent years, there has been an increased incidence of influenza-associated invasive pulmonary aspergillosis (IPA) among critically ill patients, previously fit and well, admitted to the intensive care unit. These patients developed IPA shortly after admission to the ICU, indicating a superinfection rather than hospital acquired. Influenza causes an inflammatory response that damages the bronchial mucosa, disrupts mucous ciliary clearance mechanisms and has immunomodulatory effects, all which may facilitate IPA. The use of steroids further increases the risk of IPA.

Therefore, in critically ill patients with influenza who are not responding to antiviral treatment and broad-spectrum antibiotics and on steroids, clinicians should be aware of the possibility of IPA (see Chapter 4.34 for diagnosis and treatment). It is not known if prophylactic antifungal therapy is indicated in critically ill patients with influenza.

BIBLIOGRAPHY

Public Health England. PHE guidance on use of antiviral agents for the treatment and prophylaxis of seasonal influenza. 2019. https://assets.publishing.service.gov.uk/government/uploads/system/uploads/attachment_data/file/833572/PHE_guidance_antivirals_influenza_201920.pdf
Schauwvlieghe AFAD, Rijnders BJA, Philips N et al. Invasive aspergillosis in patients admitted to the intensive care unit with severe influenza: A retrospective cohort study. *Lancet Respir Med.* 2018;6(10):782–792.
Uyeki TM, Bernstein HH, Bradley JS et al. Clinical practice guidelines by the infectious diseases society of america: 2018 update on diagnosis, treatment, chemoprophylaxis, and institutional outbreak management of seasonal influenzaa [published correction appears in *Clin Infect Dis.* 2019 May 2;68(10):1790]. *Clin Infect Dis.* 2019;68(6):e1–e47.

4.31 Intra-Abdominal Infections

Firza Alexander Gronthoud

CLINICAL CONSIDERATIONS

Intra-abdominal infection (IAI) is an umbrella term for a wide range of infections involving any organ in the abdomen and/or the peritoneum (peritonitis). IAI can be classified as uncomplicated or complicated IAI. Peritonitis can be classified as primary or secondary peritonitis. Management of IAI depends on the anatomical location of the infection, the extent of infection and suspected pathogen involved. It is therefore worthwhile to consider the following.

UNCOMPLICATED VERSUS COMPLICATED IAI

Uncomplicated IAI is a localized organ infection without peritonitis. Examples are liver abscess, splenic abscess or diverticulitis or appendicitis which has not perforated. In complicated IAI, in addition to an infected organ, there is also peritoneal involved with one or more multiple intra-abdominal abscesses or fecal soiling; examples are perforated appendicitis, perforated diverticulitis or intestinal perforation or anastomotic leakage.

PERITONITIS

Peritonitis in itself can occur without organ involvement. Primary bacterial peritonitis can be seen in patients with liver cirrhosis and ascites where the ascitic fluid becomes infected, usually with one organism. This is also called spontaneous bacterial peritonitis or SBP. Primary bacterial peritonitis can also occur in patients with an indwelling peritoneal dialysis catheter where, through an infected catheter, bacteria can infect the peritoneum.

Secondary peritonitis is the most common form of peritonitis and occurs where there is an intestinal perforation with intestinal spillage into the peritoneum. This can occur after a trauma or anastomotic leakage or after local necrosis as can be seen in a burst appendicitis or diverticulitis. Typical signs of peritonitis are fever, abdominal pain, rebound tenderness and abdominal guarding.

RELAPSED PERITONITIS

Relapses may occur after >48 h after apparently successful and adequate surgical source control of secondary peritonitis. This is more common in immunocompromised or critically ill patients and is associated with multidrug-resistant bacteria.

MICROBIOLOGY

The most common bacteria involved in intra-abdominal infections are intestinal flora such as *Escherichia coli*, *Klebsiella* spp., streptococci and anaerobes (see Chapter 2.1). There is still some debate on whether enterococci and *Candida* spp. should be covered with initial empirical treatment. During later stages of treatment, more drug-resistant bacteria start to emerge, such as *Pseudomonas aeruginosa* and *Enterococcus faecium* as well as *Candida* spp. *Candida* spp. may also initially be involved in the case of an oesophageal or gastric perforation. Drain fluids may at some point start to grow coagulase-negative staphylococci and *Stenotrophomonas maltophilia*, but initially, these organisms represent colonization. With prolonged antibiotic treatment, they are selected out and may cause a retrograde drain infection. In peritoneal-dialysis-associated peritonitis, the predominant bacteria involved are staphylococci. Of special note are viridans streptococci belonging to the milleri (or anginosus) group: *S. intermedius*, *S. constellatus* and *S. anginosus*). These streptococci are associated with abscess formation, including intraperitoneal abscesses, liver abscess and empyema.

MANAGEMENT OF IAI

Management of IAI consists of source control and empiric antimicrobial therapy broad enough to cover all likely organisms. Adequate source control is mandatory in the management of complicated IAIs.

SOURCE CONTROL

The goal of source control is to eliminate the source of infection, reduce the bacterial burden and correct or control anatomic derangements to restore normal physiologic function. Inadequate source control increases mortality in patients with complicated IAI and prolongs antibiotic therapy (see Chapter 3.9). Examples of source control in IAI are drainage, resection or debridement of necrotic tissue, as is the case in necrotizing pancreatitis.

Source control also enables collection of specimens from the site of infection and culture and sensitivity results can be used to guide antibiotic therapy. It is important to avoid sending drain fluid that has been sitting in the collection bag for hours as contaminating flora have started to overgrow, and anaerobes may not have survived. A primary peritonitis can be confirmed with ascitic fluid polymorphonuclear leukocyte (PMN) count of ≥ 250 cells/mm^3 (0.25×10^9/L) and a positive ascitic fluid bacterial culture.

EMPIRICAL THERAPY

The main goal of empirical antibiotic therapy is to prevent local and haematogenous spread, and to reduce late complications. Antibiotic therapy should cover most likely microbes involved and, if possible, informed by local antibiotic-resistance rates and previous positive microbiology culture results. Local hospital antibiotic guidelines should therefore be followed.

Risk factors for multidrug-resistant organisms should also be taken into account (see Chapter 3.1). If a patient has recently finished a course of antibiotics, it may be reasonable to use different antibiotic agents depending on the previous course length and time interval.

It is important to use the right dose, frequency and mode of administration, i.e. in critically ill patients, an extended infusion or continuous infusion for β-lactam agents may be used, a higher intravenous doses for ciprofloxacin or aminoglycosides should be used, and a higher pre-dose level for glycopeptides should be aimed for.

Therapeutic drug monitoring should be performed for aminoglycosides and glycopeptides, and antibiotic allergy status should be critically reviewed (see Chapter 3.3). Before starting antibiotics, it is important to review the drug chart for any potential drug-drug interactions.

Empirical therapy is usually initially only targeted towards bacteria, but antifungal cover against *Candida* spp. may be started if risk factors are present (see chapter 4.32) or if there is no clinical response after 48 hours of broad-spectrum antibacterial treatment despite source control. In this case, it is reasonable to start an echinocandin (ideally in critically ill or immunocompromised patients) or fluconazole and discontinue if the 1,3-β-D-glucan test is negative.

Antibiotic treatment should be reviewed daily and de-escalated based on clinical response, microbiology results and source control. During treatment, the patient should also be monitored for known drug side effects or interactions.

A randomized clinical trial showed no difference in outcome comparing a 4-day versus 10-day treatment duration when successful source control was achieved.

CLINICAL APPROACH

Spontaneous Bacterial Peritonitis (SBP)

SBP occurs almost always in patients with a cirrhotic liver and ascites. Patients may be asymptomatic or present with fever, abdominal pain, or altered mental status. Ascites WBC cell count in SBP is $\geq$250 mm^3. It may be useful to do a CT abdomen to rule out a secondary peritonitis.

SBP is usually a monomicrobial infection. It is reasonable to start amoxicillin/clavulanic acid or a third-generation cephalosporin such as ceftriaxone or cefotaxime. Treatment duration is 5 days. In patients who have multiple ascitic taps for recurrent ascites, coagulase negative staphylococci may be involved as well. A combination of vancomycin and gentamicin is reasonable. If there is a suspicion of traumatic puncture of the gut, then metronidazole may be added, or if there is no concern for coagulase negative staphylococci, but gut flora cover is needed, then amoxicillin/clavulanic acid +/− gentamicin or piperacillin/tazobactam.

A follow-up ascitic tap is not needed. In patients who present with few symptoms of infection and are haemodynamically stable, consider holding off antibiotics until ascitic culture results are back.

Secondary peritonitis should be suspected if the ascitic fluid contains total protein >1 g/dL (10 g/L), glucose <50 mg/dL (2.8 mmol/L) LDH > the upper limit of normal for serum (2 out of 3 parameters) as well as multiple bacteria in the ascitic fluid.

Peritoneal Dialysis-Associated Infections

Peritoneal dialysis (PD) can be complicated by infection of the peritoneum, subcutaneous tunnel and catheter exit site. A cloudy peritoneal dialysate fluid can have non-infectious causes such as chemical inflammation, hemoperitoneum, eosinophilia of the effluent, malignancy, or chylus.

A cell count should be performed on the dialysis fluid, and PMNs of $\geq$100 mm^3 is seen in PD peritonitis. Bacterial culture should be performed, and sensitivity of culture can be enhanced by enrichment broth.

The most frequently involved bacteria are *Staphylococcus aureus* and coagulase-negative staphylococci, but *Enterobacterales* and enterococci have also been reported. Initial therapy consists of vancomycin with gentamicin which can be given intravenously or intraperitoneally. In either case, it is recommended to monitor the pre-dose levels. Duration of treatment is 2–3 weeks.

Candida albicans is the predominant cause of fungal PD peritonitis and risk is increased after multiple antibacterial courses. Duration of antifungal treatment is at least 3 weeks.

Indications for PD catheter removal are:

- Persistent cloudy PD fluid or no clinical improvement after 5 days
- Difficult to treat organism such as *S. aureus*, *P. aeruginosa* or *Candida* spp.
- Relapsing peritonitis
- Concurrent exit site or tunnel infection

If the PD catheter is removed, then dialysis is converted to haemodialysis. Prophylactic antibiotics before PD catheter placement reduces risk of infection, and eradication of *S. aureus* nasal carriage may be indicated.

Perforation of the Colon or Anastomotic Leak in Post-Operative Patients

Patient may go back to theatre for a washout and closure of the leak or conservative management. If there is a drainable collection and anatomically approachable, this should be performed as soon as possible. Fresh drain fluids should be sent to the microbiology laboratory for culture and sensitivity testing. When adequate source control has been achieved and patient is clinically and biochemically improving, antibiotics should be stopped after 4–5 days. If a patient is not improving despite antibiotic treatment and drainage, then it may be useful to repeat a CT abdomen and consider changing the size and/or location of the drain or place a second drain. In addition, send new microbiology cultures, review the drug chart to ensure optimal dose and administration of antibiotics and consider other sources of infection or other non-infectious causes of fever.

INTRA-ABDOMINAL CANDIDIASIS

Clinical features of intra-abdominal candidiasis are non-specific. Echinocandins or fluconazole may be indicated in cases where there is no clinical response after 48 hours of antibacterial treatment and adequate source control and there is no other source of infection. Alternatively, the *Candida* scoring system may be used. Clinical scoring parameters used are severe sepsis, total parenteral nutrition, surgery and multifocal *Candida* colonization. Higher score indicates increased risk of invasive candidiasis. *Candida* score has a high sensitivity but low positive predictive value and may be more useful if the *a priori* likelihood of intra-abdominal candidiasis is high, for example, patients not responding to antibacterial treatment with a gastric perforation, recent intra-abdominal surgery, or necrotizing pancreatitis. Cultures should be obtained from blood, central lines, abdomen and probable sites of metastatic infection. The duration of therapy should be determined by adequacy of source control and clinical response.

NEUTROPAENIC ENTEROCOLITIS

Neutropaenic enterocolitis is also known as typhlitis and is seen in neutropaenic patients. It is characterized by severe colitis with bleeding which can progress to necrosis. Typhlitis should be suspected in patients with fever and abdominal pain. Imaging can show bowel thickening and pneumatosis intestinalis, which is the presence of gas in the mucous lining of the small or large intestine.

The differential diagnosis consists of *Clostridioides difficile*-associated colitis, graft-versus-host disease or cytomegalovirus colitis.

Initial management consists of broad-spectrum antimicrobial therapy, for example, amoxicillin/ clavulanic acid with gentamicin or piperacillin/tazobactam. Antifungal cover with fluconazole or an echinocandin can be considered. Platelet transfusions may be necessary in patients with severe thrombocytopenia, total parenteral nutrition and intravenous fluid support.

Surgical resection is indicated if there is persistent gastrointestinal bleeding, bowel perforation and clinical deterioration despite optimal medical management.

PYOGENIC LIVER ABSCESS

Fever is almost always present; other signs and symptoms are right upper quadrant pain, nausea, vomiting, weight loss, malaise, enlarged liver, deranged LFTs and jaundice. Bacteria can cause a liver abscess via haematogenous spread, via direct biliary spread and or translocate from the gut and reach the liver through the portal circulation. Liver abscess is the most common type of intra-abdominal organ abscess. Risk factors include diabetes mellitus, hepatobiliary or pancreatic disease, liver transplant, and regular use of proton-pump inhibitors. The main pathogens involved in liver abscess are *E. coli*, *K. pneumoniae* and viridans streptococci (especially the milleri group) and anaerobes.

The mainstay of treatment is drainage. A common empirical antibiotic treatment regimen is ceftriaxone + metronidazole. Classically, a liver abscess is treated for 4–6 weeks but is not based on strong evidence. It may be reasonable to repeat imaging after 3 weeks of drainage and antibiotic treatment and decide further management on a case-by-case basis. Differential diagnosis of a pyogenic liver abscess is *Candida* liver abscess, amoebic liver abscess and echinococcal abscess. Hepatosplenic candidiasis with multiple small abscesses is a rare phenomenon and occurs in patients with haematologic malignancies during recovery of neutrophil counts following a neutropaenic episode. Surgical drainage may be indicated if there is an inadequate response to percutaneous drainage. Abscesses smaller than 5 cm may be too small to be drained. Discuss with the radiologist if instead a needle aspiration can be performed.

BIBLIOGRAPHY

Akoh JA. Peritoneal dialysis associated infections: An update on diagnosis and management. *World J Nephrol.* 2012 August 6;1(4):106–122.

Gee MS, Kim JY, Gervais DA, Hahn PF, Mueller PR. Management of abdominal and pelvic abscesses that persist despite satisfactory percutaneous drainage catheter placement. *AJR Am J Roentgenol.* 2010 March;194(3):815–820.

Ng FH, Wong WM, Wong BC, Kng C, Wong SY, Lai KC, Cheng CS, Yuen WC, Lam SK, Lai CL. Sequential intravenous/oral antibiotic vs. continuous intravenous antibiotic in the treatment of pyogenic liver abscess. *Aliment Pharmacol Ther.* 2002 June;16(6):1083–1090.

Sartelli M, Catena F, Ansaloni L, Coccolini F, Di Saverio S, Griffiths EA. Duration of antimicrobial therapy in treating complicated intra-abdominal infections: A comprehensive review. *Surg Infect (Larchmt).* 2016 February;17(1):9–12.

Sartelli M, Weber DG, Ruppé E et al. Antimicrobials: A global alliance for optimizing their rational use in intra-abdominal infections (AGORA) [published correction appears in *World J Emerg Surg.* 2017 Aug 2;12 :35]. *World J Emerg Surg.* 2016;11:33. Published 2016 Jul 15.

Sawyer RG, Claridge JA, Nathens AB et al. Trial of shortcourse antimicrobial therapy for intraabdominal infection. *N Engl J Med.* 2015;372:1996–2005.

Vergidis P, Clancy CJ, Shields RK, Park SY, Wildfeuer BN, Simmons RL, Nguyen MH. Intra-abdominal candidiasis: The importance of early source control and antifungal treatment. *PLOS ONE.* 2016 April 28;11(4):e0153247.

4.32 Invasive Candidiasis

Firza Alexander Gronthoud

CLINICAL CONSIDERATIONS

Candida spp. are part of the commensal flora and normally do not cause disease. In the presence of certain risk factors, *Candida* spp. can cause local disease (i.e. thrush) or invasive disease which is often caused by any combination of increased colonization, damage to mucosa or skin, presence of an intravascular device and immunocompromise. Fungal diagnostic tests have relatively low sensitivity and specificity, and particularly blood cultures, have a long turnaround time, resulting in delays in starting effective antifungal treatment or unnecessary use of antifungals with risk of drug toxicities and emergence of resistance. It is therefore worthwhile to consider the following.

Risk factors for invasive candidiasis:

- Mucositis due to chemo- or radiotherapy (damage to mucosa allowing for translocation)
- Intravascular catheter (i.e. patients on dialysis, total parenteral nutrition or chemotherapy)
- Intravenous drug use
- Intra-abdominal surgery (intra-abdominal contamination with *Candida* spp.)
- Immunosuppression (particularly neutropaenia facilitates *Candida* dissemination)
- Broad-spectrum antibacterial agents (promotes *Candida* overgrowth)

CLINICAL PEARL

Clinical *Candida* prediction rules have good negative predictive value to exclude risk factors for candidiasis in the ICU, but low positive predictive value.

CANDIDIASIS AND THE IMMUNE SYSTEM

- T lymphocytes are important in preventing oral or vulvovaginal thrush.
- Neutrophils, monocytes, macrophages and dendritic cells are important in preventing invasive candidiasis.

COMMON SPECIES INVOLVED

- Most cases of candidiasis are caused by *Candida albicans*. The non-albicans *Candida* spp. are found in almost half of the cases: *Candida glabrata*, *Candida tropicalis*, *Candida parapsilosis* and *Candida krusei*.
- *Candida parapsilosis* is less virulent than other *Candida* spp. and is generally associated with lower all-cause mortality.
- *Candida krusei* is more often found in patients with underlying haematological malignancies who have received antifungal prophylaxis with fluconazole.
- Multidrug-resistant *Candida auris* has now emerged globally as a major pathogen.

COMMON CLINICAL MANIFESTATIONS

- Candidaemia—Fourth leading cause of bloodstream infections
- Intra-abdominal abscess

COMPLICATIONS OF CANDIDAEMIA

- Chorioretinitis
- Endocarditis
- Osteomyelitis
- Brain abscess
- Hepatosplenic candidiasis—Very difficult to diagnose; blood cultures and fungal biomarkers in most cases are negative

CLINICAL PEARL

Timely diagnosis of invasive candidiasis is key to ensure a favourable outcome. A 1–2-day delay in initiation of effective antifungal therapy is associated with a doubling of mortality.

LABORATORY METHODS FOR DETECTION

Candida spp. can be detected on the mucosal surfaces of ~50%–70% of healthy humans and often represent colonization in superficial swabs, urine cultures and respiratory tract specimens.

- *Microscopy*: Rapid detection; not able to provide species identification or antifungal susceptibility.
- *Culture (any sample type)*: Allows identification and susceptibility testing.
  - Blood culture—Takes 48–72 hours to flag positive; sensitivity ~50%.
  - Tissue and sterile body fluid—Needs to use a selective agar (Sabouraud) to avoid bacterial overgrowth; takes 48–72 of incubation.
- *Serology*
  - 1,3-β-D-glucan detection (serum or EDTA blood)—Sensitivity +/−80%, variable specificity. High negative predictive value. General fungal biomarker, not specific for candidiasis. Prone to contamination; needs repeat testing to confirm.
  - Mannan antigen in combination with mannan antibodies (serum, EDTA blood or CSF)—Combined sensitivity 55% and specificity 60%. Heavy colonization can also cause formation of mannan antibodies.
- *PCR (EDTA blood)*: Diagnosis <24 hours possible. Not routinely used; more expensive. Commercial assays only detect limited species.

CLINICAL PEARL

Serology generally has moderate sensitivity and specificity. To increase the diagnostic value, only perform serology in patients with risk factors for invasive candidiasis.

ANTIFUNGAL RESISTANCE

- Antifungal resistance is an emerging problem worldwide, and this further complicates the selection of appropriate antifungal therapy.

- *Candida krusei* is intrinsically resistant to fluconazole. Echinocandin resistance is emerging, particularly in *C. glabrata* and is often accompanied by fluconazole resistance.
- *Candida auris* is an emerging multidrug-resistant pathogen of increasing concern. It is almost always resistant to fluconazole and can display reduced susceptibility to all antifungal classes. Empirical treatment consists of an echinocandin.

ANTIFUNGAL TREATMENT

- Most common antifungal agents used to treat invasive candidiasis are the group of azoles (mostly fluconazole, voriconazole and itraconazole and the group of echinocandins; amphotericin B is an alternative).
- All azoles except fluconazole require therapeutic drug monitoring.
- If candidaemia or invasive candidiasis with no clear source, empirical treatment is usually an echinocandin.
- If no previous exposure to azoles, clinically stable and low prevalence of azole resistance, alternatively start fluconazole.
- If no IV access, start oral fluconazole or voriconazole.
- Azole therapy is preferred in case of endophthalmitis, meningitis and lower UTI (for UTI fluconazole only).
- If multidrug-resistant *Candida* spp. is suspected, first-line treatment is with amphotericin B formulation, preferably liposomal amphotericin B.
- Heavy use of fluconazole can result in emergence of fluconazole-resistant *C. krusei* or *C. glabrata*. Heavy use of echinocandins could select for increased incidence of *C. parapsilosis* infections.

ANTIFUNGAL PROPHYLAXIS

Indicated in solid organ recipients (i.e. liver or lung) or haematopoietic stem cell transplant recipients.

BIOFILMS

Any infected foreign bodies and intravascular devices should be removed as *Candida* spp. readily form biofilms. Echinocandins and amphotericin B should be used for biofilm infections.

PREVENTING CANDIDIASIS

- Hand hygiene
- Restricted use of antibiotics
- Catheter care bundles
- *Antifungal prophylaxis:* MDS/AML undergoing induction chemotherapy, intensive/dose-escalated therapy for lymphoma; HSCT, pancreas or intestinal transplant recipients

CLINICAL APPROACH

- Invasive candidiasis should be suspected if known risk factors are present and there is no response to antibacterial treatment.
- Cornerstone of management is source control and appropriate antifungal treatment.
- Choice of antifungal agent depends on the infecting *Candida* spp., site of infection, previous exposure to antifungals and any potential drug-drug interaction (i.e. azoles interact with rifampicin, cyclosporine and tacrolimus) but usually involves an echinocandin or fluconazole.

Management of suspected invasive candidiasis with no clear source:

- Collect blood cultures from intravascular devices and peripheral sets, drain cultures or aspirates from any pus collection and serum 1,3-β-D-glucan.
- Source of infection should be actively pursued, i.e. CT thorax, abdomen, fundoscopy, echocardiogram, ultrasound urinary tract.
- Distant sites of infection are uncommon among non-neutropaenic patients with candidaemia.
- Start empirical treatment with an echinocandin and review with microbiology results.
- If blood cultures, pus fluid cultures, imaging and biomarkers are negative, stop antifungal treatment.

CLINICAL PEARL

It is important to take frequent blood cultures with large volumes (optimally ≥40–60 mL daily) because:

- Blood culture has a sensitivity of 50%–70% because of low number of circulating *Candida* spp. (1 colony-forming unit/mL).
- Prolonged time to positivity (48–72 hours) because *Candida* spp. are slow growers.

If the site of infection is known or if *Candida* spp. has been isolated from a clinical culture, a targeted approach can be followed.

CANDIDAEMIA

- Remove any lines and catheters.
- Take repeat blood cultures every other day.
- A dilated fundoscopy should be performed by an experienced ophthalmologist and repeated at the end of treatment.
- Consider performing an echo, especially in the presence of IV drug abuse, pre-existing valvular disease or the presence of a prosthetic cardiac valve.
- Start treatment with an echinocandin or fluconazole IV (800 mg loading dose followed by 400 mg once daily) and review treatment with blood culture results. Echinocandins have better biofilm penetration. Fluconazole should be avoided in the presence of foreign bodies or if intravascular catheters cannot be removed.
- Consider switching to oral fluconazole after 3–7 days. If fluconazole resistant, switch to oral voriconazole.
- In the absence of organ involvement, total treatment duration is 14 days from the first negative blood culture with resolution of clinical symptoms.

ENDOCARDITIS

- Liposomal amphotericin B 3–5 mg/kg IV with or without flucytosine, 25 mg/kg 4 times daily OR high dose echinocandin.
- Stepdown to fluconazole if susceptible isolate and candidaemia cleared.
- Valve replacement recommended.
- Duration of treatment is at least 6 weeks from surgery.
- If valve replacement not possible, long-term suppression with fluconazole 400–800 mg once daily.

Chronic Disseminated Candidiasis

- Also called hepatosplenic candidiasis.
- Disease usually occurs after recovery of neutrophils due to previous chemotherapy.
- Three sets of blood cultures with a total volume of 40–60 mL, 1,3-β-D-glucan, combined mannan and anti-mannan, tissue biopsy.
- Treatment: liposomal amphotericin B 3–5 mg/kg IV OR an echinocandin for at least 8 weeks followed by oral fluconazole 400 mg once daily.
- Therapy should continue until lesions resolve on repeat imaging, which is usually several months.
- Chronic disseminated candidiasis is not a reason for delaying chemotherapy or hematopoietic stem cell transplantation.

Intra-Abdominal Candidiasis

- Mainstay of treatment is source control, i.e. drainage or relaparotomy with washout.
- First-line treatment is an echinocandin or alternatively fluconazole.
- Duration of treatment is at least 4 days from when source control is achieved and patient is clinically and biochemically improving.

Antifungal Suppressive Treatment

- Indicated foreign bodies that cannot be removed, i.e. prosthetic valves, prosthetic joint or intravascular devices left ventricular assist devices and intracardiac pacemakers or defibrillators.
- Chronic suppressive treatment consists of an oral azole with frequent monitoring of liver function.
- Regularly revisit possibility of removal and replacement of infected foreign bodies or debridement, resection or drainage of persistent sources of infection.

CLINICAL PEARL

In neutropaenic patients, funduscopy should be delayed until neutrophil recovery because characteristic inflammatory retinal and choroidal changes might not become clinically evident during periods of profound neutropenia.

BIBLIOGRAPHY

Alfouzan WA, Dhar R. Candiduria: Evidence-based approach to management, are we there yet? *J Mycol Med.* 2017 September;27(3):293–302.
Breazzano MP, Day HR Jr, Bloch KC et al. Utility of ophthalmologic screening for patients with candida bloodstream infections: A systematic review. *JAMA Ophthalmol.* 2019;137(6):698–710.
Cuenca-Estrella M, Verweij PE, Arendrup MC et al. ; ESCMID Fungal Infection Study Group. ESCMID* guideline for the diagnosis and management of Candida diseases 2012: Diagnostic procedures. *Clin Microbiol Infect.* 2012 December;18(Suppl 7):9–18.

Fleming S, Yannakou CK, Haeusler GM et al. Consensus guidelines for antifungal prophylaxis in haematological malignancy and haemopoietic stem cell transplantation, 2014. *Intern Med J.* 2014 December;44(12b):1283–1297.

Pappas PG, Kauffman CA, Andes DR et al. Executive summary: Clinical practice guideline for the management of candidiasis: 2016 Update by the Infectious Diseases Society of America. *Clin Infect Dis.* 2016 February 15;62(4):409–417.

Pappas PG, Lionakis MS, Arendrup MC, Ostrosky-Zeichner L, Kullberg BJ. Invasive candidiasis. *Nat Rev Dis Primers.* 2018 May 11;4:18026.

4.33 Invasive Group A Streptococcal Infections

Firza Alexander Gronthoud

CLINICAL CONSIDERATIONS

Group A *Streptococcus* (GAS; *Streptococcus pyogenes*) is a facultative anaerobic, Gram-positive coccus (meaning it can grow both aerobically and anaerobically) and the main cause of bacterial pharyngitis (see Chapter 4.1). The most common portals of entry for GAS are the skin, vagina and pharynx. It can however also cause severe invasive disease with high mortality rates and can cause sporadic outbreaks. Invasive GAS infection may occur in patients of any age and most patients are not immunosuppressed. It is therefore worthwhile to consider the following.

MICROBIOLOGY

GAS has a capsule with an M protein which is encoded by *emm* genes. Both the M protein and the *emm* genes are used for typing. M1 and M2 proteins are associated with toxic shock syndrome. Both the M protein and hyaluronic acid capsule protect GAS from phagocytosis. In addition, GAS produces several toxins and superantigens contributing to invasive disease.

> ### CLINICAL PEARL
>
> *Streptococcus dysgalactiae* subspecies *equisimilis* is a β-haemolytic *Streptococcus* and has Lancefield groups A, C and G antigens and can be mistaken for GAS.
>
> Streptococci belonging to the anginosus (or milleri) group can be β-haemolytic, α-haemolytic or nonhemolytic and can have Lancefield groups A, C, G and F antigens. These streptococci can be differentiated from GAS by their characteristic sweet smell and their small colony size (≤0.5 mm).

NON-INVASIVE DISEASE

GAS is the most common cause of bacterial pharyngitis and impetigo. These are not typically associated with invasive infection.

INVASIVE DISEASE

GAS causes invasive disease (iGAS), which is defined as isolation of GAS from a sterile site.
- *Bloodstream infection*: Most common form of iGAS. Sources are usually soft tissue infections such as cellulitis. GAS can also cause superinfections of varicella zoster vesicles and burns. A source is not always found.
- *Pneumonia*: Occurs less often. Multiple lobes may be involved. Can be accompanied by empyema. GAS bacteraemia occurs in approximately 80% of cases.
- *Necrotizing soft tissue infection*: Acute life-threatening infection with septic shock rapidly developing within hours to days. Usually the lower extremities are involved. Shock syndrome occurs as a complication of necrotizing soft tissue infection in approximately half of cases.

- *Pregnancy-associated infection*: Puerperal GAS sepsis or postpartum GAS infection. Most cases of puerperal GAS sepsis occur during the first 48–72 hours after delivery but may also occur during late pregnancy (prior to onset of labour or rupture of membranes). Postpartum endometritis can be caused by a number of organisms, including GAS; GAS endometritis can progress to puerperal sepsis. Postpartum endometritis should be suspected in the setting of fever and uterine tenderness following childbirth.
- Severe neonatal infections.

Clusters and outbreaks of invasive GAS infection have occurred in nursing homes and among patients treated in inpatient and outpatient settings.

TOXIC SHOCK SYNDROME

Toxic shock syndrome (TSS) occurs as a complication of invasive GAS disease in approximately one-third of cases. Risk factors that have been linked to TSS are young children, particularly those with varicella, the elderly, diabetes mellitus, chronic cardiac or pulmonary diseases, HIV infection and intravenous drug or alcohol abuse.

TSS should be suspected in patients with iGAS and who present with hypotension and multiorgan failure, which may manifest as renal failure, respiratory failure, thrombocytopaenia, DIC, liver failure or skin manifestations such as a desquamating rash. Differential diagnosis of TSS is staphylococcal toxic shock syndrome, Gram-negative sepsis, meningococcaemia or typhoid fever or leptospirosis in returning travellers with fever.

CLINICAL APPROACH

Invasive streptococcal infection should be suspected in patients with skin or soft tissue infection or pregnant and postpartum women in the setting of high fever or rapid onset of fever.

LABORATORY DIAGNOSIS

- GAS can be recognized by β-haemolytic colonies which may be α-haemolytic on day 1 of culture. GAS grows best in an anaerobic or CO_2-enriched atmosphere. β-haemolytic colonies >0.5 mm which are positive for Lancefield group A, should be confirmed with MALDI-ToF or alternatively the bacitracin or PYR test.
- Blood cultures (at least two sets) should be obtained prior to antibiotic administration from all clinically relevant sites, i.e. wound culture, debrided material sent for culture, endometrial aspiration, throat and sputum culture or pleural fluid.
- Susceptibility testing should be performed for penicillin, clarithromycin, clindamycin, linezolid and vancomycin although macrolide resistance is increasing.

CLINICAL DIAGNOSIS

The diagnosis of invasive GAS infection is established via positive culture for GAS from a normally sterile site (most commonly, blood; less commonly, pleural, pericardial, joint or CSF).

TREATMENT

Treatment consists of intravenous benzylpenicillin. All GAS strains isolated from invasive infections produce toxins, and antibiotic treatment should also include an antibiotic that inhibits toxin production. Clindamycin or linezolid are often added to intravenous benzylpenicillin. Intravenous immunoglobulin (IVIG) may be considered in toxic shock syndrome.

BIBLIOGRAPHY

Batalis NI, Caplan MJ, Schandl CA. Acute deaths in nonpregnant adults due to invasive streptococcal infections. *Am J Forensic Med Pathol.* 2007 March;28(1):63–68.

Bennett JE, Dolin R, Blaser MJ. *Mandell, Douglas, and Bennett's Principles and Practice of Infectious Diseases.* Philadelphia, PA: Elsevier/Saunders, 2015.

Jorgensen JH, Pfaller MA, Carroll KC, Funke G, Landry ML, Richter Sandra S, Warnock DW. (eds) *Manual of Clinical Microbiology*, 11th ed. American Society of Microbiology, 2015.

Walker MJ, Barnett TC, McArthur JD, Cole JN, Gillen CM, Henningham A, Sriprakash KS, Sriprakash KSSanderson-Smith ML, Nizet V. Disease manifestations and pathogenic mechanisms of group A streptococcus. *Clin Microbiol Rev.* 2014 April;27(2):264–301.

4.34 Invasive Pulmonary Aspergillosis

Firza Alexander Gronthoud

CLINICAL CONSIDERATIONS

Inhalation of *Aspergillus* spores is a common occurrence and harmless for healthy humans. In immunocompromised individuals, inhaled spores are not cleared by the immune system and cause invasive pulmonary aspergillosis. *Aspergillus* can also exacerbate underlying lung conditions, cause chronic pulmonary infection without angioinvasion (chronic pulmonary aspergillosis) or severe allergic reactions (allergic bronchopulmonary aspergillosis). This chapter discusses invasive pulmonary aspergillosis (IPA).

Management of invasive pulmonary aspergillosis requires an individualized approach; treatment takes weeks to months, and even with adequate therapy, invasive aspergillosis causes significant morbidity and mortality. It is therefore worthwhile to consider the following.

INDIVIDUALS AT RISK OF INVASIVE PULMONARY ASPERGILLOSIS

- Profound neutropaenia, most often seen in patients with haematological malignancies, i.e. allogeneic HSCT recipients, induction chemotherapy for AML and ALL treatment
- High-dose corticosteroids
- Solid organ transplant recipients (mainly lung and heart)
- Critically ill patients (immune paralysis post-sepsis, prior influenza infection, Child–Pugh C hepatic cirrhosis and mechanical ventilation)
- Chronic granulomatous disease

DEVELOPMENT OF INVASIVE PULMONARY ASPERGILLOSIS

- In the absence of macrophages and neutrophils, spores germinate into hyphae which invade and damage the lung parenchyma. They can also invade the blood vessels (angioinvasion), cause thrombosis, septic emboli and disseminate to other organs such as skin, brain or eyes.
- Angioinvasion occurs in neutropaenic patients.
- IPA has a rapid onset of symptoms including fever.

ASPERGILLUS SPECIES

- *Aspergillus fumigatus*: The most common cause of pulmonary aspergillosis
- *Aspergillus flavus*: More common cause of allergic rhinosinusitis, post-operative aspergillosis and fungal keratitis
- *Aspergillus terreus*: Resistant to amphotericin B
- *Aspergillus niger*: Most common fungal cause of otitis externa

DIAGNOSTIC METHODS

- Microscopy and culture on deep respiratory samples including BAL and sputum. Sensitivity for both is ~50%.
- PCR on blood and respiratory samples has higher sensitivity.

- Best sample is tissue; positive microscopy confirms IPA.
- A positive BAL/sputum indicates colonization or infection.
- Serology can be performed using galactomannan and 1,3-β-D-glucan.
- 1,3-β-D-glucan is a cell wall component of many fungi and not specific for aspergillosis.
- Both 1,3-β-D-glucan and galactomannan are detectable in blood days before clinical symptoms develop.
- Especially 1,3-β-D-glucan, but also the galactomannan test, is prone to contamination, and positive results require confirmation with a second sample.
- The main value of 1,3-β-D-glucan is to rule out infection.
- In contrast to galactomannan in BAL, galactomannan in blood has reduced sensitivity in solid organ transplant recipients and non-neutropaenic patients.
- Galactomannan is released by growing hyphae and not by conidia that colonize the airways. Its detection in an individual is therefore thought to more likely indicate invasive disease rather than simple colonization.
- Galactomannan in BAL has higher sensitivity than fungal culture.

RADIOLOGY OF INVASIVE PULMONARY ASPERGILLOSIS

- The halo sign is the earliest radiological feature of IPA and lasts for about 5 days, after which it rapidly disappears.
- A reversed halo sign may also be seen less commonly but is not specific for IPA (focal rounded area of ground-glass opacity surrounded by a crescent or complete ring of consolidation).
- Vessel occlusion seen on HR CT angiography is highly sensitive for IPA.
- Cavitating lesions and the air crescent sign are both late signs of IPA, and both are good prognostic markers.
- Complete radiological improvement takes longer when cavitating lesions are present.
- Most patients with IPA present with more than 1 macro-nodule (>1 cm).
- Size and number of IPA lesions increase within the first 7–10 days irrespective of antifungal treatment, and this does not indicate treatment failure.
- The size of the lesions then plateaus for a few days followed by slow decrease in size and number.
- Re-appearance of the halo sign together with increase in the size of existing nodules indicates relapse.

CLINICAL PEARL

- Angioinvasion in neutropaenic patients causes thrombosis and ischaemic necrosis of lung parenchyma and is surrounded by haemorrhage.
- This is visible on imaging as a pulmonary nodule or mass surrounded by ground-glass opacity and is called the halo sign.
- The halo sign has a high positive predictive value for IPA in patients with a haematological malignancy who have profound neutropaenia, are not on mould-active prophylaxis and in areas with low incidence of mucormycosis.
- If patient is on mould-active azole prophylaxis with prophylactic levels, the halo sign may be more likely caused by a different organism, i.e. Mucorales or bacteria.
- In non-neutropaenic patients, angioinvasion is less likely to occur and the halo sign has a lower incidence and lower specificity for IPA and may indicate a different infectious or non-infectious cause.
- Antifungal treatment started as early as the appearance of a halo sign is associated with significant improved outcome of IPA.

CLINICAL PEARL

- The air crescent sign develops when the neutrophil count has recovered, occurs in ~50% of patients with IPA and is a good prognostic finding because it marks the recovery phase of the infection.
- Neutrophil infiltration and peripheral reabsorption of necrotic tissue form a cavitating lesion. The air in the cavitating lesion is called the air crescent sign.
- Cavitating lesions and air crescent signs are thus markers of bone marrow recovery.

ANTIFUNGAL TREATMENT OF ASPERGILLOSIS

- All azoles have activity against aspergillosis except fluconazole. Azoles most used for first-line treatment of IPA are voriconazole and isavuconazole.
- Treatment with azoles requires therapeutic drug monitoring to ensure therapeutic levels and minimize risk of toxicity (visual disturbances, hepatotoxicity, encephalopathy).
- Azoles are cytochrome P450 inhibitors and have many drug-drug interactions.
- Second-line agent is liposomal amphotericin B 3 mg/kg IV. It is only available as IV formulation and the main side effects are infusion-related reactions, nephrotoxicity, hypokalaemia and deranged liver function tests.
- Caspofungin is fungistatic against *Aspergillus* species and should be reserved for salvage therapy.

PROPHYLAXIS OF INVASIVE PULMONARY ASPERGILLOSIS

- Indications for primary prophylaxis are profound and prolonged neutropenia or active graft-versus-host disease (GvHD).
- Preferred prophylactic agent is posaconazole suspension 200 mg 8-hourly PO OR posaconazole tablet 300 mg 12-hourly on the first day, thereafter 300 mg once-daily PO.
- Secondary prophylaxis with the same agent used for treatment is indicated if persistent immunosuppression after resolution of IPA. Continue until neutrophil count has recovered, there are functional T cells, immunoglobulin level is within normal range and immunosuppressive drugs have been discontinued.

CLINICAL APPROACH

Invasive pulmonary aspergillosis should be suspected in individuals at risk for IPA, i.e. patients with profound neutropaenia who present with:

- Persistent sepsis despite ≥36 hours of antibiotics *or*
- New pulmonary symptoms or new infiltrates on chest X-ray *or*
- A positive galactomannan, culture or PCR *or*
- CT chest with findings suggestive of fungal infection

DIAGNOSTIC WORK-UP

- If patient is on azole prophylaxis other than fluconazole, review latest pre-dose level and order a new level if indicated.
- Request high-resolution CT chest if not yet performed.
- Request blood cultures from any intravascular device and peripheral set.

- *Depending on CT finding:* Bronchoscopy for PCR for cytomegalovirus, *Pneumocystis jirovecii*, respiratory viruses AND microscopy + culture: bacteria, fungi, and mycobacteria.
- Aspergillus PCR on BAL, sputum or blood should be considered.
- Request serology:
  - Preferably galactomannan on bronchoalveolar lavage. Alternatively, galactomannan or 1,3-β-D-glucan on serum.
  - If *Pneumocystis jirovecii* is in the differential diagnosis, request serum 1,3-β-D-glucan on blood with LDH if respiratory sample for PCR not possible.
  - If travel to endemic region, consider histoplasma antigen in urine or serum for *Coccidioides* antibody.
  - Positive galactomannan or 1,3-β-D-glucan need to be repeated to rule out false positivity.

CLINICAL PEARL

- Persistently negative serum or sputum galactomannan, 1,3-β-D-glucan, aspergillus PCR, and CT chest have a high negative predictive value for ruling out IPA.
- Positive 1,3-β-D-glucan or galactomannan on repeat serum warrants extensive diagnostic testing, and antifungal therapy should be started.

EMPIRICAL TREATMENT OF NEUTROPAENIC PATIENTS

- If a patient is on antifungal prophylaxis, a different antifungal class should be used for treatment.
- If result from CT and serology not available, start an echinocandin or liposomal amphotericin B and stop antifungal prophylaxis.
- If CT shows abnormalities not specific for IPA and no other result available, start an echinocandin or liposomal amphotericin B 3 mg/kg IV and stop antifungal prophylaxis.
- If both CT and galactomannan/1,3-β-D-glucan are negative, stop antifungal treatment, resume antifungal prophylaxis and look for other sources of infection. Use therapeutic drug monitoring to ensure prophylactic serum levels.
- If CT shows typical findings of IPA but serology is negative, start voriconazole or liposomal amphotericin B and review with culture results. Note: mucormycosis may present similar to IPA. If mucormycosis is a possibility, then start liposomal amphotericin B 5–10 mg/kg IV and review with culture results. If low threshold for biopsy, use platelet transfusion if necessary.
- If galactomannan is positive on repeat testing, regardless of CT finding, start voriconazole or liposomal amphotericin B. If patient was on azole prophylaxis, start liposomal amphotericin B 3 mg/kg IV instead. Look for other sources, i.e. sinuses.

EMPIRICAL TREATMENT OF IPA IN NON-NEUTROPAENIC PATIENTS

- Start voriconazole or isavuconazole if galactomannan is positive and/or CT chest is suspicious for IPA.
- If CT chest and respiratory cultures are negative, stop treatment for IPA and consider other infections, i.e. invasive candidiasis especially if 1,3-β-D-glucan is positive on two separate occasions.

Targeted Treatment for IPA

- Rationalize empirical treatment based on antifungal susceptibility.
- In general:
  - First-line treatment of IPA is either voriconazole or isavuconazole.
  - Second-line treatment is liposomal amphotericin B.
  - Caspofungin is reserved for salvage treatment.
- Treatment duration should be based on clinical, radiological and microbiological improvement and tailored to individual risk factors, but generally is 6–12 weeks.

BIBLIOGRAPHY

Brodoefel H, Vogel M, Hebart H, Einsele H, Vonthein R, Claussen C, Horger M. Long-term CT follow-up in 40 non-HIV immunocompromised patients with invasive pulmonary aspergillosis: Kinetics of CT morphology and correlation with clinical findings and outcome. *AJR Am J Roentgenol.* 2006 August;187(2):404–413.

Colombo AL, de Almeida Júnior JN, Slavin MA, Chen SC, Sorrell TC. *Candida* and invasive mould diseases in non-neutropenic critically ill patients and patients with haematological cancer. *Lancet Infect Dis.* 2017 November;17(11):e344–e356.

Georgiadou SP, Sipsas NV, Marom EM, Kontoyiannis DP. The diagnostic value of halo and reversed halo signs for invasive mold infections in compromised hosts. *Clin Infect Dis.* 2011 May;52(9):1144–1155.

Kosmidis C, Denning DW. The clinical spectrum of pulmonary aspergillosis. *Thorax.* 2015 March;70(3):270–277.

Ullmann AJ, Aguado JM, Arikan-Akdagli S et al. Diagnosis and management of *Aspergillus* diseases: Executive summary of the 2017 ESCMID-ECMM-ERS guideline. *Clin Microbiol Infect.* 2018;24(Suppl 1):e1–e38.

4.35 Keratitis

Firza Alexander Gronthoud

CLINICAL CONSIDERATIONS

Keratitis is an infection of the cornea, caused by a broad range of organisms, and clinical diagnosis relies on a history of infectious exposure and morphologic features of corneal inflammation. It is therefore worthwhile to consider the following.

INFECTIOUS EXPOSURE

Contact lens wear is a well-known risk factor for *Pseudomonas aeruginosa* and *Acanthamoeba* keratitis and is increasingly becoming an important risk factor for mycotic keratitis. Water exposure is also a risk factor for *Acanthamoeba* keratitis. Trauma is the main predisposing factor for keratitis due to filamentous fungi such as *Aspergillus* and *Fusarium* and is most often seen in young males doing outdoor work or working in agriculture. Other risk factors are previous ocular surgery, ocular surface disease and previous use of corticosteroids. Humidity, rainfall and wind may also increase risk of infection. Systemic or local defect is a risk factor for *Candida* keratitis. Local defects (i.e. insufficient tear secretion or defective eyelid closure) or systemic conditions (i.e. diabetes mellitus, immunosuppression) predispose to infection with *Candida* spp.

CLINICAL PEARL

Knowledge of epidemiology may predict the type of microbes causing keratitis; North America, Australia, the Netherlands and Singapore have the highest proportion of keratitis caused by bacteria whereas the highest proportion of fungal keratitis is seen in India and Nepal. The proportion of corneal ulcers caused by filamentous fungi has shown a tendency to increase towards tropical latitudes, whereas in more temperate climates, fungal ulcers appear to be uncommon and to be more frequently associated with *Candida* species than filamentous fungi.

CLINICAL FEATURES

A large suppurative infiltrate corresponds well with a *P. aeruginosa*. A stromal ring infiltrate which may not be present in the early stages of infection and can occur in bacterial and fungal keratitis has a high sensitivity and specificity for *Acanthamoeba* keratitis, as does disease confined to the epithelium. It is possible that the immune ring is simply an indicator of prolonged untreated infections, which would be consistent with the longer duration of symptoms in the acanthamoeba group.

Compared to bacterial and fungal keratitis, patients with acanthamoeba keratitis are younger and have a longer duration of symptoms. This may be explained by the fact that younger individuals tend to wear contact lenses more often than older individuals.

Fungal keratitis is characterized by severe inflammation, the formation of a corneal ulcer and hypopyon, with the presence of fungal hyphae within the corneal stroma. Another feature is multifocal granular (or feathery) grey-white 'satellite' stromal infiltrates.

PATHOGENS

The most common bacterial causes are *Streptococcus pneumoniae* and *P. aeruginosa*. Fungal keratitis is caused by filamentous fungi including *Fusarium* spp. and *Aspergillus* spp. and by yeast-like fungi such as *Candida* spp. The most common parasitic cause is *Acanthamoeba*, albeit this is less often seen than bacteria or fungi. Less common causes are *Mycobacterium* and *Nocardia* spp. The most common viral cause is herpes, with adenovirus being the cause less often.

CLINICAL APPROACH

DIAGNOSIS

Material collected in one scraping is used to inoculate culture plates, and material collected in an additional scraping is used to prepare smears or mounts for direct microscopic examination. Corneal biopsy may have to be performed where scrapings yield negative results; aqueous humour may also have to be obtained from the anterior chamber.

Corneal scrapings should be obtained for microscopy and to inoculate blood agar, chocolate agar and sabouraud plates. Corneal material is usually inoculated on culture plates in the form of multiple 'C's. Acanthamoeba can also be cultured on a non-nutrient agar overlaid with *Escherichia coli*. A Gram stain can show bacterial pathogens and fungal hyphae. A potassium hydroxide (KOH) wet film can be used to detect *Acanthamoeba* cysts or fungal elements. Alternatively, for fungal elements, a calcofluor fluorescent dye or wet film stained with lactophenol cotton blue can also be used. Fungal growth usually occurs within 3–4 days, but culture media may require incubation for up to 4–6 weeks. Polymerase chain reaction (PCR) is a newer technique with a rapid turnaround time of 1–2 days. Disadvantages of PCR is it cannot differentiate between viable and non-viable organisms and therefore is not an ideal method for monitoring treatment response. It may also be associated with higher costs compared to culture.

TREATMENT

Bacterial keratitis can be treated with hourly topical eyedrops with quinolones or aminoglycosides and review after 48 hours. Dual therapy with fortified cephalosporin (5% cefuroxime or cefazolin 50 mg/mL) with gentamicin is also effective but less well tolerated.

Prolonged use of a fortified aminoglycoside such as gentamicin is toxic and may delay epithelial recovery or cause epithelial necrosis.

Treatment of *Acanthamoeba* keratitis is mainly aimed at killing the amoebic cysts as opposed to the more sensitive trophozoites and consists of eye drops with two or three agents:

- Chlorhexidine 0.02%–0.06%
- Polyhexanide or polyhexamethylene biguanide (PHMB) 0,02% (most effective against the cysts)
- Propamidine isethionate (Brolene) of hexamidine

This is a complicated regimen whereby on day 1 and 2 eyedrops should be applied every hour day and night, on days 3–5 eyedrops every hour during the day; on weeks 2–5 eyedrops every 2 hours during the day; thereafter 4–6 times a day for 6–12 months.

Topical steroid may be indicated later if there is progressive vascularization, stromal melt, scleritis or marked anterior uveitis. Oral non-steroidal agents (e.g. flurbiprofen 50 mg TDS) can help control pain, and immunosuppression should be considered if there is an associated scleritis.

Fungal keratitis is difficult to treat. Management consists of antifungal therapy and surgical intervention such as corneal transplantation. There is no evidence to suggest that any particular drug, or combination of drugs, is more effective than any other.

CLINICAL PEARL

The drug must be non-irritating and non-toxic in the eye, must penetrate the eye well and have a high level of antimicrobial activity against at least one significant ocular pathogen.

BIBLIOGRAPHY

Dahlgren MA, Lingappan A, Wilhelmus KR. The clinical diagnosis of microbial keratitis. *Am J Ophthalmol.* 2007 June;143(6):940–944.
Mascarenhas J, Lalitha P, Prajna NV et al. Acanthamoeba, fungal, and bacterial keratitis: A comparison of risk factors and clinical features. *Am J Ophthalmol.* 2014 January;157(1):56–62.
Thomas PA, Kaliamurthy J. Mycotic keratitis: Epidemiology, diagnosis and management. *Clin Microbiol Infect.* 2013;19:210–220.

4.36 Lung Abscess

Patrick Lillie

CLINICAL CONSIDERATIONS

Lung abscess develops most commonly in patients with a predisposing factor such as aspiration from the oropharynx. In the majority of cases, it is polymicrobial oropharyngeal flora, with anaerobes being a common finding; however it may also complicate infection with particular organisms such as *Staphylococcus aureus*, *Fusobacterium* spp. or *Klebsiella pneumoniae* or as a consequence of embolic disease (particularly in patients with right-sided endocarditis or infected deep venous thrombosis from intravenous drug use). Presentation is with systemic features such as fever and weight loss, together with cough, shortness of breath and possibly chest pain. It may present acutely after a severe/necrotizing pneumonia or as a more chronic presentation. Important differential diagnoses are tuberculosis and lung cancer.

CLINICAL APPROACH

INVESTIGATIONS

Diagnosis of lung abscess is generally made by radiological appearances of an air-fluid level on a chest X-ray/CT scan, together with compatible symptoms. The foul-smelling sputum that is often produced should be sent for standard culture, together with investigations for tuberculosis if this is a possible cause. Sputum culture may well not be helpful, as the polymicrobial nature of lung abscesses derived from the oropharynx will lead to the cultures being reported as mixed oral flora. Blood cultures are rarely positive, except in those patients with septic pulmonary emboli from either the deep veins or tricuspid valves, e.g. patients who inject intravenous drugs. Radiological monitoring of response to treatment can be with standard chest radiographs or CT scanning depending on the extent of the original radiological findings.

ANTIMICROBIAL THERAPY

Sputum cultures should be obtained to look for the more unusual causes of infection. After they have been taken, antibiotic therapy should be started, with drugs used that cover the commonest isolated organisms and also have activity against anaerobes. Several studies have been performed and all have similar outcomes, with clindamycin perhaps being the most useful agent. In hospitalized patients, IV therapy initially is prudent to achieve high drug concentrations and obtain clinical improvement. Broad-spectrum cover is needed, so piperacillin/tazobactam, ceftriaxone together with metronidazole or co-amoxiclav are suitable options. After 7–14 days, the IV regime can be switched to oral treatment provided that there has been clinical improvement. Suitable oral antibiotics would include clindamycin, co-amoxiclav or moxifloxacin. These should be carried on until clinical and radiological resolution of the abscess, which may take 4–8 weeks of therapy.

SURGERY/BRONCHOSCOPY/INTERVENTIONAL RADIOLOGY

As most lung abscesses drain via the large airways, surgery is rarely required to achieve source control. Concern over creating fistula between the bronchi and pleura are another reason for not operating too early in these patients. In those failing medical therapy, especially if there are large cavities and concern over significant haemoptysis, surgical resection may be needed.

CLINICAL PEARL

Surgical intervention and CT-guided drainage may be required in cases of very large abscesses and those at high risk of significant haemorrhage.

CLINICAL VIGNETTES

A 31-year-old woman with Crohn's disease presented with a 4-week history of fever, night sweats and purulent sputum. She was taking infliximab for her Crohn's. Blood tests showed a raised white cell count and CR, while CXR and CT scanning of the chest showed 2 large cavitating lesions in the right middle and lower lobes. Sputum smear and PCR was positive for Mycobacterium tuberculosis, *and she was commenced on standard 4-drug therapy with resolution of her symptoms.*

A 24-year-old man was diagnosed with acute T-cell lymphoblastic leukaemia. He lived on a farm, kept horses and had been on holiday to the Mississippi delta region one year earlier. After his first round of chemotherapy, he developed a fever, and a CT scan of his chest showed bilateral cavitating abscesses. He underwent a bronchoscopy and was found to have re-activated pulmonary Histoplasmosis and was commenced on IV liposomal amphotericin B with a good response, before being converted to oral itraconazole long term.

In immunocompromised patients, consideration should be given to a more diverse array of pathogens. In addition to standard bacterial pathogens, mycobacteria, *Nocardia* and *Actinomyces* should be included in the differential diagnosis and actively looked for. A detailed travel and exposure history may reveal risks for unusual organisms such as *Burkholderia pseudomallei*, *Rhodococcus equi*, geographically restricted dimorphic fungi such as *Histoplasma* and parasites such as *Entamoeba histolytica* and *Paragonimus westermani*.

BIBLIOGRAPHY

Fernández-Sabé N, Carratalà J, Dorca J et al. Efficacy and safety of sequential amoxicillin-clavulanate in the treatment of anaerobic lung infections. *Eur J Clin Microbiol Infect Dis.* 2003;22(3):185–187.

Gudiol F, Manresa F, Pallares R et al. Clindamycin vs penicillin for anaerobic lung infections: High rate of penicillin failures associated with penicillin-resistant *Bacteroides melaninogenicus. Arch Intern Med.* 1990;150(12):2525–2529.

Ott SR, Allewelt M, Lorenz J, Reimnitz P, Lode H; German Lung Abscess Study Group. Moxifloxacin vs ampicillin/sulbactam in aspiration pneumonia and primary lung abscess. *Infection.* 2008;36(1):23–30.

Perlino CA. Metronidazole vs clindamycin treatment of anaerobic pulmonary infection. Failure of metronidazole therapy. *Arch Intern Med.* 1981;141(11):1424–1427.

Wali SO. An update on the drainage of pyogenic lung abscesses. *Ann Thorac Med.* 2012;7(1):3–7.

4.37 Measles

Firza Alexander Gronthoud

CLINICAL CONSIDERATIONS

Measles is a double enveloped RNA virus and one of the most contagious viruses, with a basic reproduction number (R_0) estimated around 15–20. It may not always present in a classical way. The best protection is two MMR vaccinations, with a 95% protection rate. The most effective way to control measles is by achieving high uptake of two doses of measles, mumps, rubella (MMR) vaccine. A high herd immunity prevents transmission of measles and helps achieve elimination of measles. Measles is a notifiable disease. With increasing progress towards measles elimination, physicians are less likely to have experience of clinically diagnosing measles cases, and especially, immunocompromised individuals are at risk of severe complications. It may therefore be worthwhile to consider the following.

INCUBATION PERIOD

The incubation period is usually 10–12 days from exposure to onset of symptoms, but can be up to 21 days.

MODE OF TRANSMISSION

Measles is spread airborne via small respiratory droplets (aerosols) transmitted by coughing and sneezing, close personal contact or direct contact with infected nasal or throat secretions.

SYMPTOMS

Measles starts with a 2–4-day prodromal illness before the rash appears, which typically includes high fever, coryzal symptoms, cough and conjunctivitis. Fever peaks around 39°C–40°C around the time of rash onset. The morbilliform rash, which is caused by a cell-mediated reaction, classically starts behind the ears and progresses downwards to the face and trunk and can be generalized as well.

The rash, which is non-itching, lasts for 3–7 days. Koplik's spots may appear around the time of the rash, sometimes one day before, and last for 2–3 days after the rash appears. Koplik's spots are small white or bluish- white lesions with erythema on the buccal mucosa.

> **CLINICAL PEARL**
>
> Classic measles symptoms are conjunctivitis, Koplik's spots and a rash.

PERIOD OF INFECTIOUSNESS

The period of infectiousness generally starts from about 4 days before the rash and lasts up to 4 days after the onset of rash.

COMPLICATIONS

The most frequent complications include viral pneumonitis and otitis media, as well as diarrhoea. Measles infection often leads to a temporary reduction in immune responses in the few weeks following infection, which may increase the risk of severe secondary bacterial and viral infections. Tracheobronchitis ('measles croup') and pneumonia due to secondary bacterial infection are frequent complications of measles. The most frequent CNS complication of measles is an acute immune-mediated, post-measles encephalitis occurring within 2–30 days. A CSF analysis shows a lymphocytic pleocytosis and increased protein. Differential diagnosis consists of enterovirus, herpes simplex 1 and varicella zoster. Other CNS manifestations are a primary measles encephalitis, measles inclusion body encephalitis and subacute sclerosing panencephalitis (SSPE), which is a very rare but very severe complication, occurring in about 0.01% of cases. Cases of SSPE present a few years after measles infection with progressive neurocognitive symptoms, which in most cases lead to coma and death. The risk of SSPE is increased in children who acquire measles before the age of 1 year.

REINFECTION

Cases of measles reinfection are generally mild, have a shorter duration and may not have typical measles symptoms such as coryza and conjunctivitis. In some cases, the rash may not be typical. Reinfections are usually seen in patients who have received two doses of measles-containing vaccine, and initial antibody testing may be misleading. The infectivity of these cases is low, and the initial diagnosis is usually made by PCR detection of low levels of measles virus RNA. Transmission from reinfection is rare, probably due to low and transient infectivity.

POST-MEASLES IMMUNOSUPPRESSION

Measles infects dendrocytes and lymphocytes, causing a lymphocytopaenia and affecting the humoral and cellular immune deficiency causing a period of immunosuppression after a measles infection.

CLINICAL APPROACH

DIAGNOSING MEASLES

IgM and IgG testing on either serum or oral fluid. Oral fluid is more sensitive, and antibodies can be detected several days sooner than in serum. Oral fluid can be collected by rubbing the swab along the gum line. Throat swabs/nasopharyngeal aspirate/urine/EDTA blood can be used for PCR for detection of measles RNA within 6 days after onset of symptoms. RNA can also be detected in oral fluid. Sputum samples are not adequate samples. In case of encephalitis, measles RNA can be detected in CSF.

It is also important to rule out other viral causes; therefore, a viral respiratory PCR panel on a respiratory specimen should be performed.

TREATMENT OF MEASLES

The World Health Organization advises taking vitamin A to prevent severe complications of measles deficiency such as pneumonia and Bitot's spots. The dose of vitamin A is 100,000 IU (children) or 200,000 IU (adults) per day for 2 days. In the developed world, there is a lower risk for vitamin A deficiency; nonetheless, a low threshold to administer vitamin A should exist.

Treatment of acute post-measles encephalitis consists of corticosteroids; intravenous immunoglobulins may be considered.

There is limited evidence for ribavirin, but oral ribavirin 600 mg twice daily for 7–10 days can be considered for severe complications such as pneumonia and encephalitis.

POST-EXPOSURE PROPHYLAXIS

- Risk assessment likelihood of measles in index case
- Laboratory testing index case
- Assessing risk of exposure for contacts
- Assessing need for post-exposure prophylaxis in contacts

RISK ASSESSMENT LIKELIHOOD OF MEASLES IN INDEX CASES

The risk assessment of any suspected case requires consideration of a range of factors including the age of the case, vaccination history, clinical presentation and epidemiological features such as local outbreaks or an epidemiological link to a confirmed case.

RISK OF EXPOSURE

- Close contacts including household contact
- Face-to-face contact of any length
- More than 15 minutes in a small, confined area, e.g. room in a house

ASSESSING NEED FOR POST-EXPOSURE PROPHYLAXIS IN CONTACTS

Susceptible healthy contacts, including unimmunized children and adults, are unlikely to benefit from post-exposure vaccination, unless offered rapidly following exposure.

Vulnerable contacts (immunosuppressed individuals, pregnant women and infants) are at risk of complicated measles and need to be considered for post-exposure prophylaxis.

Immunosuppressed contacts should be tested for measles IgG. If the measles IgG titre is equivocal or negative, then intravenous immunoglobulins should be administered.

Effectiveness of IVIG is likely to be higher when administered as early as possible following exposure (ideally within 72 hours) although it can be given up to 6 days following exposure. The IVIG dose is 0.15 g/kg. If measles IgG testing cannot be performed within 6 days, then it is reasonable to administer IVIG.

Individuals who have received IVIG in the past 3 weeks do not require post-exposure prophylaxis.

Individuals can be considered immunosuppressed if they have received immunosuppressive chemotherapy or monoclonal antibodies in the past 6 months, are taking high-dose steroids, are HIV positive with CD4 count <200 cells/μL (<500 cells/μL if <5 years). These individuals need to be tested for measles IgG. If negative, IVIG needs to be offered.

Contacts who have a primary immunodeficiency or who had a hematopoietic stem cell transplant within the past 12 months do not require IgG testing and need to be offered IVIG.

Pregnant women with a history of measles infection or who have received two measles vaccinations are considered to be immune and do not need to be tested for IgG and do not require post-exposure prophylaxis.

In all other cases, IgG testing needs to be done within 6 days post-exposure. If negative, IVIG needs to be offered.

BIBLIOGRAPHY

Fisher DL, Defres S, Solomon T. Measles-induced encephalitis. *QJM*. 2015 March;108(3):177–182.

Forni AL, Schluger NW, Roberts RB. Severe measles pneumonitis in adults: Evaluation of clinical characteristics and therapy with intravenous ribavirin. *Clin Infect Dis*. 1994 September;19(3):454–462.

Moss WJ. Measles. *Lancet*. 2017 December 2;390(10111):2490–2502.

Rafat C, Klouche K, Ricard JD et al. Severe measles infection: The spectrum of disease in 36 critically ill adult patients. *Medicine (Baltim)*. 2013 September;92(5):257–272.

Rota PA, Moss WJ, Takeda M, de Swart RL, Thompson KM, Goodson JL. Measles. *Nat Rev Dis Primers*. 2016 July 14;2:16049.

4.38 Meningitis

Firza Alexander Gronthoud

CLINICAL CONSIDERATIONS

Meningitis can have a variety of clinical presentations and remains a challenging diagnosis despite advances in molecular methods. Diagnosing a specific pathogen can reduce length of antimicrobial use or even prevent unnecessary use and reduce mortality and number of additional diagnostic tests requested. It can be beneficial to consider the following.

POPULATION AT RISK

Age groups at risk are young children, in whom protective antibodies are not yet produced, and the elderly, whose humoral and cellular immunity functions diminish.

Patients with asplenia or sickle cell disease are unable to activate the alternative complement pathway, rendering them susceptible to infection with encapsulated bacteria. Alcohol abuse is a risk factor for pneumococcal meningitis because it decreases cough reflex, reduces ciliary clearance and impairs bacterial killing. Impairment of neutrophil adherence, chemotaxis and bacterial killing is seen in poorly controlled diabetes. Patients living with HIV have a higher risk of invasive pneumococcal infection even if on HAART. Cryptococcal meningitis occurs if CD4 T-lymphocyte cell counts are lower than 100 cells/μL. Another group at risk for cryptococcal meningitis are solid organ transplant recipients. Cancer may cause dysfunction of the immune system, increasing risk of meningitis.

COMPLICATION OF PRIMARY INFECTION

Bacteria can reach the subarachnoid space via haematogenous spread, contiguous spread as a complication of otitis media, sinusitis or orbital cellulitis through bone erosion or thrombophlebitis. A third mechanism is via septic emboli in the case of endocarditis. Severe complications of meningitis are ventriculitis and brain abscess.

CLINICAL FINDINGS

Bacterial meningitis has a rapid onset, within days. The classical triad of fever, neck stiffness and altered mental status are only present in less than half of the cases. Other symptoms may include photophobia, vomiting and headache. Almost all adults present with at least two of the four signs and symptoms of headache, fever, neck stiffness, and altered mental status. One-third of adults may present with focal neurological deficits. In contrast, in children and elderly populations the clinical symptoms often can be ambiguous.

Kernig and Brudzinski's signs are low sensitive physical findings and often absent in children. In young children, additional symptoms include bulging fontanelle, apnoeas, purpuric rash, irritability and convulsions. Genital lesions are seen in 10% of patients with HSV-2 meningitis.

CLINICAL PEARL

Complications of meningococcal sepsis:

- Meningococcal sepsis has a rapid onset and is characterized by purpuric or petechial rash, DIC, thrombocytopenia and shock leading to multiorgan failure.
- Meningococcal sepsis can also lead to Waterhouse–Friderichsen syndrome, which is defined as haemorrhage of the adrenal glands leading to adrenal gland failure.
- Without antimicrobial treatment and glucocorticosteroids, death commonly occurs within 12–24 hours.

AETIOLOGY

The majority of community acquired bacterial meningitis cases are caused by *Streptococcus pneumoniae* and *Neisseria meningitidis*. *Haemophilus influenzae* has become a much less frequent cause since the introduction of the *H. influenzae* type b conjugate vaccines. The overall efficacy of the 23-valent pneumococcal polysaccharide vaccine against pneumococcal meningitis is about 50%. *Streptococcus agalactiae* (group B) and *Escherichia coli* are the main causes of neonatal meningitis. *Listeria monocytogenes* can be seen in patients aged 50 years or older. Its incidence is decreasing, presumably due to better awareness, increased hygiene and a decrease in food contamination.

Head trauma with or without skull fracture or chronically draining ears are risk factors for pneumococcal meningitis. The most common pathogens in immunocompromised patients are *S. pneumoniae*, *L. monocytogenes*, *E. coli*, *Salmonella* spp., and *S. aureus*.

Viral meningitis is the most common form of meningitis and, in the Western world, is mainly caused by enterovirus, herpes simplex virus type 2 and varicella zoster virus. In specific geographic areas, viral meningitis is caused by arboviruses such as West Nile virus, tick-borne encephalitis (TBE) virus and Zika virus.

The most common causes of fungal meningitis are *Cryptococcus neoformans* and *Cryptococcus gattii*, most often seen in immunocompromised patients, especially patients living with HIV with a CD4 count of less than <100 cells/µL. In countries with a high prevalence of HIV such as South Africa, cryptococcal meningitis is the most common cause of community-acquired meningitis. Cerebral toxoplasmosis and progressive multifocal leukoencephalopathy caused by JC virus are other causes of meningitis in immunocompromised individuals. Tuberculous meningitis most often occurs in children under 4 years of age who have had contact with persons with infectious tuberculosis.

RECURRENT MENINGITIS

Conditions associated with recurrent meningitis are congenital anatomical defects, remote head trauma, CSF leakage, complement component deficiencies, asplenism and HIV. Clinical presentation is similar to a first episode meningitis.

CHRONIC MENINGITIS

- *Viral*: HIV, CMV, herpes simplex virus types 1 and 2
- *Bacterial*: *Actinomyces*, *Nocardia*, *Treponema pallidum*, *Borrelia burgdorferi*
- *Fungal*: Histoplasmosis and *Cryptococcus*
- *Mycobacterium tuberculosis*

CLINICAL APPROACH

THE CHOICE TO DO AN LP

- *When*: As soon as possible, before the start of empirical therapy to maximize the sensitivity of microbiological investigations.
- *When not to*: Recent or prolonged seizures, lowered consciousness, papilledema, focal neurological signs, shock, stroke or coagulopathy.
- *Which tests*: Cell count, bacterial culture and antimicrobial susceptibility testing and, dependent on CSF analysis, also PCR for viruses and tuberculosis; cryptococcal antigen screening if patient has (suspected) HIV or has had a solid organ transplant.
- *Rationale*: CSF cell count and microbiological investigations can rule out meningitis. CSF analysis may help distinguish bacterial meningitis from other causes, although often there is substantial overlap (see Chapter 2.8).

CLINICAL PEARL

Neonates often present with nonspecific symptoms, and CSF examination cannot rule out the possibility of meningitis due to low sensitivity of WBC count and low diagnostic accuracy of glucose and protein. Gram staining has a sensitivity of 60%. Late-onset neonatal meningitis can occur up to 2–3 months of age.

CLINICAL PEARL

When an LP cannot be performed, it can be useful to take two sets of blood cultures as they are positive in more than 80% of bacterial meningitis, throat and rectal swab for PCR for enterovirus as enteroviruses are shed in the stool for 3 weeks and EDTA blood for PCR for herpes viruses.

MICROBIOLOGICAL INVESTIGATIONS

Traditionally, the gold standard for diagnosis of bacterial meningitis is CSF culture. It allows for identification and antimicrobial susceptibility testing. The sensitivity of Gram stain is around 60%–80%. Polymerase chain reaction (PCR) is a molecular method more frequently used by laboratories. Its sensitivity is higher (>90%) and allows for rapid diagnosis. The sensitivity of PCR for diagnosis may be reduced if it is performed very early in the course of disease (HSV-2), if the clinical manifestations occur after the virus has left the blood (TBE) or with low viral load (enteroviral meningitis). Multiplex PCR has the advantage of detecting several pathogens in one test, albeit there is a limit to the number of pathogens. Disadvantages are higher costs, additional laboratory and personnel requirements and bacterial culture is still required for antimicrobial susceptibility testing. Cryptococcal antigen testing on CSF or blood is a rapid point-of-care test with high sensitivity and specificity, >90%.

EMPIRICAL TREATMENT

For the treatment of community-acquired bacterial meningitis, intravenous ceftriaxone 2 g IV BD or cefotaxime 2 g 4-hourly IV are the antibacterial agents of choice. Cefotaxime has a better CNS penetration but is administered more frequently. Amoxicillin 2 g 4-hourly IV can be added if risk factors for *L. monocytogenes* are present. Viral meningitis is a benign condition and does not require treatment. Cryptococcal meningitis is treated with liposomal amphotericin B 3 mg/kg OD + flucytosine 25 mg/kg QDS for at least 2 weeks, followed by consolidation therapy with fluconazole 400 mg OD for at least 8 weeks. In patients with HIV, secondary prophylaxis with oral fluconazole 200 mg OD is indicated until CD4 count >100 cells/mm^3 for at least 3 months with undetectable viral load.

CLINICAL PEARL

Time between hospital admission and first antibiotic dose should be less than 1 hour. The risk for complications may increase by up to 30% per hour of treatment delay.

CORTICOSTEROIDS

Corticosteroids can play a supportive role due to reduction of oedema, inflammation and intracerebral vasculitis, reducing the risk of hydrocephalus and stroke. They also suppress the immune system and reduce meningeal inflammation. Negative effects include reducing the CNS concentration of antimicrobial agents, reducing permeability of the blood–CSF and blood–brain barriers, further lowering the CSF concentrations of hydrophilic antibiotics. Dexamethasone reduces the CSF concentration of vancomycin and ceftriaxone by 30% and 40%, respectively, whereas methylprednisolone reduces the CSF concentration of gentamicin and ampicillin by 30% and 50%, respectively. With highly drug-susceptible bacteria, the antibacterial CSF concentrations during adjunctive dexamethasone treatment may still remain far above the minimum inhibitory concentration. If the decision is made to start dexamethasone, the general dose and duration is 10 mg 6-hourly IV for 4 days.

POST-EXPOSURE PROPHYLAXIS

Post-exposure prophylaxis may be indicated for close contacts with invasive meningococcal infection. Chemoprophylaxis is indicated if there was direct contact with respiratory secretions or saliva from sneezing, coughing and talking. Household contacts are considered close contacts.

Post-exposure prophylaxis should ideally be given within 24 hours and consists of one dose of ciprofloxacin 500 mg (adults) or 250 mg (children 5 to 11 years) or rifampicin 600 mg twice daily for 2 days for adults. For children aged 1–11 years, the rifampicin dose is 10 mg/kg BD for 2 days (maximum dose 600 mg). Azithromycin 500 mg single dose may be considered for pregnant women.

BIBLIOGRAPHY

Brouwer MC, Thwaites GE, Tunkel AR, van de Beek D. Dilemmas in the diagnosis of acute community-acquired bacterial meningitis. *Lancet*. 2012 November 10;380(9854):1684–1692.

Brouwer MC, Tunkel AR, van de Beek D. Epidemiology, diagnosis, and antimicrobial treatment of acute bacterial meningitis. *Clin Microbiol Rev*. 2010 July;23(3):467–492.

McGill F, Griffiths MJ, Solomon T. Viral meningitis: Current issues in diagnosis and treatment. *Curr Opin Infect Dis*. 2017 April;30(2):248–256.

Nau R, Djukic M, Spreer A, Ribes S, Eiffert H. Bacterial meningitis: An update of new treatment options. *Expert Rev Anti Infect Ther*. 2015;13(11):1401–1423.

Rahimi J, Woehrer A. Overview of cerebrospinal fluid cytology. *Handb Clin Neurol*. 2017;145:563–571.

4.39 Near-Drowning-Associated Pneumonia

Firza Alexander Gronthoud

CLINICAL CONSIDERATIONS

Near drowning is an episode of submersion causing hypoxemia, acidosis and hypoperfusion leading to neurological and pulmonary damage. The most common infectious complication is pneumonia. Knowledge of the risk of pneumonia, type of water exposure and its associated bacterial and fungal flora (Table 4.39.1) is essential for choosing the right microbiological tests and empirical therapy. It is therefore worth considering the following.

CAUSE OF NEAR DROWNING

Common causes of near drowning are seizures, syncope, trauma (may be accompanied by alcohol use) or sudden death. These individuals do not have a voluntary apnoea and, as a consequence, may aspirate larger volumes of water. Potentially, this could have an increased risk of pneumonia.

CLINICAL PEARL

Complications of near drowning are pre-hospital cardiac arrest, impairment of consciousness, acute respiratory failure and cardiovascular failure. Near drowning occurs mainly in healthy young male adults and is most commonly a result of accidental fall, trauma or sporting activities.

Factors that are associated with pneumonia are aspiration, water temperature, chemical composition of the water and nosocomial pneumonia.

ASPIRATION

Following submersion, voluntary apnoea occurs until the $PaCO_2$ and PaO_2 reach a threshold, after which involuntary breathing takes over resulting into aspiration of water. Only less than 10% of near-drowning victims do not aspirate, protecting them from developing pneumonia. In case of aspiration, more than 85% aspirate <22 mL/kg water. It is unknown if this correlates with increased risk of pneumonia.

Swallowing significant amounts of water increases risk of vomiting with subsequent aspiration of vomit. This particularly can occur during resuscitation. Aspiration of gastric contents causes inflammation to the pulmonary parenchyma, increasing the risk of pneumonia not only with oropharyngeal flora, but also microorganisms found in the aquatic environment.

CONTAMINATED WATER

Water contaminated with, e.g. sewage further increases the risk of pneumonia as it contains more human pathogens. Seventy percent of near-drowning victims aspirate mud, sand and vegetation. Near-drowning victims in a shallow environment are more likely to aspirate particles such as dust.

TABLE 4.39.1

Water Exposure and Associated Pathogens That Have Been Implicated in Near-Drowning Pneumonia

Type of Water	Bacterial Flora	Fungal Flora
Freshwater	*Aeromonas* spp. *Burkholderia pseudomallei* *Chromobacterium violaceum* *Streptococcus pneumoniae* *Legionella* spp. *Pseudomonas aeruginosa*	
Saltwater	*Francisella philomiragia* *Klebsiella pneumoniae* *Aeromonas* spp. *Neisseria mucosa* *Shewanella putrefaciens* *Vibrio* spp.	*Aspergillus* spp.
Contaminated stagnant water	*Chromobacterium violaceum* *Pseudomonas aeruginosa* *Aeromonas* spp. *Burkholderia pseudomallei*	*Pseudallescheria boydii/Scedosporium apiospermum* *Aspergillus* spp.

WATER TEMPERATURE

Water temperature is an important factor for the type of organisms found as bacteria and fungi have a narrow temperature in which they can survive. As a result, pneumonia following near drowning in cold water is less common as bacteria found in cold water, e.g. *Vibrio marinus*, are unable to survive in environments with a temperature >25°C such as the human body.

NOSOCOMIAL PNEUMONIA

Pulmonary damage caused by near drowning enhances the risk of pulmonary infection. Victims of near drowning may require mechanical ventilation in the intensive care unit, placing them at risk for a nosocomial pneumonia.

CLINICAL APPROACH

Because the literature with respect to near-drowning pneumonia is based on case reports or retrospective descriptive studies, clinical information might be limited. It is difficult to ascertain whether common pathogens such as *Enterobacterales* or *Pseudomonas aeruginosa* are true causes of near-drowning pneumonia or nosocomial pneumonia as a complication of hospital admission due to near drowning. Similarly, if a near-drowning victim develops a pneumonia early on during their hospital stay, it can be difficult to differentiate between a nosocomial pneumonia and a near-drowning pneumonia. Finally, many pathogens have been cultured from water without being associated in the literature with near-drowning pneumonia.

Nevertheless, empirical therapy should target pathogens found to inhabit the aquatic environment involved in the near-drowning accident and local hospital pathogens (Table 4.39.1). There is no clear evidence supporting the use of antimicrobial prophylaxis to prevent near-drowning pneumonia. A low threshold for empirical therapy should exist as most victims of near drowning have pulmonary signs and symptoms, chest X-rays may be difficult to interpret, and near-drowning pneumonia can be severe and difficult to treat. There is no role for antifungal agents in the initial management of near-drowning pneumonia. Antifungal therapy is indicated if there is slow response to antibiotic therapy, pneumonia occurs weeks after near drowning or the victim develops a brain abscess. The most common fungal cause of near-drowning pneumonia is *Scedosporium apiospermum*.

Pneumonia caused by *Aeromonas* spp., *Burkholderia pseudomallei* and *Pseudallescheria boydii* can have a mortality rate of 60%. These organisms are difficult to treat, and the clinician should have a low threshold of suspicion of these organisms.

BIBLIOGRAPHY

Assink-de Jong E, Douma M, Beishuizen A, Hoogewerf M, Debets-Ossenkopp YJ, de Waard MC, Girbes AR. Microbiological findings and adequacy of antibiotic treatment in the critically ill patient with drowning-associated pneumonia. *Intensive Care Med.* 2014 February;40(2):290–291.

Cerland L, Mégarbane B, Kallel H, Brouste Y, Mehdaoui H, Resiere D. Incidence and consequences of near-drowning-related pneumonia-A descriptive series from Martinique, French West Indies. *Int J Environ Res Public Health.* 2017 November 17;14(11).

Ender PT, Dolan MJ. Pneumonia associated with near-drowning. *Clin Infect Dis.* 1997 October;25(4):896–907.

Tadié JM, Heming N, Serve E et al. . Drowning associated pneumonia: A descriptive cohort. *Resuscitation.* 2012 March;83(3):399–401.

Wood C. Towards evidence based emergency medicine: Best BETs from the Manchester Royal Infirmary. BET 1: Prophylactic antibiotics in near-drowning. *Emerg Med J.* 2010 May;27(5):393–394.

4.40 Neutropaenic Sepsis

Patrick Lillie

CLINICAL CONSIDERATIONS

Patients with febrile neutropaenia are at high risk of infection and also of poor outcomes from this. These patients can progress rapidly to life-threatening sepsis and prompt broad-spectrum antimicrobial therapy is needed. The risk of infection is related to both the duration and the extent of the neutropaenia, and other factors to be taken into account when assessing these patients are shown in Table 4.40.1.

CLINICAL APPROACH

INVESTIGATION AND INITIAL MANAGEMENT OF THE PATIENT WITH NEUTROPAENIC SEPSIS

Table 4.40.2 provides an outline for the initial investigation and antimicrobial drug selection for patients with neutropaenic sepsis.

In patients with previous episodes of infection with documented resistant pathogens/known to be colonized with resistant organisms (e.g. MRSA/ESBL or carbapenemase-producing organisms), then the empirical regimen should include antimicrobials to cover these.

In patients who are improving, a randomized trial of stopping antibiotics after 72 hours of the patient being afebrile had comparable results to those treated until the resolution of neutropaenia.

PROPHYLAXIS

Prevention of febrile episodes in neutropaenic patients with either haematological malignancy or those receiving chemotherapy for solid tumours can be attempted with either antimicrobial prophylaxis or by the use of growth factors to stimulate neutrophil recovery. In terms of antibacterial prophylaxis, levofloxacin has a good level of evidence to support its use in patients whose neutropaenia is likely to be profound ($<0.1 \times 10^9$/L) and prolonged (>7 days), with this most likely to occur in those receiving induction chemotherapy for acute leukaemia or recipients of stem cell transplants. These patients should also be considered for antifungal and antiviral prophylaxis. Routine administration of granulocyte stimulating factor is not recommended but can be considered on a case-by-case basis.

> ### CLINICAL PEARL
>
> Although G-CSF reduces the time to neutrophil recovery and the length of hospitalization, it may affect outcome and may in fact increase risk of ARDS in patients with pulmonary infiltrates.

CLINICAL VIGNETTES

A 26-year-old woman was receiving chemotherapy for newly diagnosed acute myeloid leukaemia (AML). Five days after commencing chemotherapy, she became febrile and hypotensive, and empirical piperacillin/tazobactam was prescribed and blood cultures (peripheral and from the

264

TABLE 4.40.1
Risk of Infections Associated with Neutropaenia

	Higher Risk of Infection	Lower Risk of Infection
Cause of neutropaenia	Haematological malignancy	Non-chemotherapy/malignancy-related neutropaenia, e.g. viral reactivation such as cytomegalovirus
Physiological/clinical features	Evidence of sepsis/shock. Organ dysfunction	Febrile but no other adverse physiology

TABLE 4.40.2
Management of Neutropaenic Sepsis

Duration of Febrile Neutropaenia	Investigations	Empirical Antimicrobials
0–72 hours	Blood cultures, urine culture, basic imaging, e.g. CXR	Piperacillin/tazobactam (for penicillin allergic patients: meropenem/ceftazidime if not anaphylaxis; glycopeptide + ciprofloxacin if anaphylaxis)
72–96 hours	Repeated cultures, fungal biomarkers (galactomannan, 1,3-β-D-glucan), viral PCR (CMV/adenovirus), respiratory viruses	Carbapenem +/− glycopeptide if venous catheter present
>96 hours	CT scanning of chest/sinuses to assess for fungal infection	Empirical antifungal treatment to cover *Candida* spp. and *Aspergillus* spp., continued carbapenem

Abbreviations: CMV, cytomegalovirus; CT, computed tomography; CXR, chest X-ray; PCR, polymerase chain reaction.

indwelling venous catheter) were taken. She remained febrile despite changing her antimicrobials to meropenem, and a serum 1,3-β-D-glucan was elevated on two occasions and she commenced caspofungin. Subsequently, Candida albicans *was isolated from her venous catheter and urine. You advise removal of the catheter, ophthalmological assessment and an echocardiogram. Her empirical caspofungin was changed to fluconazole to achieve better renal tract penetration and she was treated for 14 days after which posaconazole was started as an antifungal prophylaxis. She subsequently had further fevers but was generally improving and was found to have CMV reactivation with a viral load of 7000 IU/mL. She was treated with oral valganciclovir and continued on this as secondary prophylaxis prior to further chemotherapy and stem cell transplant.*

In patients not responding to standard empirical therapy, other causes should be sought and in high-risk patients, early antifungal treatment should be considered. It should be remembered that although echinocandins are very good agents for candidaemia, their penetration into the renal tract and central nervous system is poor and, if possible, alternative agents should be used. Secondary prophylaxis for those at risk of recurrent disease during further episodes of neutropaenia is a sensible precaution.

A 43-year-old woman was being treated for metastatic breast cancer and 9 days after her chemotherapy presented with a fever of 38.1°C, but was otherwise stable and had no other comorbidities. Her neutrophil count was 0.7 × 10⁹/L and the rest of her blood tests were normal. As she was stable, she was commenced on oral ciprofloxacin and co-amoxiclav and allowed home, to be reviewed as an outpatient the next day.

Low-risk patients, in whom the duration of neutropaenia is expected to be short (<7 days), who have no significant physiological derangement or comorbidities, can be considered for outpatient oral treatment but they must have access to urgent review should they worsen.

BIBLIOGRAPHY

Aguilar-Guisado M, Espigado I, Martín-Peña A et al. Optimisation of empirical antimicrobial therapy in patients with haematological malignancies and febrile neutropaenia (How long study): An open-label, randomised controlled phase 4 trial. *Lancet Haematol.* 2017;4(12):e573–e583.

Bucaneve G et al. Levofloxacin to prevent bacterial infection in patients with cancer and neutropaenia. *N Engl J Med.* 2005;353:977–987.

Freifeld AG, Bow EJ, Sepkowitz KA et al. Clinical practice guideline for the use of antimicrobial agents in neutropenic patients with cancer: 2010 Update by the Infectious Diseases Society of America. *Clin Infect Dis.* 2011;52(4):e56–e93.

National Institute for Health and Care Excellence. Neutropaenic sepsis: Prevention and management in people with cancer. Clinical guideline CG151, Sept 2012.

Taplitz RA, Kennedy EB, Bow EJ et al. Outpatient management of fever and neutropenia in adults treated for malignancy: American Society of Clinical Oncology and Infectious Diseases Society of America clinical practice guideline update. *J Clin Oncol.* 2018;36(14):1443–1453.

4.41 Non-Resolving Pneumonia

Firza Alexander Gronthoud

CLINICAL CONSIDERATIONS

Non-responsive pneumonia or persistence or progression of the pneumonia despite antibiotic treatment is a relatively frequent occurrence and can be due to difficult to treat organisms, host factors and antibiotic factors. In some patients, however, pneumonia improves slower than others and it is more difficult to ascertain whether there is a non-resolving pneumonia or the patient simply needs more time to recover. It is therefore worthwhile to consider the following.

NORMAL-COURSE PNEUMONIA

- Patients typically note subjective improvement within 3–5 days of treatment.
- Tachycardia and hypotension should usually improve in 2 days.
- Fever, tachypnea, and arterial oxygenation (PaO_2) are expected to improve within 3 days.
- Cough and fatigue may take 14 days or longer to improve.
- It can take over a month for infiltrates to improve on chest X-ray.

CLINICAL PEARL

It takes around 3–4 weeks for radiographic signs to resolve in mild to moderate pneumonia, whilst it may take longer in severe pneumonia, elderly and patients with underlying comorbidities.

MOST COMMON REASONS OF NON-RESOLVING PNEUMONIA

- Difficult to treat pathogens (i.e. tuberculosis)
- Host factors (e.g. older age, immunocompromised, airway disease, cancer or chemotherapy, alcoholism and cigarette smoking)
- Complications
- Non-infectious causes including malignancy (i.e. carcinoma or lymphoma); airway obstruction due to malignancy which can lead to accumulation of secretions predisposing to infection

---

CLINICAL PEARL

Patients with a pneumonia without underlying lung conditions can be considered clinically stable (Halm's criteria) if temperature $\leq 37.8°C$, heart rate ≤ 100 beats/minute, respiratory rate ≤ 24 breaths/minute, systolic blood pressure ≥ 90 mmHg, O_2 saturation $\geq 90\%$ or arterial O_2 tension ≥ 60 mmHg, normal mental status, and normal oral intake.

DIFFICULT-TO-TREAT OR UNCOMMON PATHOGENS

- Consider drug-resistant organisms: *Streptococcus pneumoniae* (pneumococcus) is the organism of most concern, multidrug-resistant *H. influenzae* and *Pseudomonas aeruginosa* as well as Panton–Valentine leucocidin (PVL) producing *Staphylococcus aureus*
- *Atypical: Mycoplasma pneumoniae* (3–5 year cycle), *Chlamydia psittaci* (birds) and *Legionella pneumophila* (infected water source)
- *Travel:* Mississippi area (*Histoplasma*), southern part of United States (Coccidioidomycosis), Southeast Asia (*Burkholderia pseudomallei*)
- If the patient has AIDS, profound neutropenia or is on steroids for underlying lung disease, consider pulmonary aspergillosis (see Chapter 4.34)
- If there is a cavitary lesion, consider *Nocardia* or *Actinomyces* or *Aspergillus*
- Consider pulmonary cryptococcosis and *Pneumocystis jirovecii* in patients with CD4 count <200/μL or in allogeneic bone marrow transplant recipients

CONSIDER HOST FACTORS

- HIV
- Primary humoral immune deficiencies including hypogammaglobulinaemia, common variable immune deficiency and selective immunoglobulin (Ig)G subset deficiency
- *Asplenia:* Significant risk factor for infections caused by polysaccharide-encapsulated bacteria: *S. pneumoniae, H. influenzae, N. meningitidis*
- *Alcohol abuse:* Increased risk of *S. pneumoniae* and aspiration (anaerobes)
- *COPD or bronchiectasis: Pseudomonas aeruginosa, Enterobacterales*

CONSIDER COMPLICATIONS

- Community-acquired pneumonia complicated by parapneumonic effusion or empyema
- Aspiration pneumonia and lung abscess
- Risk factors: Alcoholism, seizures, poor oral hygiene and previous aspiration

NON-INFECTIOUS CAUSES

- Pulmonary embolism
- *Malignancy*: Carcinoma or lymphoma
- Pulmonary vasculitis syndromes
- Sarcoidosis
- Bronchiolitis obliterans organizing pneumonia
- Eosinophilic pneumonia
- Acute interstitial pneumonia
- Diffuse alveolar damage of various aetiologies with or without intercurrent infection treated with current antibiotic course
- *Drug induced*: Long-term nitrofurantoin, amiodarone, methotrexate, bleomycin

STREPTOCOCCUS PNEUMONIAE

In immunocompetent individuals without comorbidities, clinical improvement is relatively rapid and precedes radiographic improvement. It may take several days for the temperature to completely settle, with a minority remaining febrile beyond 20 days.

- Clinical improvement is delayed in severe presentation, multilobar disease and infection with drug-resistant organisms.

- Radiographic improvement is often much slower, with 20%–30% of patients demonstrating no radiographic improvement after one week. Initial worsening of the chest radiograph is common. Risk factors for delayed radiographic resolution include bacteraemia, persistent fever or leucocytosis beyond 6 days, advanced age, chronic obstructive pulmonary disease, alcoholism and HIV.
- Radiographic clearing occurs by 1–3 months in nonbacteraemic cases and 3–5 months in bacteraemic cases. Residual radiographic abnormalities are rare in nonbacteraemic cases but are present in up to 35% of bacteraemic cases.

LEGIONELLA

- Many of the risk factors for development of *Legionella* are also risk factors for delayed resolution. These include cigarette smoking, alcoholism, age greater than 65 years, immunosuppression (especially glucocorticoid use), chronic kidney disease and hematopoietic stem cell and solid organ transplantation.
- As a result, the rate of resolution for *Legionella* infection is usually slower than for other organisms.
- Radiographic, but not necessarily clinical, deterioration despite treatment is common, occurring in up to two-thirds of patients with *Legionella*, compared with 4% of patients with nonbacteraemic pneumococcal pneumonia. In addition, after this initial deterioration, resolution is slow, with clearing beginning only after 2–3 weeks, and approximately one-half of patients demonstrating residual abnormalities at 10 weeks. Resolution may take as long as 6–12 months, and residual fibrosis may be evident in up to 25% of patients.

CLINICAL APPROACH

- If stable or slowly improving pneumonia and patient has comorbidities or host factors known to delay the resolution of pneumonia, carefully monitor patient for 4–8 weeks.
- If there is no resolution or progression of disease, a more aggressive diagnostic approach is appropriate:
  - Repeat history, physical examination and review of the medical record. Ensure full travel history, occupational exposures, diet, animal contact and hobbies.
  - If a patient is on a penicillin (i.e. amoxicillin/clavulanic acid or piperacillin/tazobactam), consider changing to a second- or third-generation cephalosporin to take into account a penicillin intermediate, resistant *S. pneumoniae*, *S. aureus* and β-lactam/β-lactamase inhibitor resistant *H. influenzae* (BLNAR or BLPACR).
  - Based on risk factors and previous culture results, consider antipseudomonal and/or MRSA cover.
  - Looking for systemic features of malignancy (lymphadenopathy, possible distant metastasis, weight loss, night sweats).
  - Repeat chest X-ray OR more detailed imaging:
    - High-resolution chest CT for more detailed visualization of parenchymal abnormalities, including emphysema, airspace disease, interstitial disease and nodules
    - CT pulmonary angiogram to exclude pulmonary embolism
  - If HR CT is compatible with mycobacterial or fungal infection, discuss with respiratory team the possibility of bronchoscopy for bacterial, mycobacterial and fungal microscopy and culture. If patient is clinically stable, preferably stop antibiotics few days prior to procedure.
  - If HR CT shows lymphadenopathy, discuss with respiratory team possibility of aspiration or biopsy of suspect lesions for mycobacterial and fungal microscopy and culture.
- With a worsening chest radiograph and progressive symptoms accompanied by a negative bronchoscopy, further evaluation with thoracoscopic or open lung biopsy.

CLINICAL PEARL

Neoplastic lesions are an important cause and may result in non-resolving pneumonia through a variety of mechanisms including blocking the airway directly or through extrinsic compression of an airway.

BIBLIOGRAPHY

Arab T, Malekzadegan MR, Morante J, Cervellione KL, Fein AM. Nonresolving pneumonia in the setting of malignancy. *Curr Opin Pulm Med.* 2019 July;25(4):331–335.
Chalmers JD, Hill AT. Investigation of 'non-responding' presumed lower respiratory tract infection in primary care. *BMJ.* 2011 October 13;343:d5840.
Finch S, Chalmers JD. Brief clinical review: Non-responding pneumonia. *EMJ Respir.* 2014;2:104–d5111.

4.42 Norovirus

Firza Alexander Gronthoud

CLINICAL CONSIDERATIONS

Infection with norovirus leads to temporary immunity after which individuals are susceptible again to new infections. Norovirus mostly causes self-limiting disease, but in the immunocompromised, elderly and children younger than 5 years, it can cause severe disease and death potentially. Although much is known about the clinical manifestation and complication of norovirus, there are many knowledge gaps in norovirus biology, and consequently, there is no antiviral treatment or vaccines on the market which is of great clinical concern. Norovirus requires a small infective dose to cause disease in humans (100 viral particles). It is therefore worthwhile to consider the following.

NOROVIRUS BIOLOGY

Norovirus belongs to the *Caliciviridae* family, which is a group of non-enveloped, positive-sense, single-stranded RNA (ssRNA) viruses. Another member of this family which causes human infections is sapovirus. The norovirus genus can be subdivided into at least seven genogroups and >40 genotypes. Genogroups II (mostly GII.4), I and infrequently genogroup IV cause human infections. Infections occurring during outbreaks of GII.4 strains are associated with more severe outcomes, including mortality, than infections during outbreaks of non-GII.4 strains.

The norovirus genome encodes six non-structural proteins and two structural proteins, which are major capsid protein VP1 and minor capsid protein VP2. Norovirus particles display an icosahedral symmetry.

SYMPTOMS

The main symptoms are nausea and vomiting, abdominal cramps, lethargy, diarrhoea and fever. Symptoms usually last 2 days (range 1–3 days). The illness may be more severe and prolonged in individuals with medical comorbidities. Those that are younger than 2 years and older than 65 years and immunocompromised individuals are at increased risk of severe symptoms and death. Incubation period is 48 hours.

TRANSMISSION

The fecal-oral route is the main mode of transmission, although several other modalities have been described. These modalities include transmission via aerosolized viral particles in vomitus and through food, water and environmental contamination (norovirus can survive for up to 7 days on fomites). GII.4 is more likely to be associated with person-to-person transmission, especially in long-term care facilities (LTCFs) and hospital settings, whereas GI.7 and GII.12 are associated with food-borne disease.

PERIOD OF SHEDDING AND PERSISTENCE IN THE ENVIRONMENT

The ability to cause major outbreaks is promoted by prolonged viral shedding and ability to survive in the environment. Fecal excretion of norovirus infection in asymptomatic individuals is common, especially in children. Transplant recipients can have a prolonged period of shedding of several years. Similarly, symptoms may last for 2 weeks in bone marrow recipients, whilst in renal transplant recipients, persistent symptoms lasting 3 years have been described in the literature.

DIAGNOSING NOROVIRUS

Kaplan's criteria:

- Vomiting in more than half of symptomatic cases
- Mean (or median) incubation period of 24–48 h
- Mean (or median) duration of illness of 12–60 h
- No bacterial pathogen isolated in stool culture

LABORATORY DIAGNOSIS

Specimens should be collected in a closed container within 48–72 h of the onset of symptoms, although norovirus may be detected in stool samples for 7–10 days or longer. Specimens should be refrigerated at 4°C prior to testing and frozen at −20°C or −70°C for long-term storage.

Vomitus is an alternative specimen type that may be used to supplement stool sample testing during outbreak investigations. Collection and handling are the same as for stool specimens. Serum specimens are not recommended for routine diagnosis.

Various commercial EIA assays exist with sensitivities for each assay ranging from 30% to 90% and specificity 60% to 100%. Factors influencing this are the viral load and genotype. To increase the sensitivity of the EIAs, it is recommended to take multiple samples. Because of the modest performance of these commercial kits, particularly their poor sensitivity, they are not recommended for clinical diagnosis of norovirus infection in sporadic cases of gastroenteritis. Besides EIAs, there now also exist lateral-flow immunochromatographic assays with sensitivities also showing a wide range between 19% and 90%. Real-time RT-PCR is the gold standard for diagnosis.

CLINICAL PEARL

Asymptomatic excretion of norovirus has diagnostic implications. Diarrhoea due to another cause in an asymptomatic carrier may be misdiagnosed as being due to norovirus infection. Especially in outbreaks, it is therefore worthwhile to also test for other common causes of gastroenteritis such as sapovirus and adenovirus.

TREATMENT

There is no clear proven effective treatment. There are some reports showing a reduction in duration of symptoms in patients administered nitazoxanide. The mainstay of management is supportive treatment maintaining hydration fluids and electrolytes. In immunocompromised individuals with persistent symptoms, reduction of immunosuppressive therapy should be attempted.

CHALLENGES FOR VACCINE DEVELOPMENT

The viral capsid protein VP1 has three structural domains, with the shell (S) being the core from which two other domains, P1 and P2, protrude. P2 is the most exposed portion and is likely the major point of contact with histo-blood group antigen (HBGA) ligands and with neutralizing antibody. Mutations and recombination events involving P2 can significantly affect antigen properties and interactions with HBGAs. GII.4 strains, in particular, are undergoing rapid evolution that affects receptor binding by changes in surface-exposed P2 and antigenic expression, resulting in the emergence of new epidemic strains of the virus. In contrast, there has been only limited evolution of GI viruses over the last four decades.

GII.4 undergoes epochal evolution characterized by periods of stasis followed by the emergence of a new epidemic strain. There have been seven different GII.4 variants associated with global epidemics since the 1990s, which occurred in 1996, 2002, 2004, 2007–2008 (2 variant strains), 2009–2012 and 2012 onward (the Sydney strain). Thus, on average, new variants of GII.4 have appeared every 2–3 years.

Natural susceptibility to norovirus can vary between individuals and genotypes; the duration and degree of cross-protection of acquired immunity is not well understood, and there is no single, well-established correlate of protection for norovirus infection or illness that can be used in vaccine development.

Evidence indicates that new variants emerge under positive selection, likely as a result of the pressure exerted by the development of herd immunity as larger portions of the population experience infection, with resultant viral antigenic drift.

CLINICAL PEARL

Reasons why no norovirus vaccine exists:

- Inability to cultivate norovirus *in vitro*.
- Inability to directly measure neutralizing antibody.
- Susceptibility to norovirus infection can vary based on an individual's fucosyltrans-ferase-2 (*FUT2*) gene. This gene regulates the expression of histo-blood group anti-gens (HBGAs), which serve as infection binding ligands on cells needed for infection.
- Multiple viral genogroups and genotypes and their continued evolution.
- Limited heterotypic immunity.
- Likely need for continuing vaccine reformulation.
- Uncertain duration of immunity.
- Incomplete understanding of the role of cellular immunity.
- Possible acceleration of viral evolution in response to a vaccinated population.
- Uncertain efficacy in most vulnerable individuals, including young children, the elderly and the immunocompromised.

CLINICAL APPROACH

Outbreak Management

Detection of an Outbreak

An outbreak of acute gastroenteritis is considered to be laboratory confirmed as attributable to norovirus if stool or vomitus specimens from two or more ill persons are positive for norovirus by RT-PCR, EIA. It has been estimated that at least six samples must be tested by EIA to achieve a 90% probability of detecting a norovirus outbreak. In order to detect an outbreak, whole-stool specimens from at least five ill persons should be tested, reflecting the poor sensitivity of the rapid tests.

Hygiene and Environmental Decontamination

During outbreaks, hands should be washed with soap and running water for a minimum of 20 seconds after providing care for patients with suspected or confirmed infection. Alcohol-based hand sanitizers can be used in addition to water and soap. For disinfection, a bleach concentration of 1000 ppm sodium hypochlorite prepared fresh daily should be used. Unaffected areas should be cleaned first followed by cleaning of affected areas. Similarly, cleaning should start in low contamination areas and move to high contamination areas.

Isolation Precautions

Patients with proven norovirus should placed in a single room with contact precautions until they are 48 hours symptom free. Patients with norovirus infection can be cohorted if there are not enough single rooms available. A mask should be worn when patients are vomiting or when cleaning up vomit. Needless to say, personal protective equipment should be disposable and single use.

Patients on an outbreak ward should be symptom free for 48 hours before they can be transferred to another ward or facility. Outbreaks can be closed if there are no more new cases for at least 48 hours.

Staff

Members of staff should care for one patient cohort at a time, and movement of staff between patient cohorts should be limited. Members of staff with GI symptoms should stay at home until 48 hours after symptoms have resolved.

BIBLIOGRAPHY

Barclay L, Park GW, Vega E, Hall A, Parashar U, Vinjé J, Lopman B. Infection control for norovirus. *Clin Microbiol Infect.* 2014;20:731–740.
Robilotti E, Deresinski S, Pinsky BA. Norovirus. *Clin Microbiol Rev.* 2015 January;28(1):134–164.

4.43 Onychomycosis

Firza Alexander Gronthoud

CLINICAL CONSIDERATIONS

Onychomycosis is a fungal disease of the nail and the most common nail disorders in adults, accounting for 15%–40% of all nail diseases. Up to 70% of patients have a long history of recurrent infections. It is therefore worthwhile to consider the following.

AETIOLOGY

Onychomycosis occurs in 10% of the general population. A higher prevalence in older adults is related to peripheral vascular disease, immunologic disorders and diabetes mellitus. Other risk factors are trauma and hyperhidrosis.

Fungal nail disease is more prevalent in men and in individuals with other nail problems such as psoriasis, in persons with immunosuppressive conditions such as diabetes mellitus or HIV infection and in those taking immunosuppressive medications. Onychomycosis affects toenails more often than fingernails because of their slower growth, reduced blood supply and frequent confinement in dark, moist environments. It may occur in patients with damaged nails, a history of nail trauma, genetic predisposition, hyperhidrosis, concurrent fungal infections and psoriasis. It is also more common in smokers and in those who use occlusive footwear and shared bathing facilities.

CAUSATIVE AGENTS

Most infections are caused by dermatophytes and about 5% are due to nondermatophyte moulds. The most common dermatophytes are *Trichophyton rubrum*, followed by *Trichophyton interdigitale*.

CLINICAL MANIFESTATION

Nails infected with fungi look discoloured, deformed, hypertrophic or hyperkeratotic. Onychomycosis can be confused with dystrophic toenails from repeated low-level trauma.

CLINICAL APPROACH

LABORATORY DIAGNOSIS

Good nail specimens are difficult to obtain but are crucial for maximizing laboratory diagnosis. The affected area should first be cleaned with 70% isopropyl alcohol to prevent overgrowth of bacteria.

Material should be taken from any discoloured, dystrophic or brittle parts of the nail. In cases of superficial involvement, nail scrapings may be taken with a curette. To improve accuracy, 8–10 nail shards should be collected. Samples should also be taken from associated skin lesions.

Clinical diagnosis can be challenging and should be confirmed with laboratory tests. The most widely used test is a KOH preparation. KOH will dissolve keratin, leaving the fungal cell intact. Microscopy can also be done using a calcofluor stain, which has an increased sensitivity compared to KOH. Periodic acid-Schiff (PAS) can be applied to histological sections and smears. For species identification, a culture is needed which may grow the causative agent within 2–6 weeks.

TABLE 4.43.1
Treatment Options

Agent	Dose	Side Effects
Terbinafine	250 mg orally once per day for 6 weeks (fingernails) or 12 weeks (toenails)	Liver function should be monitored in patients with pre-existing hepatic dysfunction and in all patients being treated for longer than 1 month
Itraconazole	Pulse dosing: 200 mg orally two times per day for 1 week per month, for 2 months (fingernails) or 3 months (toenails)	Prolonged QT interval, elevated transaminase
	Continuous dosing: 200 mg orally once per day for 6 weeks (fingernails) or 12 weeks (toenails)	
Fluconazole	100–300 mg orally every week for 3–6 months (fingernails) or 6–12 months (toenails)	Prolonged QT interval, elevated transaminase

TREATMENT

If the microscopy shows fungal elements, treatment should be started. If microscopy is negative, consider awaiting culture results before start of antifungal treatment.

Topical agents poorly penetrate the nail bed, and treatment therefore consists of an oral azole. Terbinafine and oral itraconazole is considered first-line treatment, whereas fluconazole and griseofulvin are reserved for second-line treatment. (See Table 4.43.1.)

Mycotic cure rates are highest for terbinafine (76%), followed by itraconazole pulse dosing (63%), continuous itraconazole (59%) and 48% for fluconazole. Clinical cure rates were 66% for terbinafine, 70% for itraconazole with pulse dosing, 70% for itraconazole with continuous dosing and 41% for fluconazole. Generally, onychomycosis caused by nondermatophytic moulds does not respond to oral antifungal therapy, and current effective management options are limited.

CLINICAL PEARL

- Because of the slow growth pattern of the toenails, up to 18 months is required for the nail plate to grow out fully.
- Therapeutic success of antifungal therapy of onychomycosis depends on the newly grown-out nail plate being fungus free.

RECURRENCES

After treatment of onychomycosis, relapse or reinfection occur in of 20%–25% of the cases. Risk factors are concomitant disease, >50% nail involvement at baseline, genetic factors, immunosuppression, incorrect dosing or duration of treatment, occlusive footwear, older age, poor hygiene, tinea pedis and trauma. Topical antifungal for prophylaxis after completed treatment has been shown to reduce the recurrence rate significantly. Duration is unknown but could be lifelong.

BIBLIOGRAPHY

Ameen M, Lear JT, Madan V, Mohd Mustapa MF, Richardson M. British Association of Dermatologists' guidelines for the management of onychomycosis 2014. *Br J Dermatol.* 2014 November;171(5):937–958.

Lipner SR, Scher RK. Onychomycosis clinical overview and diagnosis. *J Am Acad Dermatol.* 2019 April;80(4):835–851.

Lipner SR, Scher RK. Onychomycosis: Treatment and prevention of recurrence. *J Am Acad Dermatol.* 2019 April;80(4):853–867.

Westerberg DP, Voyack MJ. Onychomycosis: Current trends in diagnosis and treatment. *Am Fam Physician.* 2013 December 1;88(11):762–770.

4.44 Osteomyelitis

Caryn Rosmarin

CLINICAL CONSIDERATIONS

HOW DOES BONE BECOME INFECTED?

There are two primary routes for infection to reach bone.

- Local extension from a neighbouring contaminated source (contiguous spread), such as following trauma or bone surgery, or spread from infected soft tissue infection, most commonly diabetic foot or decubitus ulcers.
- Spread from a distant site via the bloodstream (haematogenous spread). This is seen most often in young children and in the elderly, or when prosthetic material is present in the bone following surgery.

WHAT ARE THE COMMON PATHOGENS CAUSING OSTEOMYELITIS?

Staphylococcus aureus is the commonest aetiological agent. *Staphylococcus epidermidis*, in its ability to form biofilms, is a pathogen common in osteomyelitis secondary to prosthetic material. Chronic osteomyelitis secondary to contiguous spread from infected soft tissue, as in diabetic foot infection, may be polymicrobial in nature and include Gram-negative bacilli, anaerobes and streptococci. In haematogenous osteomyelitis, the infecting organism reflects the frequency of age-specific bacteraemia, including group B strep in neonates and Gram-negative bacilli in the elderly. Other pathogens to consider related to specific circumstances include *Salmonella* spp. in sickle cell disease, *Brucella* spp. in travellers from the Middle East and Mediterranean regions and tuberculosis in populations from high-risk areas.

> ### CLINICAL PEARL
> - Osteomyelitis occurs via contiguous or haematogenous spread of infection to bone.
> - Chronic osteomyelitis is characterized by the formation of sinuses and sequestra.
> - *Staphylococcus aureus* is the commonest infecting organism.

CLINICAL APPROACH

HOW IS OSTEOMYELITIS DIAGNOSED?

Clinically

Acute osteomyelitis presents with fever and pain, swelling and tenderness over the affected bone. Other causes of symptoms such as cellulitis, soft tissue abscess, septic arthritis, infarction or malignancy need to be considered.

Chronic osteomyelitis is characterized by relapsing or persistent low-grade fever and pain, which eventually lead to abscesses and fistula formation. It should be suspected in any patient with an underlying risk factor.

Laboratory

Investigations to determine the underlying cause depend on the source of infection. For haematogenous osteomyelitis, blood cultures are the test of choice. For contiguously spread osteomyelitis, blood cultures may well be negative and direct bone biopsy and culture is the gold standard. Swabs of surrounding areas of infection should be avoided as they tend to grow a multitude of contaminating organisms. Biopsy samples for histology should be sent to confirm inflammation and unusual organisms and exclude malignancy, especially in vertebral or disseminated osteomyelitis.

Radiology

Diagnosis of chronic osteomyelitis can often be made on plain X-rays. In acute infection, however, plain X-rays may be normal or only show soft tissue swelling or joint space changes, and diagnosis will require a more sensitive MRI scan. Plain X-rays should be performed in all cases, as they are more sensitive than other imaging modalities in assessing response to treatment. Other imaging modalities such as CT, bone, white cell or PET scans may be used under special circumstances when the above tests are inconclusive or contraindicated, or if osteomyelitis is more disseminated.

CLINICAL PEARL

- Diagnosis requires clinical suspicion confirmed radiologically by plain X-ray and/ or MRI.
- Blood culture and culture of bone are the gold standards for determining the infecting pathogen.
- Swabs of surrounding tissue are to be discouraged as they are likely to grow organisms contaminating the area.

WHAT ARE THE TREATMENT OPTIONS FOR MANAGING OSTEOMYELITIS?

Osteomyelitis should be managed with advice from both orthopaedics and microbiology. Despite best treatment, recurrent and persistent infections occur in a significant number of cases.

ANTIBIOTIC THERAPY

In acute osteomyelitis, early antibiotic therapy, before extensive destruction of bone or necrosis, leads to the best response. As the possible causative organisms in chronic osteomyelitis are broad, antibiotic treatment should ideally be delayed until a microbiological diagnosis is made.

Despite much research on the treatment of osteomyelitis, the evidence is not adequate to determine the best antibiotic(s), route or duration of therapy. All hospitals will have a local policy of antibiotic treatment for osteomyelitis. Principles of antibiotic treatment are used and include:

- Initial intravenous (IV) antibiotic therapy based on the likelihood of the organism involved, modified by Gram stain and culture.
- IV therapy is commonly used for a minimum of 2 weeks.
- Switch to oral if antibiotics with good bioavailability and bone penetration are available. Oral agents are often used in combination to prevent development of resistance. Examples of these include quinolones, clindamycin, rifampicin and fusidic acid.
- For native osteomyelitis without bacteraemia and haemodynamically stable, oral antibiotics with high bone penetration and bioavailability can be directly started without an initial intravenous course.
- As a general principle, acute osteomyelitis is treated for 6 weeks. This may be prolonged in chronic osteomyelitis, especially when not accompanied by surgical debridement.

SURGERY

Surgical debridement may be necessary, especially in those infections where necrotic or dead tissue, bone, abscess or prosthetic material is present.

CLINICAL VIGNETTE

A 68-year-old man presents 10 days after having a prostate biopsy with fever and new onset of lower back pain. His temperature is 38.2°C and he is tender over his lumbar spine. Urine and blood cultures grow an Escherichia coli.

In adults, vertebral osteomyelitis occurs following haematogenous spread. One should suspect the diagnosis of vertebral osteomyelitis in patients with new or worsening back or neck pain and fever together with one or more of the following: elevated ESR or CRP, bloodstream infection or infective endocarditis, or new neurologic symptoms.

BIBLIOGRAPHY

Calhoun JH, Manring MM, Shirtliff M. Osteomyelitis of the long bones. *Semin Plast Surg.* 2009;23(2):59–72.

Conterno LO, Turchi MD. Antibiotics for treating chronic osteomyelitis in adults. *Cochrane Database Syst Rev.* 2013;(9). Art. No.: CD004439. Published 2013 Sep 6.

Lazzarini L, Lipsky BA, Mader JT. Antibiotic treatment of osteomyelitis: What have we learned from 30 years of clinical trials? *Int J Infect Dis.* 2005;9:127–138.

Li HK, Rombach I, Zambellas R et al. Oral versus intravenous antibiotics for bone and joint infections. *N Engl J Med.* 2019;380(5):425–436.

Scarborough M, Li HK, Rombach I et al. Oral versus intravenous antibiotics for bone and joint infections: The OVIVA non-inferiority RCT. *Health Technol Assess.* 2019;23(38):1–92.

Thabit AK, Fatani DF, Bamakhrama MS, Barnawi OA, Basudan LO, Alhejaili SF. Antibiotic penetration into bone and joints: An updated review. *Int J Infect Dis.* 2019 April;81:128–136. Epub 2019 February 14.

Yew DP, Waldvogel FA. Osteomyelitis. *Lancet.* 2004 July;364:369–379.

4.45 Otitis Externa

Firza Alexander Gronthoud

CLINICAL CONSIDERATIONS

Acute otitis externa (AOE) is a diffuse inflammation of the external ear canal, which may also involve the pinna or tympanic membrane. Initial management is with topical agents; however, in specific situations, systemic antimicrobial treatment is indicated, and it is then worthwhile to consider the following:

ACUTE OTITIS EXTERNA

Otitis externa usually develops within a few weeks. The main feature is rapid onset of signs or symptoms of inflammation of the external ear canal including otalgia, itching, or fullness with or without hearing loss and ear canal pain on chewing. A hallmark sign of diffuse AOE is intense tenderness of the tragus when pushed and/or tenderness of the pinna when pulled, disproportionate to what might be expected based on appearance of the ear canal. Otoscopy can reveal diffuse ear canal oedema, erythema, otorrhea or debris in the ear canal. Regional lymphadenitis or cellulitis of the pinna and adjacent skin may be present in some patients. Most common pathogens are *Pseudomonas aeruginosa* and *Staphylococcus aureus*. Otomycosis or fungal otitis externa caused by *Aspergillus niger* or *Candida* spp. is less common but may be more common in chronic otitis externa or after antibacterial treatment.

AETIOLOGY

The aetiology of AOE is multifactorial. Regular cleaning of the ear canal removes cerumen, which is an important barrier to moisture and infection. Cerumen creates a slightly acidic pH that inhibits infection (especially by *P. aeruginosa*) but can be altered by water exposure, aggressive cleaning, soapy deposits, or alkaline eardrops. Debris from dermatologic conditions may also predispose to infections. Other factors such as sweating, allergy and stress have also been implicated in the pathogenesis of AOE. AOE is more common in regions with warmer climates, increased humidity or increased water exposure from swimming.

CLINICAL PEARL

AOE can mimic the appearance of acute otitis media (AOM) because of erythema involving the tympanic membrane. Distinguishing AOE from AOM is important, because the latter may require systemic antimicrobials, whereas for AOE, topical treatment is usually sufficient. Other conditions that can mimic AEO are cholesteatoma, eczema, seborrhoea, contact dermatitis, furunculosis, viral infections of the ear such as herpes zoster causing Ramsay Hunt syndrome, measles or malignancy.

COMPLICATION

Malignant otitis externa (MOE) is a rapidly spreading, severe, invasive infection of the external ear canal and the lateral skull base and can affect the cranial nerves. Susceptible groups are the elderly, patients with diabetes mellitus and immunocompromised patients.

Symptoms include intense ear pain, persistent discharge, facial palsy, deafness, hoarseness and dysphagia.

On CT, bony erosions can be visualized. CT is limited in determining disease resolution, as changes persist for an extended time following antimicrobial treatment. Resolution of infection is based on the absence of clinical signs or symptoms of disease and the absence of radiographic progression of disease after a minimum follow-up period of 1 month after the completion of antibiotic therapy.

Other complications are sinus thrombosis, meningitis and intracranial abscesses.

CLINICAL PEARL

Otalgia radiating to the periauricular area, temple or neck in the absence of ear swelling and without apparent middle ear disease could indicate temporo-mandibular joint syndrome rather than infection. Crepitus may be present.

CLINICAL APPROACH

PREVENTION

Strategies to prevent AOE are aimed at limiting water accumulation and moisture retention in the external auditory canal and maintaining a healthy skin barrier.

TOPICAL OINTMENTS

Topical therapy remains first-line treatment of uncomplicated AOE (see Table 4.45.1). Topical ointments usually contain one or more of the following compounds: antibiotics such as an aminoglycoside, quinolone or polymyxin B; a steroid, e.g. hydrocortisone or dexamethasone or antiseptics, e.g. acetic acid or boric acid. Duration of treatment is 7–10 days as most patients experience significant clinical improvement after 48 hours and most patients have little to no symptoms after 7–10 days of treatment.

Prolonged exposure to subtherapeutic concentrations of antibiotics can be avoided as topical treatment allows for high local concentration of drugs being achieved, far exceeding the minimum inhibitory concentration. Thus, antimicrobial resistance may not impact clinical use and *in vitro* susceptibility data may be of less importance.

TABLE 4.45.1
Common Topical Ointments

Component	Dosage	Side Effects
Acetic acid 2%	4–6 times daily	May cause pain and irritation; may be less effective than other treatments if use is required beyond 1 week; often used as prophylactic agent
Ciprofloxacin 0.3%/ dexamethasone 0.1%	Twice daily	Low risk of sensitization
Hydrocortisone 2%/ acetic acid 1%	4–6 times daily	May cause pain and irritation
Neomycin/polymyxin B/ hydrocortisone, solution or suspension	3–4 times daily	Ototoxic; higher risk of contact hypersensitivity; avoid in chronic/ eczematous otitis externa
Ofloxacin 0.3%	Once to twice daily	Low risk of sensitization

Delivery of topical treatment can be enhanced by using performing aural toilet and/or placing a wick if there is obstruction of the ear canal.

In case of a known or suspected perforation of the tympanic membrane, the use of aminoglycoside or polymyxin B containing topical preparation should be avoided as they are ototoxic.

CLINICAL PEARL

Common predisposing factors for AOE are humidity or prolonged exposure to water, dermatologic conditions (eczema, seborrhoea, psoriasis), anatomic abnormalities (narrow canal, exostoses), trauma or external devices (wax removal, inserting earplugs, using hearing aids) and otorrhea caused by middle ear disease. AOE may also occur secondary to ear canal obstruction by impacted cerumen, a foreign object, a dermoid cyst, a sebaceous cyst or a furuncle.

SYSTEMIC ANTIBIOTICS

Systemic antibiotics are usually reserved for recurrent infections, those resistant to topical therapy, malignant otitis externa, extension beyond the external auditory canal, diabetics, or immunocompromised patients or a malignancy requiring chemotherapy, radiotherapy, presence of tympanostomy tubes or perforated eardrum.

Options for systemic treatment of *P. aeruginosa* AOE are ceftazidime, ciprofloxacin or piperacillin/tazobactam. First-line treatment for *S. aureus* is flucloxacillin.

Tympanostomy tube or perforated eardrum allows for purulent middle ear secretions to enter the ear canal and cause infectious eczematoid dermatitis of the ear canal. Management of the underlying otitis media requires systemic antibiotics.

Before treatment is started, a sample should be taken to guide empirical therapy.

The best sample is a tissue biopsy as organisms isolated through ear swab cultures could represent colonization.

Treatment of malignant otitis externa requires at least 6 weeks of systemic antibiotics. The duration can be extended as needed on the basis of clinical or radiographic evidence of persistent or progressive disease. Depending on the extent of inflammation and presence of collections, local debridement and drainage may be required. No clear criteria exist for when to discontinue antibiotic treatment as CT and MRI changes may persist for a prolonged time.

ANALGESIA

Mild to moderate pain responds to paracetamol or NSAIDs by mouth. For severe pain, opioids can be prescribed for a limited number of doses to prevent misuse. There is no clear role for topical analgesia.

CLINICAL PEARL

Otomycosis is mostly seen after long-term topical antibiotic therapy, in immunocompromised patients, in tropical countries and humid conditions. Most common agents are *Aspergillus* spp., especially *Aspergillus niger* causing a moist white plug dotted with black debris and *Candida* spp. causing white debris. Management consists of debridement and topical ointment: clotrimazole, fluconazole and ketoconazole. Duration ranges from a few days to several weeks.

BIBLIOGRAPHY

Courson AM, Vikram HR, Barrs DM. What are the criteria for terminating treatment for necrotizing (malignant) otitis externa? *Laryngoscope*. 2014 February;124(2):361–362.

Hobson CE, Moy JD, Byers KE, Raz Y, Hirsch BE, McCall AA. Malignant otitis externa: Evolving pathogens and implications for diagnosis and treatment. *Otolaryngol Head Neck Surg*. 2014 July;151(1):112–116.

Lee A, Tysome JR, Saeed SR. Topical azole treatments for otomycosis. *Cochrane Database Syst Rev*. 2011 September; 2011(9):CD009289.

Mahdyoun P, Pulcini C, Gahide I, Raffaelli C, Savoldelli C, Castillo L, Guevara N. Necrotizing otitis externa: A systematic review. *Otol Neurotol*. 2013 June;34(4):620–629.

Rosenfeld RM, Schwartz SR, Cannon CR, Roland PS, Simon GR, Kumar KA, Huang WW, Haskell HW, Robertson PJ. Clinical practice guideline: Acute otitis externa. *Otolaryngol Head Neck Surg*. 2014 February;150(1 Suppl):S1–S24.

Schaefer P, Baugh RF. Acute otitis externa: An update. *Am Fam Physician*. 2012 December 1;86(11):1055–1056.

4.46 Pelvic Inflammatory Disease

Firza Alexander Gronthoud

CLINICAL CONSIDERATIONS

Pelvic inflammatory disease (PID) is an ascending infection from the vagina or cervix to the upper female genital tract. The signs and symptoms of PID are not specific and can lead to chronic pelvic pain and infertility. Various organisms may be involved and there is no clear consensus regarding the optimal treatment. It is therefore worthwhile to consider the following.

LOCATION OF INFECTION

PID is a spectrum of inflammatory disorders including endometritis, parametritis (infection of the structures near the uterus), salpingitis (infection of the fallopian tubes), oophoritis (infection of the ovary) and tubo-ovarian abscess. Peritonitis and perihepatitis can also occur. Peritonitis, tubo-ovarian abscess and severe systemic illness (e.g. fever and malaise) are considered severe forms of PID.

CLINICAL PEARL

Differential diagnoses of a PID include a UTI, bacterial vaginosis and ectopic pregnancy.

SYMPTOMS

The hallmark of PID is pelvic tenderness and inflammation of the lower genital tract. Women with PID often have very subtle symptoms and signs. The most common complaint of PID is lower abdominal pain, with or without vaginal discharge, dyspareunia and abnormal menstrual bleeding. Long-term complications secondary to tubal damage occur and include chronic pelvic pain, ectopic pregnancy and infertility.

BACTERIAL AETIOLOGY

PID is often a polymicrobial infection and is caused by members of the vaginal flora including Gram-positive organisms (e.g. *Streptococcus* spp.), *Enterobacterales* anaerobic bacteria (*Peptostreptococcus* spp., *Bacteroides* spp.) and sexually transmitted organisms (*Chlamydia trachomatis*, *Neisseria gonorrhoeae* and *Mycoplasma hominis*).

COMPLICATIONS

Among women with PID, 10%–20% may become infertile, 40% will develop chronic pelvic pain and 10% of those who conceive will have an ectopic pregnancy.

ANTIBIOTIC TREATMENT

Intravenous antibiotics can usually be switched to oral therapy 24 hours clinical improvement. The optimal treatment strategy is unclear. A variety of antibiotic regimens have been used, with marked geographical variation. Current practice generally involves the use of multiple agents to cover *C. trachomatis*, *N. gonorrhoeae* and anaerobic bacteria, but the best combination of agents is unknown. Also, the background prevalence and antimicrobial resistance patterns of bacterial pathogens in different regions may influence the choice of empirical therapy.

CLINICAL APPROACH

DIAGNOSIS

PID can be considered in sexually active young women and other women at risk for sexually transmitted disease (STD) with pelvic or lower abdominal pain in which no cause other than PID can be identified, and pelvic examination shows cervical motion tenderness, uterine tenderness or adnexal tenderness. The diagnosis can be supported with a high vaginal swab for bacterial culture and PCR for *C. trachomatis* and *N. gonorrhoeae* and transvaginal ultrasound or pelvic CT to identify any abscesses. A vaginal saline wet mount with pH would assist in diagnosing bacterial vaginitis. It is also recommended to perform a urine culture to rule out a urinary tract infection and to perform a pregnancy test.

CLINICAL PEARL

Clinical symptoms of a PID have a positive predictive value for salpingitis of only 65% to 90% compared with laparoscopy.

ANTIBIOTIC TREATMENT

There are various antibiotic regimens and no significant difference in outcome has been observed. There are no clear difference outcomes between different regimens, and it is recommended to follow local hospital antibiotic formularies. Below are some examples of regimens used:

Options for intravenous treatment:

- Clindamycin 450 mg 6-hourly + gentamicin 5 mg/kg once daily
- Ceftriaxone 2 g IV once daily + doxycycline 100 mg twice daily orally

Options for oral regimens:

- One dose of ceftriaxone 250 mg intramuscularly followed by doxycycline 100 mg BD +/− metronidazole 400 mg 8-hourly (or in some countries, 500 mg twice daily or 8-hourly)
- Ofloxacin 400 mg once daily + metronidazole 400 mg 8-hourly (or in some countries, 500 mg twice daily or 8-hourly)

Total treatment duration for all regimens is 14 days. Doxycycline can be substituted with azithromycin 1 g once daily for 1 week and should be used in pregnant women.

DRAINAGE

In refractory cases, surgery to drain an abscess or hydrosalpinx may be necessary. Necrotic tissue and pus present in an abscess may prevent antibiotics reaching the infected area (see Chapter 3.9).

BIBLIOGRAPHY

Brunham RC, Gottlieb SL, Paavonen J. Pelvic inflammatory disease. *N Engl J Med.* 2015;372:2039–2048.

Chappell CA, Wiesenfeld HC. Pathogenesis, diagnosis, and management of severe pelvic inflammatory disease and tuboovarian abscess. *Clin Obstet Gynecol.* 2012 December;55(4):893–903.

Savaris RF, Fuhrich DG, Duarte RV, Franik S, Ross J. Antibiotic therapy for pelvic inflammatory disease. *Cochrane Database Syst Rev.* 2017 April 24;4:CD010285.

Sweet RL. Pelvic inflammatory disease: Current concepts of diagnosis and management. *Curr Infect Dis Rep.* 2012;14:194–203.

4.47 Perianal Abscess

Firza Alexander Gronthoud

CLINICAL CONSIDERATIONS

Although perianal abscess is clinically characterized by perianal discharge, pain and swelling, it may also be asymptomatic. It has a high recurrence rate complicated by fistulation. It is therefore worthwhile to consider the following.

RISK FACTORS

- Blocked anal gland
- Sexually transmitted infection (STI)
- Infected anal fissure
- Crohn's disease or ulcerative colitis
- HIV, diabetes mellitus and other immunocompromised conditions
- Anal sex
- Corticosteroids
- Chemotherapy
- Diverticulitis
- Chronic infections such as tuberculosis and actinomycosis

PATHOPHYSIOLOGY

Most perianal abscesses occur because of infection of obstructed anal glands. Bacteria can enter the intramuscular space via obstructed glands and form an abscess. Most occur posteriorly and in the intersphincteric space, where the anal glands are located. Abscesses are classified as superficial or deep in relation to the anal sphincter. If the infection bursts through the external sphincter, it will form an ischiorectal abscess. If it spreads laterally on both sides it can form a collection of sepsis, which forms a 'horseshoe' around the sphincters. Superior extension (supralevator abscess) beyond the puborectalis or the levators is rare and may represent iatrogenic injury (such as inadvertent injury from a fistula probe).

Up to 50% off individuals with an anal abscess develop an anal fistula which often requires surgery. Other fistulas develop secondary to trauma (i.e., rectal foreign bodies), Crohn's disease, anal fissures, carcinoma, radiation therapy, actinomycoses, tuberculosis and lymphogranuloma venereum secondary to chlamydial infection.

CLINICAL PEARL

A perianal fistula connects a primary opening inside the anal canal to a secondary opening in the perianal skin. Secondary tracts may form and can extend from the same primary opening. It should be differentiated from hidradenitis suppurativa, which does not communicate with the anal canal.

CLINICAL SYMPTOMS

Superficial abscesses present acutely as tender, localized, erythematous swellings, and some may present with discharge. Ischiorectal abscesses may take longer to become visible externally. They may present with vague pelvic or perianal pain and fever, and on examination, the buttock may be red and indurated compared with the unaffected side. Digital rectal examination can be painful in the acute setting and can be postponed until examination under anaesthesia, if appropriate.

Deep abscesses are often harder to diagnose. Patients may present with sepsis, even though there are no visible signs. Imaging may be required to confirm the diagnosis in these cases.

A combination of systemic sepsis and a clinical history of recent pelvic infections, Crohn's disease, or previous anorectal sepsis may point to an underlying deep abscess. When examining a patient with anal symptoms, look for signs suggestive of alternative pathology, including fissures or thrombosed haemorrhoids. STI can also present with anal lesions and pain, as can malignancy.

CLINICAL APPROACH

IMAGING

In patients with recurrent perianal abscesses, Crohn's disease or clinical suspicion of fistula, it is recommended to perform a pelvic MRI. MRI classifies 90% of fistulas and accurately identifies associated abscesses and extensions.

MANAGEMENT

Anal abscesses require incision and drainage. After drainage, the area is left open. Because of the risk of deep infection, sepsis and necrotizing soft tissue infection, patients who are immunosuppressed, have diabetes or have evidence of systemic sepsis or cellulitis require urgent drainage on the day of presentation. Incision and drainage can be performed under general anaesthesia or local anaesthesia. In superficial abscesses or in pregnant women, local anaesthesia is preferred. General anaesthesia, on the other hand, allows for sigmoidoscopy and detailed assessment of the anorectum. Proctitis, strictures, ulcers, fissures, recurrent abscesses and fistulas and an elevated calprotectin support diagnosis of Crohn's disease. The addition of antibiotics to drainage does not improve healing rates or reduce recurrence. In individuals who are apyrexial and clinically well, antibiotics are not indicated. Fistulas require surgical excision.

CLINICAL VIGNETTE

A 40-year-old male presents with a painful fluctuating perianal mass with redness and swelling of the surrounding soft tissue with satellite lesions. He also is pyrexic, tachycardic, clammy and hypotensive. The surgical SHO calls the on-call microbiology registrar for antibiotic advise. The registrar advises to send blood cultures, drain the abscess and send pus for culture and to start ceftriaxone 2 g OD IV, clindamycin 450 mg QDS IV and a stat dose of gentamicin 5 mg/kg IV.

- If a patient is immunocompromised, septic or if there is soft tissue infection, antibiotic therapy for several days is indicated.
- An MRI should be considered to view the extent of infection and rule out deep seat infection such as an osteomyelitis.
- Blood culture should be taken to rule out bloodstream infection, as bacteria in the abscess can translocate.

- Antibiotic therapy should be based on local epidemiology and should be targeted against coliforms (i.e., *E. coli*, *K. pneumoniae*), *Bacteroides* spp., *Staphylococcus aureus* and streptococci.

BIBLIOGRAPHY

Kaye TL, O'Connor A, Burke D, Tolan DJ. A young woman with recurrent perianal sepsis. *BMJ*. 2015 April 23;350:h1969.
Sahnan K, Adegbola SO, Tozer PJ, Watfah J, Phillips RK. Perianal abscess. *BMJ*. 2017 February 21;356:j475.

4.48 *Pneumocystis jirovecii* Pneumonia (PJP) in Patients with a Haematological Malignancy or Solid Organ Transplant

Firza Alexander Gronthoud

CLINICAL CONSIDERATIONS

Pneumocystis jirovecii (formerly *Pneumocystis carinii*) causes pneumonia in individuals with cellular immune deficiencies and is spread via aerosols from patients with pneumonia or from early-life contact with family or community members who carry the organism in their lungs.

There are significant differences in clinical features of *Pneumocystis jirovecii* pneumonia (PJP) between HIV-infected and non-HIV-infected individuals and is generally more severe in non-HIV-infected patients, with higher mortality rates. It is therefore worthwhile to consider the following.

Patient population at risk:

- Haematological or solid organ malignancy undergoing chemotherapy or transplant
- Methotrexate or high-dose corticosteroid treatment (16–25 mg of prednisolone per day or ≥4 mg dexamethasone daily for ≥4 weeks)
- CD4 cell count <200/μL

Risk factors for individuals with a haematological malignancy:

- *Highest risk*: Acute lymphoblastic leukaemia (ALL) OR allogeneic haemopoietic stem cell transplant (HSCT) OR high-dose corticosteroid treatment (16–25 mg of prednisolone per day or ≥4 mg dexamethasone daily for ≥4 weeks) OR lymphocyte-depleting agents (i.e., alemtuzumab)
- *Moderate risk*: Autologous bone marrow transplant OR high-intensity chemotherapy regimens R-CHOP (rituximab, cyclophosphamide, Adriamycin, vincristine, prednisolone chemotherapy on a 14-day cycle) OR FCR (fludarabine, cyclophosphamide, rituximab) OR AVBD (Adriamycin, vincristine, bleomycin, dexamethasone) OR gemcitabine OR high-dose methotrexate OR prolonged CD4 lymphopenia
- *Low risk*: Low-intensity chemotherapy regimens (such as R-CHOP given on a 21-day cycle)

Risk factors for individuals with a solid organ malignancy:

- Solid organ transplant, high-dose corticosteroid treatment (16–25 mg of prednisolone per day or ≥4 mg dexamethasone daily for ≥4 weeks)
- Brain tumours, particularly if temozolomide (causes significant lymphopenia) or craniospinal irradiation is planned

DIAGNOSTIC FEATURES

In HIV-infected individuals, *Pneumocystis jirovecii* pneumonia usually has an insidious onset over weeks. Main presenting symptoms are progressive dyspnoea, tiredness and later fever. However, in the extreme immunosuppression associated with bone marrow transplantation, PJP may involve rapidly over a few days. Cough is often dry and there are few chest signs. Despite treatment, mortality rates of 10%–15% have been reported. Rates are higher for those on intensive care units (ICUs). Response to treatment takes time, and failure to respond clinically cannot be decided until the end of the first week of treatment.

IMAGING

- *X-ray*: Classically a 'bat's wing' interstitial pneumonitis.
- *CT-chest*: Suggestive features for PJP are a combination of ground-glass and consolidative opacities, cystic changes, linear-reticular opacities, solitary or multiple nodules and parenchymal cavities. With treatment, most of these changes resolve. Bilateral, ground-glass changes with apical predominance and peripheral sparing and signs of consolidation are detected more frequently on CT—and cystic changes less frequently—than in HIV-positive patients with PJP.

Differences PJP in HIV non-infected immunosuppressed individuals compared to HIV-infected individuals:

- Infection in immunosuppressed HIV-negative individuals has a shorter duration of onset and fewer systemic symptoms than in HIV-infected individuals.
- Bronchoalveolar lavage fluid from immunosuppressed non-HIV-infected patients shows lower concentrations of organisms but higher inflammatory scores.
- Clinical disease is generally more severe in non-HIV-infected patients, with increased length of hospital stay and higher rates of ICU admission and mechanical ventilation, compared with HIV-infected patients.
- Significantly higher mortality rates are also observed in non-HIV-infected individuals compared to those with HIV.

Diagnostic tests:

- *Microscopy*: Methenamine silver and toluidine blue preparations (stain only cyst wall) OR Giemsa stains (detects cysts and trophozoites) OR direct and indirect immunofluorescent assays.
- *PCR*: Sputum and BAL. Highest sensitivity. Alternatively, oral washing but sensitivity unclear. High negative predictive value, moderate positive predictive value as it also detects colonization and no standardized cut-off value exists.
- *Biomarkers*: 1,3-β-D-glucan has excellent negative predictive value. LDH >350 is often seen in PJP.

CLINICAL PEARL

- Quality of microscopy depends on quality of respiratory specimen, sample processing and experience of the laboratory observer.
- Lower burden of *P. jirovecii* in non-HIV-immunocompromised patients and the likelihood that they may already be on anti-pneumocystis prophylaxis affect sensitivity of microscopy.

CLINICAL PEARL

- PCR has the highest sensitivity and specificity (99% and specificity of 92%).
- May distinguish between colonization and infection based on quantity of DNA detected, but no official fungal load thresholds exist and threshold may differ between different patient populations.
- Always correlate the quantity of PJP with the clinical picture.
- Each institution must establish and validate its own qPCR cut-off values appropriate to the molecular method used.

SEVERITY GRADING PJP

The grading system of Miller should be used to assess severity of infection in non-HIV patients (Table 4.48.1).

Treatment options:

1. *Severe PJP*: 20 mg/kg trimethoprim and 100 mg/kg sulfamethoxazole per day in two or more divided doses OR pentamidine 4 mg/kg (max 300 mg) IV slow infusion OR clindamycin + primaquine (test for G6PD deficiency before treatment with primaquine).
2. *Moderate to severe PJP*: 600 mg clindamycin 8-hourly PO PLUS 15–30 mg primaquine once-daily PO (test for G6PD deficiency before treatment with primaquine).
3. *Non-severe PJP*: Atovaquone 750 mg 12-hourly PO OR dapsone 100 mg once daily PLUS 20 mg/kg trimethoprim in 2–4 divided doses (test for G6PD deficiency before treatment with dapsone).
4. *Steroids*: Whilst the use of steroids in HIV patients with PJP is standard, it may be harmful in other immunocompromised individuals and no official recommendation exists.
5. Monitor twice weekly full blood count, urea, creatinine and liver function tests.

TABLE 4.48.1
Miller Grading System

	Mild	Moderate	Severe
Symptoms	Increasing exertional dyspnoea with or without cough and sweats	Dyspnoea on minimal exertion, occasional dyspnoea at rest, fever with or without sweats	Dyspnoea at rest, tachypnoea at rest, persistent fever, cough
Arterial oxygen tension (PaO$_2$) at rest, room air	>11.0 kPa (>82.5 mmHg)	8.1–11.0 kPa (60.75–82.5 mmHg)	<8.0 kPa (60 mmHg)
Arterial oxygen saturation (SaO$_2$) at rest, room air	>96%	91%–96%	<91%
Chest radiograph	Normal or minor perihilar shadowing	Diffuse interstitial shadowing	Extensive interstitial shadowing with or without diffuse alveolar shadowing ('white out') sparing costophrenic angles and apices

Source: Miller RF, Le Noury J, Corbett EL et al. *J Antimicrob Chemother*. 1996;37(Suppl).

PJP PROPHYLAXIS

- Individuals with haematological malignancy with high risk of PJP.
- Having completed a treatment course, patients should be put on secondary prophylaxis until immune reconstitution.
- Prophylaxis should also be considered for immunocompromised individuals who are on high-dose steroids for at least 4 weeks or individuals with severe T-cell deficiency.
- First choice: trimethoprim/sulfamethoxazole 960 mg twice-daily PO on three non-consecutive days a week OR 480 mg once-daily PO; may also confer protection against toxoplasmosis, nocardiosis and bacterial sepsis.
- Alternative options: monthly nebulized pentamidine 300 mg monthly or 150 mg fortnightly OR dapsone 100 mg once-daily PO OR atovaquone 750 mg 12-hourly PO.
- Prophylaxis should be continued for 6 weeks after the steroid tapering period (steroid dose should be lower than 15 mg/day) OR peripheral blood lymphocytes $>1 \times 10^9$/L. With some chemotherapy regimens (e.g. alemtuzumab and FCR), where there are high rates of late-onset PJP, consideration should be given to extended PJP prophylaxis for up to 12 months, particularly in pre-treated patients and, for allogeneic HSCT recipients, from engraftment until $\geq$6 months after transplant or longer in patients who continue to receive immunosuppressive drugs and/or have chronic GvHD.

TRIMETHOPRIM/SULFAMETHOXAZOLE DESENSITIZATION

Desensitization may be considered with trimethoprim/sulfamethoxazole-associated rash. It is contraindicated in those with prior history of associated drug rash with eosinophilia and systemic symptoms ('DRESS'), Stevens–Johnson syndrome or toxic epidermal necrolysis. After a grade 3 reaction, desensitization should be deferred for 2 weeks. After a grade 4 reaction, desensitization should not be attempted.

CLINICAL APPROACH

CLINICAL PICTURE IN PATIENT POPULATION AT RISK FOR PJP

Acute presentation of dyspnoea, non-productive cough, severe hypoxaemia, tachypnoea and fatigue, with or without fever in a patient with haematological or solid organ malignancy undergoing chemotherapy or transplant OR high-dose corticosteroids.

TESTS TO BE ORDERED

- Arterial blood gases and monitoring of oxygen saturation level
- Preferably CT chest OR X-thorax
- Sputum or BAL for PCR for cytomegalovirus, *Pneumocystis jirovecii*, respiratory viruses, bacterial microscopy and culture, and mycobacterial microscopy and culture
- Serum β-D-glucan and LDH

TREATMENT

- Start PJP treatment with, ideally, trimethoprim/sulfamethoxazole. Alternative options are listed under 'Clinical Considerations' and review with microbiology results.
- Early and reversible deterioration in the first 3–5 days is typical, and clinicians should wait at least 4–8 days before changing therapy due to lack of improvement.
- If after 4–8 days, no clinical improvement or improvement in arterial oxygen saturation, then switch to an alternative agent.

- If PCR on BAL or sputum is negative AND/OR negative β-D-glucan +/− LDH <350 U/L, then stop PJP treatment and look for alternative cause of infection.
- Treatment duration: 14–21 days.

BIBLIOGRAPHY

Avino LJ, Naylor SM, Roecker AM. *Pneumocystis jirovecii* Pneumonia in the non-HIV-infected population. *Ann Pharmacother.* 2016 August;50(8):673–679.

Cooley L, Dendle C, Wolf J, Teh BW, Chen SC, Boutlis C, Thursky KA. Consensus guidelines for diagnosis, prophylaxis and management of *Pneumocystis jirovecii* pneumonia in patients with haematological and solid malignancies, 2014. *Intern Med J.* 2014 December;44(12b):1350–1363.

Maschmeyer G, Helweg-Larsen J, Pagano L, Robin C, Cordonnier C, Schellongowski P. ECIL guidelines for treatment of *Pneumocystis jirovecii* pneumonia in non-HIV-infected haematology patients. *J Antimicrob Chemother.* 2016;71:2405–2413.

Miller RF, Le Noury J, Corbett EL et al. *Pneumocystis carinii* infection: Current treatment and prevention. *J Antimicrob Chemother.* 1996;37(Suppl B):33–53.

Winthrop KL, Baddley JW. Pneumocystis and glucocorticoid use: To prophylax or not to prophylax (and when?); that is the question. *Ann Rheum Dis.* 2018 May;77(5):631–633.

4.49 Pneumonia (CAP, HAP and VAP)

Patrick Lillie

CLINICAL CONSIDERATIONS

Pneumonia is a common cause of severe infection, with respiratory infection remaining one of the leading causes of death worldwide. Pneumonia is categorized by how related to healthcare/invasive procedures the case is, with community-acquired pneumonia (CAP), hospital-acquired pneumonia (HAP) and ventilator-associated pneumonia (VAP) having different microbiological profiles as shown in Table 4.49.1.

CLINICAL APPROACH

DIAGNOSTIC TESTING

As pneumonia is defined by radiological changes as well as clinical findings, all patients in secondary care should have a CXR performed, while some may require CT scanning. Imaging does not tell the clinician what organism is present, although bilateral interstitial shadowing is more commonly seen in viral infection such as primary influenza pneumonia, and it will also be of use in excluding other pathology such as malignancy.

MICROBIOLOGICAL TESTS

Identifying a pathogen in patients with pneumonia should allow for rationale choice of antimicrobials and sensitivity testing. The British Thoracic Society guidelines give a range of tests that can be performed according to the severity of the patient as defined by their CURB-65 score. Sputum cultures, while neither sensitive nor specific enough to be definitive, are of use in those patients who are expectorating purulent sputum. Blood cultures are often negative but, if positive, will allow for streamlining of therapy. Multiplex molecular testing is becoming increasingly available, both for viruses such as influenza and atypical pathogens including *Legionella* and *Mycoplasma* (see Chapter 4.4 for more information on diagnosis and management of atypical pneumonia). Urinary antigen testing for *Legionella pneumophila* only detects serotype 1 and pneumococcal urinary antigen testing has insufficient sensitivity and specificity to be relied upon for changing treatment in the severe pneumonia patient. In previously well patients who develop CAP, consideration of testing for underlying risk factors, including HIV infection, should be strongly considered. In HAP and VAP cases, as there is a broader range of pathogens and often with significant antibiotic resistance, sputum, tracheal aspirates and bronchoalveolar lavage should all be considered in an attempt to identify the causative organism.

ANTIMICROBIAL THERAPY

Both British and American guidelines are available for community-acquired pneumonia. All the guidelines recognize that pneumococcal cover is essential given the high likelihood of this organism. For most patients, this can be achieved with a β-lactam, typically amoxicillin if oral therapy is desirable, with respiratory fluroquinolones such as levofloxacin being another option. For those

TABLE 4.49.1

Aetiology of Community-Acquired Pneumonia (CAP), Hospital-Acquired Pneumonia (HAP) and Ventilator-Associated Pneumonia (VAP)

	CAP	HAP	VAP
Common causes	*Streptococcus pneumoniae, Mycoplasma pneumoniae, Legionella pneumophila, Staphylococcus aureus*, influenza virus	Gram-negative bacilli including *Pseudomonas aeruginosa* MRSA	Gram-negative bacilli including *Pseudomonas aeruginosa, Acinetobacter baumannii, Stenotrophomonas maltophilia* MRSA

TABLE 4.49.2

Empirical Therapy of Community-Acquired Pneumonia

Severity	1st-Line Treatment	Alternative Options
CURB 65 = 0–1	Amoxicillin	Clarithromycin/doxycycline
CURB 65 = 2	Amoxicillin + clarithromycin	Doxycycline/respiratory fluroquinolone
CURB 65 ≥3	Co-amoxiclav + clarithromycin	An IV cephalosporin + clarithromycin or respiratory fluroquinolone

patients with severe pneumonia agents with broader-spectrum cover to include *Staphylococcus aureus* and Gram-negative organisms is generally needed, together with cover for atypical pathogens. Table 4.49.2 shows suggested regimes stratified by severity.

Where a specific pathogen is detected, then the antibiotic regime can be adjusted accordingly. Duration of therapy is poorly defined, but there is evidence that shorter courses are not associated with poorer outcomes, and for low severity CAP, 3–5 days of treatment may be sufficient, with 5–7 days for those with more severe disease.

CLINICAL VIGNETTE

A 52-year-old man suffered a head injury while travelling in Kenya and required an emergency craniotomy and subsequent ventilation on intensive care. He received several courses of antibiotics for various infections prior to his repatriation. He was noted to have increasing oxygen requirements, new infiltrates on his CXR and purulent tracheal secretions grew a carbapenem-resistant Acinetobacter baumannii. *He was treated with high-dose intravenous colistin and nebulized amikacin, and strict infection control procedures were initiated.*

Ventilator-associated pneumonia is a serious complication of intensive care and carries a significant mortality and morbidity. Gram-negative bacilli are commonly isolated, and antibiotic resistance can be a major problem with limited therapeutic options. Local antibiotic-resistance patterns should be noted when considering empirical therapy for both HAP and VAP. Recent antibiotic therapy is recognized as a risk for resistant pathogens in both HAP and VAP. Depending on the local prevalence of MRSA, potential regimes would include piperacillin-tazobactam, meropenem with vancomycin or linezolid if MRSA cover is required. Extended sensitivity testing of isolates may be needed to guide susceptibility to agents not commonly used such as colistin, fosfomycin and newer agents such as ceftazidime/avibactam, particularly when MDR pathogens such as *Acinetobacter* are found.

BIBLIOGRAPHY

Kalil AC, Metersky ML, Klompas M et al. Management of adults with hospital acquired and ventilator associated pneumonia: 2016 clinical practice guidelines by the infectious disease society of America and the American thoracic society. *Clin Infect Dis*. 2016;63:e61–e111.

Lim WS, Baudouin SV, George RC et al. BTS guidelines for the management of community acquired pneumonia in adults: Update 2009. *Thorax*. 2009;64(Suppl 3):iii1–iii55.

Lim WS, van der Eerden MM, Laing R et al. Defining community acquired pneumonia severity on presentation to hospital: An international derivation and validation study. *Thorax*. 2003;58(7):377–382.

Mandell LA, Wunderink RG, Anzueto A et al. Infectious diseases society of America/American thoracic society consensus guidelines on the management of community acquired pneumonia in adults. *Clin Infect Dis*. 2007;44(Suppl 3):S27–S72.

National Institute for Health and Care Excellence. Pneumonia in adults: Diagnosis and management. Clinical guideline 191, December 2014.

4.50 Post-Exposure Prophylaxis for Healthcare Workers Exposed to Blood-Borne Viruses

Firza Alexander Gronthoud

CLINICAL CONSIDERATIONS

Exposure to blood-borne viruses arises from needlestick injuries and bodily fluid splashes on skin or mucosa. The risk of exposure depends on the nature of the accident and the likelihood that the source, which is usually a patient, contains a blood-borne virus. It is therefore worthwhile to consider the following:

BLOOD-BORNE VIRUSES

The three main blood-borne viruses (BBV) are human immunodeficiency virus (HIV), hepatitis B (HBV) and hepatitis C (HCV). HIV can be transmitted via penetrative sexual intercourse, contact with infected blood (e.g., blood transfusion and sharing needles in IV drug users, IVDUs), horizontal transmission during birth and breastfeeding. Hepatitis B can be transmitted via contact with infected blood, semen and vaginal fluid and perinatally from mother to child. HCV is most frequently acquired by direct blood-to-blood contact, for example, sharing of blood-contaminated injecting equipment by injecting drug users.

TYPES OF EXPOSURE

A significant exposure in which there is a risk of BBV transmission can be classified as percutaneous exposure and mucocutaneous exposure.

PERCUTANEOUS EXPOSURE

Percutaneous exposure occurs when the skin of the healthcare worker is breached by a sharp object that may contain bodily fluids infected with a blood-borne virus. This usually occurs through a needlestick injury. Sharp instruments that carry a risk of transmission are hollow and solid bore needles, sharp-edged instruments, broken glassware or any other item which may be contaminated during use by blood or body fluids and which may cause laceration or puncture wounds. Sharp tissues such as spicules of bone or teeth may also pose a risk of injury. The risk of percutaneous exposure depends on the procedure involved and type of sharp used.

MUCOCUTANEOUS EXPOSURE

Mucocutaneous exposure occurs when bodily fluid, which may contain BBV, splashes on non-intact skin, mucous membranes or eyes of the healthcare worker.

Bodily Fluids Which May Harbour a Blood-Borne Virus

These include blood, amniotic fluid, cerebrospinal fluid, human breast milk, pericardial fluid, peritoneal fluid, pleural fluid, semen, synovial fluid, unfixed tissues and organs and vaginal secretions.

Bodily Fluids That Normally Do Not Contain Blood-Borne Viruses

These include saliva, sweat, sputum, feces, nasal secretions, tears, urine and vomit. However, this must be assessed on an individual basis as, for example, saliva from a patient who had a tooth extraction earlier that day may potentially contain blood.

Risk of Transmission with BBV

In the healthcare setting, transmission most commonly occurs after percutaneous exposure to a patient's blood by a needlestick injury. Hepatitis B virus is the most infectious of the common blood-borne viruses. Most of the occupational exposure to HIV is associated with injury from hollow-bore needles in association with procedures where a needle or cannula is placed in a vein or artery, e.g. venepuncture. Others have arisen through exposure of mucous membranes or non-intact skin to blood. The transmission risks after a mucocutaneous exposure are lower than those after a percutaneous exposure. The risk of acquiring HIV after a single mucocutaneous exposure is less than 1 in 2000. Mucocutaneous exposures, however, occur more frequently than percutaneous exposures. The risk of infection after percutaneous exposure to hepatitis C virus-infected blood is estimated to be 1.8% per exposure. There is no evidence that BBVs can be transmitted by blood contamination of intact skin, by inhalation or by fecal-oral contamination.

Risk of HIV Transmission

Factors associated with HIV transmission after percutaneous exposure include deep injuries involving a hollow-bore needle (due to the higher volume of blood inoculated), with visible blood present on the device, which has been in a vein or artery of an HIV-positive source patient with advanced disease or high viral load. The risk of HIV transmission after percutaneous exposure is estimated to be 0.3%. Mucocutaneous exposures accounted for only 24% and carry a significantly lower risk of transmission (approximately one in 1000). Incidents involving a human scratch/bite were considerably less common (3%), and in these cases, transmission is dependent on injury severity, patient oral hygiene and stage of disease.

Risk of HBV Transmission

The risk of hepatitis B infection after a needlestick injury and in the absence of vaccination or post-exposure prophylaxis is 37%–62% if the source patient is hepatitis B e antigen positive, and 23%–37% if the patient is hepatitis B e antigen negative. Introduction of standard precautions and safety devices, together with increased hepatitis B vaccination of healthcare workers and post-exposure prophylaxis, has significantly reduced transmission rates over the past two decades. Hepatitis C transmission also occurs through exposure to blood, but much less efficiently than hepatitis B transmission.

CLINICAL PEARL

Risk of transmission is dependent on the prevalence in the population (e.g., IVDU), infectious status of the source (viral load) and the nature of exposure (blood–blood contact). For hollow-bore needle injuries, the risk of transmission is 1 in 3 when the patient is infected with HBV ('e' antigen positive), 1 in 30 when the patient is infected with HCV and 1 in 300 when the patient is infected with HIV.

CLINICAL APPROACH

The main steps after a potential exposure to a BBV are:

- Cleaning body part of exposure
- Assessing nature of injury and risk of exposure to blood-borne viruses
- Assessing likelihood that source is infected with HIV
- Consenting source for testing of blood-borne viruses; healthcare worker to also send baseline blood for storage
- Notifying line manager and occupational health

CLEANING BODY PART OF EXPOSURE

Free bleeding of puncture wounds should be encouraged without squeezing or sucking the wound. The site of exposure, e.g. wound, puncture site or non-intact skin should be washed liberally with soap and running water but without scrubbing. Exposed mucous membranes including conjunctivae should be irrigated copiously with water.

ASSESSING NATURE OF INJURY AND RISK OF EXPOSURE TO BLOOD-BORNE VIRUSES

The source should be identified, and the exposure should then be classified as non-significant or significant if it was a percutaneous exposure or a mucocutaneous exposure with a bodily fluid which potentially contained a BBV. The significant exposure should then be classified:
High-risk exposure:

- Deep injury with hollow-bore needle with visible blood
- Prolonged contact/heavy contamination with non-intact skin
- Deep injury with solid instrument with blood

Medium-risk exposure:

- Superficial injury with hollow-bore needle with blood
- Deep injury with hollow-bore needle with no visible blood

Low-risk exposure:

- Superficial injury with solid instrument/no visible blood
- Superficial injury with hollow-bore needle/no blood
- Mucocutaneous exposure
- Blood contact with healthy skin

ASSESSING LIKELIHOOD THAT SOURCE IS INFECTED WITH HIV

High-risk source:

- Seroconversion illness
- Patient infected with HIV and not on antiretroviral treatment
- High-risk history, i.e. IVDU

Low-risk source:

- HIV positive but on antiretroviral treatment with undetectable load
- History not known
- No high-risk history

COLLECT BLOOD FROM SOURCE PATIENT

After a significant exposure, blood should be collected from both the source patient and the healthcare worker. The source patient should be counselled regarding the incident and informed consent requested to establish evidence of hepatitis B, hepatitis C and HIV infectivity.

ASSESSING NEED FOR PEP OR HEPATITIS B IMMUNIZATION

- If the source tested HIV negative and there is no concern that the patient may be in the window period of seroconversion, then there is no indication for PEP.
- If the source tested HIV positive and there was a high-risk exposure to blood or another high-risk body fluid from a source either known to be HIV infected or considered to be at high risk of HIV infection, then PEP should be started.
- If the result of an HIV test has not or cannot be obtained, then PEP should be considered based on an individual risk assessment. Examples are:
  - Start PEP if there is a high-risk history and high-risk exposure.
  - Consider PEP if there is a high-risk history and medium-risk exposure.
  - Hold PEP if there is a low-risk history and low-risk exposure, i.e. bodily fluid on intact skin.
  - Hold PEP if there is a low-risk history and medium-risk exposure

If the source tested HIV positive but there was a low-risk exposure, then PEP could be considered. HIV-containing blood on intact skin is not an indication for PEP. PEP consists of triple therapy with tenofovir-emtricitabine 300/200 mg once daily plus raltegravir 400 mg orally twice daily OR one Truvada tablet (245 mg tenofovir and 200 mg emtricitabine [FTC]) once a day plus two Kaletra film-coated tablets (200 mg lopinavir and 50 mg ritonavir) twice a day. The duration is at least 28 days. PEP should be administered ideally within 1 hour after injury and no later than 72 hours.

Anti-HIV1/HIV2 should be tested at baseline, 6 weeks and 16 weeks post-exposure. Conduct complete blood count, urea, creatinine, liver function tests, serum glucose (if on PIs) and creatine phosphokinase (if on raltegravir) at baseline, 2 weeks and 4 weeks after initiating PEP.

A course of hepatitis B vaccination with or without hepatitis B immunoglobulins is recommended following high-risk exposure to hepatitis B if the source has serological evidence of infection (or if the HBV status cannot be determined) and if the healthcare worker has not been vaccinated to hepatitis B or did not complete the hepatitis B immunization. If the healthcare worker is a known non-responder to HBV vaccination, then it is reasonable to only administer hepatitis B immunoglobulins.

POST-EXPOSURE PROPHYLAXIS HEPATITIS C

There is no effective post-exposure prophylaxis for hepatitis C. If the patient is hepatitis C positive and there was a high-risk exposure, then the healthcare worker should be followed up at 6, 12 and 24 weeks after exposure. Serum taken at 6 and 12 weeks should be tested for hepatitis C virus (HCV) and RNA and serum taken at 12 and 24 weeks for anti-HCV. If the healthcare worker develops hepatitis C, then referral to a hepatologist or infectious diseases physician needs to be arranged.

BIBLIOGRAPHY

Bader MS, Brooks A, Kelly DV, Srigley JA. Postexposure management of infectious diseases. *Cleve Clin J Med.* 2017 January;84(1):65–80.
Department of Health, 2008. HIV Post-Exposure Prophylaxis: Guidance from the UK Chief Medical Officer's Expert Advisory Group on AIDS.

Ramsay ME. UK healthcare workers infected with blood-borne viruses: Guidance on risk, transmission, surveillance, and management.

Samaranayake L, Scully C. Needlestick and occupational exposure to infections: A compendium of current guidelines. *Br Dent J.* 2013 August;215(4):163–166.

Ward P, Hartle A. UK healthcare workers infected with blood-borne viruses: Guidance on risk, transmission, surveillance, and management. *Contin Educ Anaesthesia, Crit Care Pain.* 2014 July 6;15(2):103–108.

4.51 Post-Operative Infections

Firza Alexander Gronthoud

CLINICAL CONSIDERATIONS

Fever above 38°C is common in the first few days after major surgeries and is caused by an inflammatory response to surgery. Fever can also indicate the presence of a post-operative infection. Post-operative infections may not have any specific signs and symptoms and fever may even be absent in patients who are immunocompromised, undergoing cancer chemotherapy or post-transplant immunosuppression, elderly or in chronic renal failure. It is therefore worthwhile to consider the following.

AETIOLOGY OF POST-OPERATIVE FEVER

- The severity of the trauma is correlated with the degree of the fever response.
- A temporary bacterial translocation from the colon during surgery may be responsible for some episodes of self-limited post-operative fever not requiring antibiotic treatment.
- Fever is more likely to be due to infection as the time interval following surgery increases.
- Fever in patients may have more than one cause at the same time, and infectious and non-infectious causes may coexist.

CLINICAL PEARL

Infectious causes of post-operative fever:

- Surgical site infection
- Surgical complication, i.e. anastomotic leak, collection or infected haematoma, perforated organ
- Hospital-acquired pneumonia including VAP
- Intravascular catheter-associated bloodstream infection
- Viral respiratory tract infection, i.e. influenza
- Reactivation of herpesviruses and adenovirus in immunocompromised individuals, i.e. after bone marrow transplantation

---

CHANGE IN COMMENSAL FLORA DURING ADMISSION AND IMPACT ON ANTIBACTERIAL TREATMENT

- Post-operative infections are caused by a patient's own commensal flora.
- During the course of admission, patients are likely to become colonized with more drug-resistant hospital flora.

EPIDEMIOLOGY

- Post-operative fever will be experienced by 20%–90% of patients.
- Post-operative fever can occur after minor operative procedures but is rare and depends on the type of procedure.
- Overall, both abdominal and chest procedures result in the highest incidence of post-operative fever.

CLINICAL PEARL

- Malignant hyperthermia: High-grade fever (greater than 40°C) with metabolic acidosis and hypercalcemia.
- Occurs shortly after inhalational anaesthetics or muscle relaxant.
- If not readily recognized, it can cause cardiac arrest.
- Treatment is intravenous dantrolene, 100% oxygen, correction of acidosis, cooling blankets and watching for myoglobinuria.

TIMING OF ONSET OF POST-OPERATIVE INFECTION AND FEVER

- *Immediate*: Onset in the operating suite or within hours after surgery
  - Drugs, blood products, trauma, surgery, pre-existing infections, malignant hyperthermia.
  - Febrile non-haemolytic transfusion reaction: Fevers, chills, and malaise 1–6 hours after surgery (without haemolysis).
  - Fever due to the trauma of surgery usually resolves within 2–3 days. Fever caused by severe head trauma can be persistent and may resolve gradually over days or even weeks.
  - *Bacteraemia:* High-grade fever (greater than 40°C) occurring 30–40 minutes after the beginning of the procedure (e.g., urinary tract instrumentation in the presence of infected urine).
  - *Gas gangrene of the wound:* High-grade fever (greater than 40°C) occurring after gastrointestinal (GI) surgery due to contamination with *Clostridium perfringens*; severe wound pain.
- *Acute*: Onset within the first week after surgery
  - Catheter-associated urinary tract infection, hospital-acquired pneumonia, surgical site infection (SSI), ventilator-associated pneumonia (VAP).
  - Risk of aspiration pneumonia if depressed mental status or gag reflex due to anaesthesia and analgesia or presence of a nasogastric tube.
  - *Non-infectious:* Atelectasis, thrombophlebitis. Also, pancreatitis, myocardial infarction, pulmonary embolism, alcohol withdrawal, acute gout.
- *Subacute*: Onset from 1–4 weeks following surgery
  - SSI most often presents in the subacute period, 1 week or more after surgery. SSI caused by *Streptococcus pyogenes* (GAS) and *Clostridium perfringens* can have a rapid onset and lead to necrotizing fasciitis.
  - Catheter exit site infections and intravascular associated bloodstream infections.
  - *Clostridium difficile*-associated diarrhoea.
  - *Drug fever:* β-Lactam antibiotics and sulpha-containing products, H2-blockers, procainamide, phenytoin, and heparin.
  - Thrombophlebitis, deep venous thrombosis and pulmonary embolism.
  - Intra-abdominal abscesses, hospital acquired pneumonia, urinary tract infection, sinusitis (nasogastric tube).
- *Delayed*: Onset more than one month after surgery
  - Most delayed post-operative fevers are due to infection.
  - Infections associated with implant devices, caused by low-virulent organisms (coagulase-negative staphylococci, *Propionibacterium*).
  - Infective endocarditis due to perioperative bacteraemia more likely to present weeks or months after surgery.

CLINICAL PEARL

Non-infectious causes of post-operative fever:

* Operative site hematoma/seroma
* Suture reaction
* Deep vein thrombosis
* Pulmonary embolism
* Fat embolism
* Pancreatitis
* Stroke
* Myocardial infarction
* Bowel ischaemia
* Drug fever
* Transfusion-related reactions
* Transfusion-related acute lung injury (TRALI)
* Transplant rejection
* Hyperthyroidism (including thyroid storm)
* Hypoadrenalism
* Cancer/neoplastic fever
* Malignant hyperthermia
* Neuroleptic malignant syndrome
* Post-cardiac injury syndrome

FEVER AND CUTANEOUS REACTIONS

* Acute generalized exanthematous pustulosis
* Drug reaction with eosinophilia and systemic symptoms syndrome (DRESS)
* Cutaneous small-vessel vasculitis

CLINICAL FEATURES

* Superficial wound infections: Cellulitis with or without discharge. In sternotomy wounds, this could lead to sternal osteomyelitis with sternal dehiscence.
* Persistent serous discharge from the wound may indicate infection with or without dehiscence.
* Cellulitis: Localized redness, swelling, tenderness or heat at wound site.
* Deep wound infections: Purulent discharge from incision site often with fever and leucocytosis.
* Sternal dehiscence is present in fewer than 50% of patients with mediastinitis, systemic signs are often nonspecific and most common finding is serous discharge from the wound.
* Sternal dehiscence can be noted as instability of the sternum with or without crepitus on palpation; however, this may be present in less than 50% of the cases. A more consistent and less specific finding is ongoing discharge of serous fluid from incision. Most patients have a mild leucocytosis or fever.
* Deep-seated abscesses or pneumonia may present as fever with leucocytosis with or without organ-specific findings such as increased oxygen requirements in pneumonia or prolonged ileus in a patient with an intraperitoneal abscess.

- Post-operative mediastinitis is associated with bacteraemia in 40%–60% of the cases and can be complicated by empyema and infectious pericarditis.
- Deep sternal wound infections can be identified in up to two-thirds of patients who have bacteraemia after cardiac operation.

MICROBIOLOGY

- *Surgical site infections: Staphylococcus aureus* or streptococci. Less commonly, *Enterobacterales* in sternal infections, mediastinitis and groin infections.
- Coagulase-negative staphylococci in device-associated infections, including sternal wires.
- *Intra-abdominal and pelvic infections:* Polymicrobial in nature, often involving *E. coli, K. pneumoniae*, streptococci from the milleri group and anaerobes. In the absence of source control, ongoing antimicrobial therapy will select for enterococci, *Pseudomonas aeruginosa, Candida* species and AmpC- and ESBL-producing *Enterobacterales.*

CARDIAC SURGERY

- Graft site soft tissue infection (CABG).
- Sternal wound infection (usually occurring within the first month).
- *Mediastinitis:* Infection of central structures in the chest excluding lungs and pleural space. Presents within 1–2 weeks post-surgery, but can be as late as 4–6 months post-surgery.
- *Pneumonia:* Correlated with reintubation, hypotension, neurologic dysfunction and transfusion of more than three units of blood components.

CLINICAL PEARL

Coagulase-negative staphylococci (CoNS) have been found to be the most common pathogen involved in this post-operative infection related to implanted foreign materials, i.e. sternal fixation wires made from stainless steel.

CLINICAL PEARL

- Pleural effusion is a common occurrence in patients undergoing cardiac surgery such as a CABG or pleural effusion.
- It can develop within the first week or weeks to months later.
- Post-operative pleural effusions can also be caused by pneumonitis reaction, congestive heart failure, haemothorax, pneumonia, pleural infections, central venous catheter erosion, mediastinitis or chylothorax.
- The majority of effusions are small and resolve gradually over months and do not result in patient morbidity.
- The primary symptom of larger effusions (>25% of hemithorax) is dyspnoea without chest pain and fever.
- Large, progressive or symptomatic pleural effusions require thoracentesis with pleural fluid analysis, and, in some instances, further evaluation with serum brain natriuretic peptide (BNP), echocardiography, lung ultrasound, chest CT or other diagnostic studies.

NEUROSURGERY

Meningitis and ventriculitis and rarely brain abscess may complicate neurosurgical procedures.

VASCULAR GRAFT INFECTIONS

- Occur by direct inoculation of the operative site or, less frequently, by haematogenous spread.
- Infection is more common in grafts at inguinal and upper leg operative sites.
- Most commonly present soon after surgery but can occur months to years later.

CLINICAL PEARL

Post-implantation syndrome:

- Seen after aortic aneurysm repair with vascular stent
- Fever, leucocytosis, elevated CRP and gas around the stent
- Often fever >38.6°C
- Non-infectious in nature and fever will resolve without antimicrobial therapy

ABDOMINAL SURGERY

- Intra-abdominal abscess.
- Splenoportal thrombosis may cause fever following splenectomy. Risk factors include massive splenomegaly and myeloproliferative and haemolytic disorders.
- Identifying a fluid collection and distinguishing between abscess, haematoma and a benign fluid collection, though difficult, can be critically important.

OBSTETRIC AND GYNAECOLOGICAL SURGERY

- Postpartum endometritis
- More common in patients with pre-existing medical problems, after premature rupture of membranes or difficult deliveries and after the use of internal fetal monitoring
- UTI, cellulitis, necrotizing fasciitis, superficial abscess, deep abscess and pelvic thrombophlebitis

ORTHOPAEDIC SURGERY

Operative site infection, infected prosthesis, haematoma and deep vein thrombosis

CLINICAL APPROACH

- Deviation from expected post-operative course may be a first sign to suspect a post-operative infection.
- Patients should be expected to diurese 48–72 hours following a major surgery.
- Fever and/or raised inflammatory markers during the first 3 days after surgery are common findings, and in the absence of any localizing symptoms, it is appropriate to hold off any laboratory and radiological investigations.

IMAGING

- X-ray for suspected pneumonia: Following cardiothoracic surgery can be difficult to interpret as post-operative changes are to be expected. Following thoracic surgery, the sensitivity for diagnosis of pneumonia or mediastinitis is <50%, whilst sensitivity of CT scan is 100% 2–3 weeks after surgery when the underlying inflammatory process resulting from the operation should have subsided.
- CT scan with contrast for deep-seated infections.

TREATMENT

- Empirical antibiotic treatment should be targeted at suspected involved endogenous flora.
- Multidrug-resistant organisms should be taken into account with longer hospital stays, frequent hospital admissions and previous antibiotic courses in the past 3–6 months.
- The need for indwelling and intravascular catheters should be reviewed.
- Drugs known to cause drug fever should be discontinued or replaced with other agents.
- Primary management consists of source control (see Chapter 3.9).
- Supportive management consists of antimicrobial therapy rationalized based on culture results and fluid resuscitation if indicated.
- Antimicrobial treatment should be discontinued if, after 48–72 hours, no source has been identified, patient is afebrile and haemodynamically stable and radiological and microbiological investigations are negative.

PREVENTION

- There is weak evidence from the literature to suggest that body washing with antiseptics is better than soap or placebo before surgery and antiseptic skin preparation in theatre to reduce risk of infection, although this is common practice in many hospitals.
- Wound infections can be prevented or minimized by leaving the skin open; open wounds have lower incidence of infection than closed wounds.
- Wounds cannot be closed after they have been opened.
- Selective decontamination of the digestive tract or oropharynx can be considered as it has been shown to significantly reduce the rate of pneumonia and bacteraemia in the critically ill patient.

BIBLIOGRAPHY

Ashley B, Spiegel DA, Cahill P, Talwar D, Baldwin KD. Post-operative fever in orthopaedic surgery: How effective is the 'fever workup?' *J Orthop Surg (Hong Kong)*. 2017 September–December;25(3):2309499017727953.

Light RW, Rogers JT, Moyers JP et al. Prevalence and clinical course of pleural effusions at 30 days after coronary artery and cardiac surgery. *Am J Respir Crit Care Med*. 2002 December 15;166(12 Pt 1):1567–1571.

4.52 Prosthetic Joint Infections

Devan Vaghela and Simon Tiberi

CLINICAL CONSIDERATIONS

DEFINITION OF PROSTHETIC JOINT INFECTION (PJI)

Diagnosing PJIs is difficult and requires a low threshold for suspicion or they can be missed. PJI should be considered in patients that have a replacement joint who have an inflammatory response. The following are either definitive or highly suggestive of a PJI.
   Clinical:

- The presence of a sinus tract over a joint prosthesis is definitive evidence of infection.
- The presence of severe pain with low-grade fever is highly suggestive of a prosthetic joint infection.
- The presence of purulent discharge intraoperatively with no other local focus of infection is considered definitive evidence.

Laboratory findings:

- The presence of inflammation on periprosthetic tissue.
- Two or more intraoperative tissue samples containing the same organism or one tissue sample containing a virulent is considered definitive evidence.

ACQUISITION OF INFECTION

Any foreign body such as prosthetic implants acts as a hub for infection, and the minimal pathogen load required for infection to occur at the site of a prosthetic joint is significantly less compared to a native joint.
   Patients having a revision procedure are more likely to develop a joint infection than those having a primary procedure. Patients who are having a revision procedure because of infection are at highest risk of developing infection again and with the same bacterial species.
   Risk factors include BMI >30, ASA score greater than 3 and prolonged operation time.

CAUSATIVE AGENTS

The most common pathogens are *Staphylococcus aureus* and coagulase-negative staphylococci.
   Gram-negative species including *Pseudomonas aeruginosa* account for up to 30% of infections.
   Polymicrobial disease with both Gram-positive and Gram-negative bacteria are often associated with infections at other locations such as urine or abdomen, with translocation to the prosthetic joint.
   If infections occur within the month, it is likely because of environmental infections intraoperatively, and therefore, *S. aureus* infection should be considered as the most likely pathogen.

THE FORMATION OF A BIOFILM

Biofilm is an aggregation of bacterial cells that produces an extracellular matrix, which allows adherence to the surface of a prosthetic implant or indwelling lines. As well as providing a means of adherence to prosthetic joints, they also act as a barrier to the immune system and antibiotics. This makes treatment very difficult.

THE DIFFICULTY OF SURGERY

Many patients who have prosthetic joint infections are elderly, often with multiple comorbidities. Intraoperative risk is high. Post-operative complications are high, and often, there is need for a second-stage procedure further down the line. Many patients, however, have severely reduced mobility or significant frailty, and therefore options can be severely limited.

CLINICAL APPROACH

DIAGNOSIS

Early diagnosis allows narrowing the antibiotics and treating for the shortest duration possible. Blood cultures whenever the patient is febrile will help identify the pathogen responsible. Concurrent investigations should also include:

- Swabs for culture of any sinuses present
- Urine culture
- Joint aspiration

If *S. aureus* is cultured in the blood, then the patient will need to also have the following:

- IV flucloxacillin 2 g QDS or 2 g 6 times a day if >85kg
- Skeletal examination with imaging (i.e. MRI) of any joint or spine if any tenderness
- Repeat blood cultures in 48 hours after initiation of antibiotics to ensure no longer bacteraemic
- An echocardiogram to assess for endocarditis

The purpose of MRI imaging of the spine or any other joints and the echocardiogram is to ensure that there has been no seeding there rather than to investigate the source. If a patient develops new back pain or there is suspicion of a new murmur and the patient is still bacteraemic, then repeat investigations may be warranted.

SURGERY

Surgery has two main purposes: source control and identification of the pathogen. There are different options available; the most frequent, surgical intervention, is a two-stage exchange procedure. This consists of removal of the prosthesis with a spacer placed *in situ* (sometimes containing antibiotics) for a period of 6 weeks, followed by a second operation in which a new prosthesis is placed.

ANTIBIOTICS

Antibiotics should be guided by the microbiology that is cultured from preoperative samples. Unless clinically indicated (bacteraemia or severe sepsis), antibiotics should be held off until cultures are taken intraoperatively.

Vancomycin with gentamicin is a commonly used regimen; however, please adhere to local policies or speak to your microbiologist.

Treatment durations are long (>6 weeks). Early planning with a peripherally inserted central catheter (PICC) and organization with the local outpatient antibiotic therapy (OPAT) team should be considered.

INTRAVENOUS ANTIBIOTIC THERAPY

Monitoring is done in outpatient clinic with input from an infectious diseases expert/microbiologist and an orthopaedic surgeon. Patient parameters including fever, weight and pain are assessed, as well as monitoring the ESR and CRP. Admission should be considered if the patient is clinically deteriorating or has worsening inflammatory markers.

CLINICAL VIGNETTES

A 75-year-old woman with clinically suspected PJI is due for an exploratory hip operation, but due to theatre staff difficulties, the operation has been delayed to early next week. You are the microbiology registrar and the orthopaedic consultant contacts you as he is concerned about lack of antibiotic cover and is keen to initiate treatment. She is haemodynamically stable and has never had a fever over 37.8°C since admission 4 days ago. Her CRP is 120 mg/L. An initial joint aspirate was culture negative with no puss cells. What would you suggest?

Microbiology diagnosis here is very important and if the patient is clinically well, then empirical therapy can be delayed for a few more days until operative samples are taken. Best advice is to reassure the consultant that currently no antibiotics are indicated and to offer an 'SOS' option should the patient deteriorate in the interim, such as teicoplanin and ciprofloxacin.

You are part of the infectious diseases team and are reviewing a 67-year-old gentleman in outpatient antibiotic clinic. He has been on IV Tazocin which he has self-administered for 5 weeks now following a first-stage revision of an infected joint that cultured Pseudomonas aeruginosa *from 3 tissue samples. He reports that he has been doing well in the post-operative period but has become a bit more run down in the last week. He had a temperature of 38.1°C in the clinic. A CRP and ESR were performed and this shows an upward trend (76 mg/L and 24 mm/h respectively from 20 mg/L and 18 mm/h 2 weeks ago). He has no pain in the joint, nor any localizing symptoms, including diarrhoea. Clinical examination was unremarkable apart from fever (bp 140/80, pulse 70 sinus, sats 98% on room air). He has no other significant past medical history and is on no regular medication. A urine dip stick is negative. Repeat bloods show a mild anaemia (hb 112 dg/L, stable) with a white cell count that is on a downward trend, but of note, the eosinophil count is now 0.52% from 0.15% and an ALT of 123 IU/L which has risen from 65 IU/L.*

Drug fever is associated with penicillins and monobactams. This is characterized by a hepatitis, eosinophilia and fever, with a diffuse macular rash tending to be a later sign. Blood cultures should be taken here but the key is to identify this early and switch antibiotics, potentially even allowing a holiday for a couple of days. An alternative to Tazocin would be meropenem.

BIBLIOGRAPHY

National Joint Registry. Available from: http://www-new.njrcentre.org.uk/njrcentre/Healthcareproviders/Accessingthedata/StatsOnline/NJRStatsOnline/tabid/179/Default.aspx.

Osmon DR, Berbari EF, Berendt AR, Lew D, Zimmerli W, Steckelberg JM, Rao N, Hanssen A, Wilson WR. Diagnosis and management of prosthetic joint infection: Clinical Practice Guidelines by the Infectious Diseases Society of America. *Clin Infect Dis.* 2012;56(1):1–25.

Zimmerli W, Trampuz A, Ochsner PE. Prosthetic-joint infections. *N Engl J Med.* 2004;351:1645–1654.

4.53 Prostatitis

Firza Alexander Gronthoud

CLINICAL CONSIDERATIONS

Acute bacterial prostatitis is an acute infection of the prostate gland that may easily be misdiagnosed as a cystitis. It requires a longer treatment duration and few antibiotics reach therapeutic concentrations in the prostate. It is therefore worthwhile to consider the following.

BACTERIAL PROSTATITIS IS COMMON

- Prostatitis is the underlying cause in >90% of men with fever, urinary symptoms and absence of pyelonephritis.
- Prostatitis accounts for nearly 8% of urologist visits.

ACUTE (ABP) VERSUS CHRONIC BACTERIAL PROSTATITIS (CBP)

- ABP is an acute lower urinary tract infection with involvement of the prostate more commonly found in men between 20 and 40 years and in men >60 years of age.
- CBP is defined as recurrent UTIs with the same organism in prostatic secretions during asymptomatic periods and develops slowly over a period of 3 months or longer.
- Only 10% of men with ABP will eventually develop CBP.

> **CLINICAL PEARL**
>
> Recurrent UTIs with the same organism suggest a persistent source of urinary tract bacterial seeding and should raise the suspicion of a chronic bacterial prostatitis.

SYMPTOMS

- ABP presents with any lower urinary tract symptoms and/or pelvic or perineal pressure, suggesting prostate involvement, and may be accompanied by signs and symptoms of sepsis.
- ABP may also mimic benign prostatic hypertrophy (BPH): hesitancy, incomplete voiding, straining to urinate, weak stream.
- Prostatic massage should not be undertaken in patients with acute prostatitis because of the risk of precipitating bacteraemia.

PHYSICAL EXAMINATION

- Rectal examination shows a tender, enlarged or boggy prostate and should be performed gently to avoid inducing bacteraemia and sepsis.
- Consider postvoid residual urine volume measurement with ultrasound.
- See Table 4.53.1 for physical findings suggesting different aetiology.

TABLE 4.53.1
Differential Diagnosis

Differential Diagnosis	Symptoms
Benign prostatic hypertrophy	Obstructive voiding symptoms; enlarged, nontender prostate; affects older men
Cystitis	Normal prostate examination
Diverticulitis	Left lower-quadrant abdominal pain; acute change in bowel habits
Epididymitis	Tender epididymis
Orchitis	Swelling, pain and/or tenderness to palpation in one or both testicles
Proctitis	Tenesmus; rectal bleeding; feeling of rectal fullness; passage of mucus through the rectum

Risk Factors

Risk factors include ascending urethral infection or intraprostatic reflux, any transurethral manipulation, transrectal prostate biopsy or haematogenous spread via bacterial sepsis (i.e. bacterial endocarditis caused by *Staphylococcus aureus*).

Infectious Aetiology

- *Enterobacterales* (mainly *Escherichia coli*), *Pseudomonas aeruginosa* and *Enterococcus* spp. *Staphylococcus aureus* may be more commonly seen in CBP.
- In sexually active men, *Neisseria gonorrhoeae* and *Chlamydia trachomatis* should be considered.
- Less commonly, in immunocompromised prostatitis, also nontyphoidal *Salmonella* spp. or yeasts including *Candida* spp. and *Cryptococcus* spp.

Antibiotic Treatment

- Lipophilicity and a high pKa (acid dissociation constant) are important factors that determine whether or not an antibiotic will reach therapeutic concentrations in the prostate.
- The milieu of the infected human prostate is alkaline (pH=8.34). An alkaline environment can enhance the antibacterial activity of certain antibiotics, i.e. fluoroquinolones against Gram negatives and azithromycin against *Staphylococcus aureus*.
- Excellent prostate penetration: Ciprofloxacin and trimethoprim/sulfamethoxazole.
- Good prostate penetration: Fosfomycin, piperacillin/tazobactam, cefuroxime, ceftriaxone, cefotaxime, ceftazidime, aztreonam, carbapenems, macrolides (erythromycin, clarithromycin and azithromycin), clindamycin, doxycycline and minocycline, amikacin.
- Poor prostate penetration: Gentamicin, tobramycin, tetracycline, benzylpenicillin.

Transrectal Ultrasound-Guided Biopsy (TRUBP)-Associated Infection

- Occurs via direct inoculation of bacteria into the prostate, urinary tract or local vasculature.
- Single-dose antimicrobial prophylaxis during TRUBP of the prostate is effective at reducing risk of infection.
- In areas with high antimicrobial-resistance rates (especially against quinolones), it is cost-effective to perform rectal cultures to guide antimicrobial prophylaxis.
- Rectal disinfection prior to TRUBP using povidone iodine can significantly reduce fever, bacteriuria and bacteraemia.
- Transperineal prostate biopsy is a strategy that uses a transcutaneous approach to avoid the 'trans-fecal' route. Prophylactic agents targeting Gram-positive microorganisms are used for this method.

COMPLICATIONS OF PROSTATITIS

Prostatic abscesses occur in 2.7% of patients and require urology consultation for drainage. Risk factors for prostatic abscess include long-term urinary catheterization, recent urethral manipulation and immunocompromise. In these patients, it is recommended to perform imaging studies of the prostate with ultrasound or CT.

CLINICAL APPROACH

- Distinguish between acute and chronic bacterial prostatitis based on history
- If chronic bacterial prostatitis is suspected:
  - *Two-glass test:* Clean-catch urine before prostate massage in glass 1 and clean-catch urine after prostate massage in glass 2 and send both for culture.
  - *Meares–Stamey four-glass test:* 10 mL of urine in glass 1, 10 mL of midstream urine in glass 2, prostatic massage followed by collection of expressed prostatic secretion (EPS) glass 3 and post-massage urine in glass 4. Glass 1 is tested for *N. gonorrhoea* and *C. trachomatis*, glass 2 is cultured for uropathogens, the EPS is examined for WBCs. The post-massage urine is used to flush out bacteria in the prostate that may remain within the urethra.
  - Urine culture.
  - Perform transrectal ultrasound to look for prostatic calcification, which may serve as a source for recurrent infection. Consider performing urodynamics to document bladder problems or obstruction.

CLINICAL PEARL

Consider catheterization or a suprapubic catheter for patients with severe obstructive voiding symptoms or urinary retention.

ACUTE BACTERIAL PROSTATITIS

- Urine cultures and blood cultures in patients with systemic signs of infection and in immunocompromised patients.
- Sexually active men <35 years and men >35 years engaging in high-risk sexual behaviour: send urine for PCR for detection of *N. gonorrhoeae* and *C. trachomatis*.
- Intravenous antimicrobial treatment is indicated for patients with sepsis, failed treatment on ciprofloxacin or trimethoprim/sulfamethoxazole, recent transurethral or transrectal prostatic manipulation, immunosuppressed, elderly patients or severe voiding disorder.
- Oral treatment:
  - First-line drug of choice: ciprofloxacin 500 mg PO 12-hourly OR trimethoprim/sulfamethoxazole 960 mg PO 12-hourly.
  - Second-line drug of choice: fosfomycin trometamol 3 g PO once daily for the first week followed by 3 g every 2 days for the remaining duration of treatment.
- Intravenous treatment:
  - First-line drug of choice is ceftriaxone 2 g IV once daily OR piperacillin/tazobactam 4.5 g IV 8-hourly.
  - Consider adding amikacin 15 mg/kg IV once daily with therapeutic drug monitoring in areas with high ESBL and AmpC prevalence OR alternatively start ertapenem 1 g IV once daily.

- If *P. aeruginosa*, piperacillin/tazobactam 4.5 g IV 8-hourly may reach insufficient therapeutic concentrations; consider ceftazidime 2 g IV 8-hourly OR increase frequency of piperacillin/tazobactam to 6-hourly and add amikacin 15 mg/kg IV.
- Outpatient intravenous treatment:
  - Ceftriaxone 2 g IV once daily OR ertapenem 1 g IV once daily.
- Consider prostate imaging to rule out prostate abscess if no clinical improvement after 36 hours. Abscess drainage can be performed transurethral, through the rectum or the perineum.
- Duration of antimicrobial treatment: 2–4 weeks (4 weeks if bacteraemia and/or abscess is present).
- Consider NSAIDs and an alpha-1 blocker for pain management and lower urinary tract symptom relief.
- If no other oral option, either doxycycline 100 mg PO 12-hourly or minocycline 100 mg PO 12-hourly for 6 weeks may be considered, depending on organism and MIC result. Only CLSI has breakpoints for tetracyclines and *Enterobacterales*, with an MIC of ≤4 mg/L considered sensitive.

CLINICAL PEARL

Approximately 70% of men will have an elevated prostate specific antigen (PSA) owing to inflammatory changes, and PSA therefore has no diagnostic value.

TREATMENT OF CHRONIC BACTERIAL PROSTATITIS

- Treatment of CBP can usually be delayed until culture and susceptibility results are available.
- A transrectal ultrasound is recommended to look for signs of inflammation, presence of calcifications or an abscess.
- Start antibacterial treatment with either ciprofloxacin OR trimethoprim/sulfamethoxazole OR fosfomycin for 6 weeks.
- Review after 6 weeks.
- If CBP still present, repeat course for a further 6 weeks (25%–50% recurrence rate after first treatment).
- Discuss surgical options with urology, i.e. removal of infected prostatic tissue or stones.
- If the source of prostatic infection cannot be eliminated, consider long-term low-dose suppressive antibiotic therapy (low evidence).

BACTERIAL PROSTATITIS CAUSED BY INTRACELLULAR ORGANISMS

- *Chlamydia trachomatis*, *Ureaplasma urealyticum* and *Mycoplasma* spp.
- Either doxycycline 100 mg PO 12-hourly OR a macrolide, i.e. clarithromycin 500 mg PO 12-hourly or azithromycin 500 mg once daily on the first 3 consecutive days of each week

PROPHYLAXIS FOR TURBP

- Add single-dose gentamicin 5 mg/kg IV OR amikacin 15 mg/kg IV to either ciprofloxacin or trimethoprim/sulfamethoxazole *or*
- Oral fosfomycin trometamol 3 g 1–4 hours prior to surgery; might be ineffective if the MIC is >4 mg/L *or*
- Single-dose ceftriaxone 2 g IV *or*

- If resistant to all above, single-dose ertapenem 1 g IV
- Consider rectal culture results to guide antimicrobial therapy prior to TRUBP in areas with high antimicrobial-resistance rates

BIBLIOGRAPHY

Charalabopoulos K, Karachalios G, Baltogiannis D, Charalabopoulos A, Giannakopoulos X, Sofikitis N. Penetration of antimicrobial sgents into the prostate. *Chemotherapy.* 2003 December;49(6):269–279.

Coker TJ, Dierfeldt DM. Acute bacterial prostatitis: Diagnosis and management. *Am Fam Physician.* 2016 January 15;93(2):114–120.

Gill BC, Shoskes DA. Bacterial prostatitis. *Curr Opin Infect Dis.* 2016 February;29(1):86–91.

Karaiskos I, Galani L, Sakka V, Gkoufa A, Sopilidis O, Chalikopoulos D, Alivizatos G, Giamarellou E. Oral fosfomycin for the treatment of chronic bacterial prostatitis. *J Antimicrob Chemother.* 2019;74(5):1430–1437.

Khan FU, Ihsan AU, Khan HU, Jana R, Wazir J, Khongorzul P, Waqar M, Zhou X. Comprehensive overview of prostatitis. *Biomed Pharmacother.* 2017 October;94:1064–1076.

Zowawi HM, Harris PN, Roberts MJ, Tambyah PA, Schembri MA, Pezzani MD, Williamson DA, Paterson DL. The emerging threat of multidrug-resistant Gram-negative bacteria in urology. *Nat Rev Urol.* 2015 October;12(10):570–584.

4.54 Pyomyositis

Firza Alexander Gronthoud

CLINICAL CONSIDERATIONS

Pyomyositis is an acute bacterial infection of skeletal muscle. Clinical presentation can be similar to common conditions such as soft tissue cellulitis which can lead to a delay in treatment and potential clinical deterioration from sepsis. It is then worthwhile to consider the following.

POPULATION AT RISK

Historically, pyomyositis was described in tropical areas in children between 2 and 5 years, with malnutrition as a possible predisposing factor. In temperate zones, it is mainly seen in adult males with a history of intravenous drug use, immunosuppression such as HIV or diabetes mellitus, cirrhosis and patients with concurrent viral and parasitic infections including toxocariasis and varicella zoster. Although a rare diagnosis in temperate zones, with globalization and increased foreign travel, potentially, pyomyositis could be encountered with increasing frequency.

AETIOLOGY

The source of pyomyositis is believed to be a transient bacteraemia where bacteria get lodged in skeletal muscle causing a localized abscess. This is especially seen in *Staphylococcus aureus* which has the propensity to disseminate as a septic embolus through its production of coagulase enzyme. Because skeletal muscle is usually resistant to bacterial infection, it is hypothesized that local muscle injury such as ischaemia or trauma is a precipitating factor. Trauma facilitates haematogenous access to the muscle tissue and provides an iron-enriched environment for bacterial growth through the release of myoglobin. Another mechanism is via direct extension from a septic arthritis or osteomyelitis.

CLINICAL PRESENTATION

Pyomyositis is characterized by fever, swelling, tenderness and localized muscle pain, most often affecting the quadriceps or iliopsoas. In up to 20% of cases, multiple muscle groups are affected. Pyomyositis has three phases (see Table 4.54.1). Patients usually do not present in stage I because of the vague presentation, and when they do visit a doctor, they are often misdiagnosed as a muscle strain, contusion, cellulitis, haematoma, deep vein thrombophlebitis, osteomyelitis, septic arthritis or a soft tissue sarcoma. More than 90% of patients present in stage II or III, and in stage III, complications such as septic shock or septic emboli to other organs can be seen. Long-term sequelae are muscle scarring, residual weakness and functional impairment.

CLINICAL APPROACH

IMAGING IS KEY

- *How*: MRI, CT or ultrasound.
- *Rationale*: Clinical picture and laboratory investigation are not specific and may lead to a false diagnosis with delayed complications. MRI can identify muscle inflammation,

TABLE 4.54.1
Stages of Pyomyositis

Stage I	Stage II	Stage III
Invasive stage	Suppurative stage	Septicaemia
• Localized crampy muscle pain	• 10–21 days after onset of symptoms	• Development of severe
• Low-grade fever	• Abscess formation	sepsis or septic shock
• 'Woody' texture of affected muscle on palpation		

intramuscular abscess and confirm the presence of purulent arthritis or osteomyelitis. CT shows loss of flat surface of the muscle, fluid retention inside the muscle and contrast enhancement in the surrounding area. CT can be performed more easily than MRI, but CT has lower sensitivity than MRI and provides less anatomical information. Ultrasound can visualize purulent fluid collections in the deeper tissue planes and can easily be performed at the bedside. Especially in cases of a positive blood culture, echocardiography should be performed to rule out endocarditis (see Chapter 5.6).

Microbiological Investigation

Blood cultures are positive in 10%–35% of cases, and the most important specimen remains abscess fluid cultures. The most common pathogen is *Staphylococcus aureus*, causing up to 90% of infections in tropical areas and 75% in temperate zones, followed by *S. pyogenes*. Less frequent agents include *Pseudomonas aeruginosa* and *Enterobacterales*. *Escherichia coli* is an emerging agent of pyomyositis in patients with haematological malignancies. Rare cases of mycobacterial pyomyositis have also been reported.

Management

Patients with stage I disease can usually be conservatively managed with antimicrobial therapy. Stages II and III, in addition, require drainage of the abscess with debridement of necrotic tissue. In most cases, this will result in a complete recovery without long-term sequelae. Abscess fluid and tissue should be sent to the microbiology laboratory for culture, after which empirical therapy can be rationalized based on susceptibility results. Initial choice of antimicrobial therapy is intravenous flucloxacillin 2 g QDS. An aminoglycoside such as gentamicin 5 mg/kg IV or amikacin 15 mg/kg IV can be added in immunocompromised patients in whom a higher incidence of Gram-negative rods is seen. Alternative empirical treatment is ceftriaxone 2 g IV once daily or piperacillin/tazobactam 4.5 g 8-hourly IV if antipseudomonal coverage is needed. The duration of treatment depends on the aetiology. Four to six weeks of intravenous antibiotic therapy is indicated for an endocarditis, concomitant *Staphylococcus aureus* bacteraemia, septic arthritis or osteomyelitis. In the absence of other infectious foci, 2–3 weeks of antibiotic therapy after source control would suffice.

CLINICAL PEARL

Failure of antibiotic therapy and surgery may be due to recurrence of a previously debrided abscess or by unrecognized abscesses elsewhere. Up to half of patients require abscess drainage, and in 10% of the cases, drainage needs to be repeated. Pyomyositis may recur despite prolonged therapy, especially in HIV-infected patients.

The clinical vignettes below illustrate the insidious nature and different clinical presentations of pyomyositis.

CLINICAL VIGNETTES

A 58-year-old male was brought to the local hospital by his wife who found him febrile and confused at home. On admission, CT scan of his head was unremarkable. He was treated with intravenous amoxicillin/clavulanic acid for a presumed urosepsis, after which his mental status improved, and he was stepped down to oral antibiotics. Blood culture and urine culture taken on admission remained negative. After a few days, he noticed pain, tenderness and swelling of his right calf. A CT scan of the right calf was highly suggestive of an abscess. Irrigation and drainage was performed, and the purulent fluid grew a Streptococcus agalactiae. *A holosystolic murmur was detected and a transoesophageal echocardiogram showed a large mitral valve vegetation. High-dose benzylpenicillin was started, and he underwent valve replacement.*

- Initial presentation of pyomyositis is similar to other common infections.
- Even in the absence of a positive blood culture, the diagnosis of endocarditis should always be entertained.

A 62-year-old man is seen by his GP with right-leg cramp after running half a marathon, having lost a bet with his mates. His GP advises rest and no physical activities for the next weeks. After two weeks, he becomes systemically unwell with high fever and progressively worsening pain in his right leg. He is admitted to the ICU with septic shock. An MRI showed necrotic muscle tissue and a deep abscess. Unfortunately, due to the severity and extent of disease progression, he required an amputation of his right lower leg, after which he recovered from his infection but is now facing chronic disability and long-term rehabilitation.

- Clinical acumen and early imaging is essential in preventing long-term complications.

BIBLIOGRAPHY

Christin L, Sarosi GA. Pyomyositis in North America: Case reports and review. *Clin Infect Dis.* 1992 October;15(4):668–677.

Crum-Cianflone NF. Bacterial, fungal, parasitic, and viral myositis. *Clin Microbiol Rev.* 2008 July;21(3):473–494.

Elzohairy MM. Primary pyomyositis in children. *Orthop Traumatol Surg Res.* 2018;104(3):397–403.

Kwak YG, Choi SH, Kim T, Park SY, Seo SH, Kim MB, Choi SH. Clinical guidelines for the antibiotic treatment for community-acquired skin and soft tissue infection. *Infect Chemother.* 2017 December;49(4):301–325.

Lemonick DM. Non-tropical pyomyositis caused by methicillin-resistant *Staphylococcus aureus*: An unusual cause of bilateral leg pain. *J Emerg Med.* 2012 March;42(3):e55–e62.

Scharschmidt TJ, Weiner SD, Myers JP. Bacterial pyomyositis. *Curr Infect Dis Rep.* 2004 October;6(5):393–396.

4.55 Ringworm

Firza Alexander Gronthoud

CLINICAL CONSIDERATIONS

Ringworm, or tinea infections, are classified by the involved site. The most common infections in prepubertal children are tinea corporis and tinea capitis, whereas adolescents and adults are more likely to develop tinea cruris, tinea pedis, and tinea unguium or onychomycosis (onychomycosis will be discussed separately; see Chapter 4.43). Tinea infections can mimic other conditions and can be difficult to treat. It is therefore worthwhile to consider the following.

PATHOGENS

Tinea infections are caused by dermatophytes with the exception of tinea versicolor which is caused by *Malassezia*. Dermatophytes include three genera: *Trichophyton*, *Microsporum* and *Epidermophyton*.

CLINICAL MANIFESTATIONS

Tinea corporis (ringworm) typically presents as a red, annular, scaly, pruritic patch with central clearing and an active border. Lesions may be single or multiple, and the size generally ranges from 1 to 5 cm, but larger lesions and confluence of lesions can also occur. Worsening after empiric treatment with a topical steroid for eczema should raise the suspicion of a dermatophyte infection.

Tinea cruris (jock itch) most commonly affects adolescent and young adult males and involves the portion of the upper thigh opposite the scrotum. The scrotum itself is usually spared in tinea cruris but involved in candidiasis. A Wood's lamp examination may be helpful to distinguish tinea from erythrasma because the causative organism of erythrasma (*Corynebacterium minutissimum*) exhibits a coral red fluorescence. However, results of the Wood's lamp examination can be falsely negative if the patient has bathed recently.

Tinea pedis (athlete's foot) typically involves the skin between the toes, but can spread to the sole, sides and dorsum of the involved foot. The acute form presents with erythema and maceration between the toes, sometimes accompanied by painful vesicles. The more common chronic form is characterized by scaling, peeling and erythema between the toes; however, it can spread to other areas of the foot. Involvement of the plantar and lateral aspects of the foot with erythema and hyperkeratosis is referred to as the 'moccasin pattern' of tinea pedis.

Tinea capitis is a ringworm infection of the scalp and most commonly affects children. The main symptoms are itching, redness and dryness of the scalp. Sometimes bald patches can occur as infected hairs are brittle and break easily. There are three types of tinea capitis: grey patch, black dot and favus. It may progress to kerion, which is characterized by boggy tender plaques and pustules. The child with tinea capitis will generally have cervical and suboccipital lymphadenopathy, and the physician may need to broaden the differential diagnosis if lymphadenopathy is absent.

CLINICAL APPROACH

DIAGNOSIS

Tinea corporis, tinea cruris and tinea pedis can often be diagnosed based on appearance, but a KOH preparation should be performed when the appearance is atypical (see Table 4.55.1).

TABLE 4.55.1
Differential Diagnosis Tinea Infections

Tinea	Differential Diagnosis
Tinea corporis	Eczema, psoriasis, seborrheic dermatitis, erythema multiforme
Tinea capitis	Alopecia areata, eczema, seborrheic psoriasis, seborrheic dermatitis
Tinea cruris	Candida intertrigo, erythrasma, inverse psoriasis, seborrheic dermatitis

Cultures are usually not necessary. Skin biopsy with periodic acid-Schiff (PAS) stain may rarely be indicated for atypical or persistent lesions. For tinea capitis, a KOH preparation can be performed by scraping the black dots (broken hairs) and looking for fungal spores. The spores of *T. tonsurans* will be contained within the hair shaft, but for the less common *Microsporum canis*, the spores will coat the outside of the hair shaft. Culture, which is more sensitive than the KOH preparation, can be performed by moistening a cotton applicator or toothbrush with tap water and rubbing it over the involved scalp.

TREATMENT

Tinea corporis, tinea cruris and tinea pedis generally respond to topical agents such as terbinafine cream or butenafine cream, but oral antifungal agents may be indicated for extensive disease, failed topical treatment, immunocompromised patients or severe moccasin-type tinea pedis.

Patients with chronic or recurrent tinea pedis may benefit from wide shoes, drying between the toes after bathing and placing lamb's wool between the toes. Patients with tinea gladiatorum, a generalized form of tinea corporis seen in wrestlers, should be treated with topical therapy for 72 hours before a return to wrestling.

Tinea capitis must be treated with systemic antifungal agents because topical agents do not penetrate the hair shaft. However, concomitant treatment with 1% or 2.5% selenium sulfide (Selsun) shampoo or 2% ketoconazole shampoo should be used for the first 2 weeks because it may reduce transmission. Terbinafine may be superior to griseofulvin for *Trichophyton* species, whereas griseofulvin may be superior to terbinafine for the less common *Microsporum* species. Most cases are caused by *Trichophyton* spp., making terbinafine a reasonable first choice. Once treatment has started, the child may return to school, but for 14 days should not share combs, brushes, helmets, hats or pillowcases, or participate in sports that involve head-to-head contact, such as wrestling. Consider treating household members with a sporicidal shampoo, such as 2.5% selenium sulfide or 2% ketoconazole, for 2–4 weeks.

CLINICAL PEARL

Kerion is a fungal abscess and should be treated with griseofulvin unless *Trichophyton* has been documented as the pathogen.

BIBLIOGRAPHY

Ely JW, Rosenfeld S, Seabury Stone M. Diagnosis and management of tinea infections. *Am Fam Physician*. 2014 November 15;90(10):702–710.
Kelly BP. Superficial fungal infections. *Pediatr Rev*. 2012 April;33(4):e22–e37.
Hay RJ. Tinea capitis: Current status. *Mycopathologia*. 2017 February;182(1–2):87–93.

4.56 *Salmonella* Carriage

Firza Alexander Gronthoud

CLINICAL CONSIDERATIONS

Salmonella species are subdivided into subspecies which can cause typhoid and paratyphoid fever, invasive nontyphoidal *Salmonella* (NTS) disease or non-invasive NTS disease. Immunocompromised individuals such as individuals living with HIV are especially at risk of extra-intestinal disease or relapses. *Salmonella* infection can be complicated by prolonged shedding in the stool and *Salmonella* Typhi infection may be complicated by a chronic carriage state. It is less clear if nontyphoidal *Salmonella* species can cause a chronic carriage state, as this is a less well studied area. It is therefore worthwhile to consider the following.

PERIOD OF SHEDDING

- The median duration of excretion following infection is approximately 5 weeks.
- Routine follow-up cultures are not recommended after uncomplicated *Salmonella* gastroenteritis in immunocompetent patients, particularly if symptoms have resolved.
- Antibiotic treatment is also not indicated for patients incidentally found to have continued *Salmonella* isolation from the stools following an episode of gastroenteritis.
- Immunocompromised patients may warrant special consideration; infectious disease consultation is advised.
- Age younger than 5 years is associated with a longer duration of excretion, with a median of approximately 7 weeks. Among this age group, 2.6% excrete *Salmonella* bacteria for more than 1 year, compared with less than 1% among all age groups.
- The duration of excretion may be longer after symptomatic versus asymptomatic infection.
- *Salmonella typhimurium* is more rapidly cleared than other serotypes.
- Intermittent shedding is common, so a single negative culture is not that reassuring.
- Antibiotic therapy of symptomatic diarrhoeal illness does not prevent or shorten the duration of carriage and, in some studies, is associated with a longer duration of excretion.
- Furthermore, short-course antibiotic treatment of asymptomatic carriage is not effective in eradicating it and may promote resistance.
- Non-fluoroquinolone antibiotics have been associated with an increased risk of subsequent *Salmonella* carriage.

SALMONELLA CHRONIC CARRIAGE

Following the resolution of disease, approximately 2%–5% of typhoid patients fail to clear the infection fully within 1 year of recovery, and instead progress to a state of carriage. Fecal carriage is more frequent among individuals with gallbladder disease and is most common among women over 40 years of age. In the Far East, there is an association between fecal carriage and opisthorchiasis, and urinary carriage is associated with schistosomiasis and nephrolithiasis. Chronic carriage can occur with both *Salmonella* serovar Typhi and Paratyphi A. There is less data on the association between NTS infections and chronic carriage, but the incidence may be around 0.5%.

Chronic carriage with typhoidal *Salmonella* is more common in young children, older individuals, women and those with biliary tract abnormalities, especially gallstones. Eradication is indicated for immunosuppressed patients, particularly those with advanced HIV infection, who are at higher risk of complications from infection.

PATHOGENESIS

Salmonella Typhi can pass the intestinal epithelial barrier, evade the innate immune system and adhere to gallbladder epithelia and cause a chronic inflammation, which may progress to gallbladder cancer. In addition, it can form biofilms on gallstones, further contributing to a chronic carriage state. About 90% of *Salmonella* Typhi carriers have gallstones.

CLINICAL PEARL

Asymptomatic shedding of *Salmonella* spp. in the stool is common after either symptomatic or asymptomatic nontyphoidal *Salmonella* infection.

CLINICAL PEARL

Antibiotic treatment does not facilitate clearance of intestinal carriage of *Salmonella* and may induce super-shedding and increase duration of shedding as it suppresses the colonization resistance of the microbiota, which plays a protective role in limiting gut infection.

CLINICAL APPROACH

LABORATORY DETECTION

The detection of chronic carriers depends on persistent positive stool or urine cultures. Shedding can be intermittent, and at least three negative stool cultures are required for patients to be considered free of infection. It may be possible to prospectively detect chronic carriers through their abnormally high anti-Vi IgG antibody titres. The specificity of anti-Vi IgG for detecting chronic carriers is lower in areas where *Salmonella* is endemic or where the Vi vaccine is used widely.

CLINICAL PEARL

Unlike typhoid fever, NTS have a dramatically more severe and invasive presentation in immunocompromised adults, such as HIV.

TREATMENT OF CHRONIC CARRIAGE

Treatment of chronic *Salmonella* Typhi carriage is aimed at eradication from the gallbladder. Various antimicrobials have been used to treat chronic carriers; however, no treatment is completely effective in the resolution of chronic colonization of the gallbladder. The drug of choice for treatment of chronic carriage is a fluoroquinolone such as ciprofloxacin 500 mg or 750 mg BD PO for 4 weeks. Increasing drug resistance and increased risk of *Clostridium difficile* remain important challenges. Failure to treat carriers effectively with antimicrobials may be dependent on resistant organisms being selected in the gallbladder or the protective effect of biofilm formation. In the presence of severe cholelithiasis, antimicrobial therapy in combination with source control (cholecystectomy) may be required because biofilm infections usually persist until the colonized surface is surgically removed from the body. Cholecystectomy alone raises the cure rate to 85% but does not guarantee elimination of the carrier state. Additional foci of infection can persist in the biliary tree, mesenteric lymph nodes or the liver.

Second-line treatment includes:

- Trimethoprim/sulfamethoxazole (160 mg/800 mg orally twice daily) for 3 months.
- Ampicillin or amoxicillin (3–5 g orally in four divided doses) for 6 weeks (depending upon susceptibilities of the isolate).
- A combination of cholecystectomy plus antibiotic therapy is probably most effective but does not guarantee carriage will be eradicated.

SUPPRESSIVE THERAPY

Suppressive prophylactic therapy to prevent a relapse after a primary *Salmonella* infection may be warranted in HIV-infected individuals, particularly, if (1) gastroenteritis was complicated by a bloodstream infection indicating invasive disease, (2) low CD4 cell counts or (3) poor response to antiretroviral therapy.

PUBLIC HEALTH MEASURES FOR ENTERIC FEVER

The introduction of public health principles such as sanitary infrastructure, pasteurization of milk and water-supply chlorination has led to the virtual elimination of typhoid fever from most developed countries in the 20th century. Strategies for enteric fever prevention include improving sanitation, ensuring the safety of food and water supplies, identification and treatment of chronic carriers of *Salmonella* serovar Typhi and the use of typhoid vaccines to reduce the susceptibility of hosts to infection or disease. Reducing the proportion of people without access to safe drinking water is a component of Millennium Development Goal 7. Several vaccines exist: an oral vaccine containing a live, attenuated virus, *Salmonella* serovar Typhi strain Ty21a, and the parenteral Vi vaccine based on the *Salmonella* serovar Typhi Vi capsular polysaccharide antigen. For both vaccines, the protective efficacy over 3 years is about 50%. Newer Vi conjugate vaccines which are still in development have shown an efficacy of 90%. However, Vi-based monovalent vaccines do not offer protection against most paratyphoid fever, because only *Salmonella* serovar Typhi, Paratyphi C and Dublin carry the Vi antigen. Ty21a may provide limited protection against *Salmonella* serovar Paratyphi B.

CLINICAL VIGNETTE

You receive a call from an SHO who is calling regarding a 38-year-old asymptomatic male on the ward. He is receiving chemoradiotherapy for colorectal cancer. A stool screen for multidrug-resistant organisms coincidentally yielded an ESBL producing nontyphoidal Salmonella, *also resistant to quinolones. He is wondering if this requires antibiotic treatment. You advise that antibiotic treatment at this point is not indicated, that the patient can shed this organism in the stool for a prolonged time and strict hand hygiene is important to reduce the likelihood of transmission to his environment.*

- Antibiotic treatment can lead to prolonged shedding.
- Unlike typhoidal *Salmonella*, it is less clear if NTS can cause chronic gallbladder infection.
- Antibiotic treatment of asymptomatic NTS carriage in both immunocompetent and immunocompromised individuals has not been studied.
- Prolonged antibiotic treatment can lead to adverse events, and especially quinolones are associated with increased rates of *Clostridium difficile* infections.

BIBLIOGRAPHY

Crump JA, Sjölund-Karlsson M, Gordon MA, Parry CM. Epidemiology, clinical presentation, laboratory diagnosis, antimicrobial resistance, and antimicrobial management of invasive salmonella infections. *Clin Microbiol Rev.* 2015 October;28(4):901–937.

Dekker JP, Frank KM. *Salmonella*, *Shigella*, and *Yersinia*. *Clin Lab Med.* 2015 June;35(2):225–246.

Gal-Mor O. Persistent infection and long-term carriage of typhoidal and nontyphoidal salmonellae. *Clin Microbiol Rev.* 2018 November 28;32(1). pii: e00088-18.

Gunn JS, Marshall JM, Baker S, Dongol S, Charles RC, Ryan ET. *Salmonella* chronic carriage: Epidemiology, diagnosis, and gallbladder persistence. *Trends Microbiol.* 2014 November;22(11):648–655.

Marzel A, Desai PT, Goren A, Schorr YI, Nissan I, Porwollik S, Valinsky L, McClelland M, Rahav G, Gal-Mor O. Persistent infections by nontyphoidal *Salmonella* in humans: Epidemiology and genetics. *Clin Infect Dis.* 2016 April 1;62(7):879–886.

4.57 Septic Arthritis

Caryn Rosmarin

CLINICAL CONSIDERATIONS

Presentation of septic arthritis is most often acute and monoarticular, with the knee being the commonest joint affected in adults and the hip in young children. In up to 20% of cases, the disease can be oligo- or polyarticular, especially in those with underlying rheumatoid arthritis or other systemic connective tissue disease. Axial joint (e.g. sacroiliac, costochondral and sternoclavicular) septic arthritis is rare, although it has an association with intravenous drug use.

HOW DOES A JOINT BECOME INFECTED?

Acute septic arthritis develops most commonly via the haematogenous route. The associated bacteraemia may be transient, self-limited or recurrent and the risk of deposition of bacteria in a joint is increased in those with pre-existing joint disease, especially disease affecting the synovium. The offending microorganism can also reach the joint space by direct inoculation through surgical interventions such as arthroscopy, intra-articular injection, or open joint trauma including bites.

WHAT ARE THE COMMON PATHOGENS CAUSING SEPTIC ARTHRITIS?

Most cases of septic arthritis are monomicrobial, with *Staphylococcus aureus* being the most common pathogen. This includes both methicillin-sensitive *S. aureus* (MSSA) and methicillin-resistant *S. aureus* (MRSA). This is followed by other Gram-positive organisms, most often streptococci including *Streptococcus pyogenes* (associated with skin and soft tissue infection, IV drug users and trauma), *Streptococcus agalactiae* (more common in diabetics and immune compromised individuals) and *Streptococcus pneumoniae* (associated with alcoholism). *Staphylococcus epidermidis*, in its ability to form biofilms, is the most common agent associated with prosthetic joint infection. Other bacteria increase in importance in certain risk groups, but even in these groups, *Staphylococcus aureus* and streptococci are the most frequently isolated pathogens. The exception to this is in children under 2 years of age, where *Kingella kingae* is the most common pathogen.

Gram-negative coliforms may be causally associated with the elderly, a history of recent gastrointestinal surgery, recurrent urinary tract infections and immune suppression. In particular, those on disease-modifying agents have increased risk of Gram-negative and intracellular organisms such as *Listeria* spp. and *Salmonella* spp.

Intravenous drug users are more likely to have a polymicrobial infection caused by common and unusual Gram-positive, Gram-negative and fungal pathogens.

In sexually active adults, *Neisseria gonorrhoea* needs to be considered, especially if the symptoms include an oligoarthritis.

Bites as a cause of septic arthritis have an additional range of potential pathogens. *Pasteurella multocida* and *Capnocytophaga* spp. are associated with cat or dog bites; while the HACEK (*Haemophilus* spp., *Aggregatibacter* spp., *Cardiobacterium* spp., *Eikenella corrodens* and *Kingella* spp.) group of organisms found in oral flora can result in infection following a human bite to or near a joint.

Unusual pathogens known to be associated with particular geographic locations or epidemiologic risk factors include *Brucella* spp., mycobacteria, spirochaetes and fungi.

WHO IS AT RISK OF DEVELOPING SEPTIC ARTHRITIS?

Predisposing factors can be divided into three main groups, with combinations of these independent risk factors substantially increasing the risk:

- *Risk of bacteraemia*: Intravenous drug use, indwelling intravenous catheters, haemodialysis, skin and soft tissue infection, immune suppression and endocarditis.
- *Risk of seeding the joint*: Recent joint surgery, presence of a prosthetic joint, intra-articular procedure especially steroid injection, and pre-existing arthropathy. Rheumatoid arthritis, in particular, is associated with a significant increased risk of septic arthritis.
- *Immune suppression*: Elderly patients, those with chronic underlying diseases or malignancies, alcoholism and those on immune suppressant, cytotoxic or disease-modifying agents.

HOW DO YOU KNOW IF A HOT SWOLLEN JOINT IS SEPTIC ARTHRITIS OR NOT?

The presentation with one or more hot and swollen joints is a common medical condition, and deciding whether or not septic arthritis is present is challenging. While the differential diagnosis of this condition is broad, septic arthritis is the most serious, as it has a significant associated morbidity and mortality.

The differential diagnosis of acute septic arthritis is broad and includes the following.

Inflammatory Arthritis

This group is the most common cause of an acutely hot swollen joint in adults and includes:

- Crystal arthropathy (gout and pseudogout) may mimic septic arthritis in presentation. Clues suggesting crystal arthritis include involvement of the first metatarsophalangeal joint, prior similar attacks and the presence of tophi. Diagnosis is confirmed by seeing crystals in the synovial fluid; however, the presence of crystals doesn't rule out a concomitant septic arthritis.
- Reactive arthritis secondary to an infection elsewhere in the body, such as urogenital (*Chlamydia* spp.) or gastrointestinal (e.g.. *Campylobacter* spp., *Yersinia* spp.). It may occur in the presence of recent conjunctivitis, mucus membrane lesions and urogenital or gastrointestinal symptoms.
- Rheumatoid arthritis is more often a symmetrical polyarthritis, but exacerbation of disease in a single joint can occur. The fact that patients with rheumatoid arthritis are at increased risk of developing septic arthritis makes the differentiation all the more difficult.

Systemic Viral Infections

Many present with a polyarthritis including HIV, dengue, Zika, parvovirus, rubella and chikungunya.

Osteonecrosis

Secondary to glucocorticoid treatment.

Rheumatologic Presentations of Systemic Diseases

For example, Rheumatic fever, Still's disease, hepatitis C, sarcoidosis, malignancy.

Haemarthrosis

Usually a history of trauma, although may be minor and not reported, especially in haemophilia.

CLINICAL PEARL

Differentiating acute septic arthritis from other causes of a hot swollen joint is challenging and may not be possible until appropriate samples are taken and analyzed.

CLINICAL CONSIDERATIONS

A 48-year-old woman presents with a 2-day history of a hot, swollen knee. She has no fever. She has underlying diabetes and rheumatoid arthritis for which she takes methotrexate. You are called by the emergency doctor and asked whether you think this is septic arthritis.

How Is Septic Arthritis Diagnosed?

Clinically

The classic presentation is an acutely swollen, painful and hot joint with restricted movement in the joint. Fever may be present but its absence does not exclude the diagnosis, especially if anti-inflammatory painkillers have been used.

As discussed above, the differential diagnosis is wide, and the prevalence of septic arthritis in an adult presenting with an acutely hot swollen joint being estimated at less than 20%.

Despite this, as septic arthritis is associated with destructive changes in the affected joint and has a not insignificant mortality, all hot swollen joints should be managed as septic until proven otherwise.

Early diagnosis and treatment is therefore essential to prevent permanent damage of the joint and associated complications.

Laboratory

Definitive diagnosis of acute septic arthritis relies on finding evidence of bacteria in the synovial fluid or membrane. Arthrocentesis (aspiration of synovial fluid) is mandatory for establishing the diagnosis and ideally should be taken before antibiotic therapy is started. The fluid should be sent for microscopy, culture and sensitivity (M,C&S), as well as assessment for crystals. Remember the presence of crystals does not rule out a concomitant septic arthritis.

In septic arthritis, the synovial fluid is likely to look turbid and have a raised WCC, which is predominantly neutrophils. While this is suggestive, it is not diagnostic as this may also be present in non-infectious arthritis. A synovial fluid WCC of >50 000/μL is thought to predict bacterial over non-infectious arthritis, although this has not been conclusively evidenced. The Gram stain is positive in up to 50% of cases. Despite the low sensitivity of the Gram stain, culture is positive in most cases if the patient has not received antibiotics before the sample is taken. Culture negative samples in the absence of antibiotics should raise the possibility of fastidious organisms or an inflammatory arthritis.

Molecular-based techniques such as a polymerase chain reaction (PCR) may be useful when antibiotics are taken prior to sampling or in culture negative arthritis with a high index of suspicion of a septic joint.

Blood cultures are another important diagnostic sample as most septic arthritis is haematogenously spread. They are positive in about 50% of cases and should be taken even in the absence of a fever.

Additional cultures, or tests for an infectious aetiology, should be performed depending on clinical scenario. These may include wound swabs of infected looking skin lesions, urine for M,C&S, or testing for suspected gonococcal or chlamydial infection.

Routine blood inflammatory markers (WCC, CRP, ESR) and uric acid levels should be performed even though raised levels do not distinguish infective from non-infective causes. They are important for monitoring response to therapy if a diagnosis of septic arthritis is confirmed.

Radiologically

Imaging studies can assess the presence and extent of inflammation and destruction, but cannot accurately distinguish infective from non-infective inflammatory causes. X-ray of the affected joint(s) should be obtained as baseline, and the presence of an underlying arthropathy, foreign bodies or complicating osteomyelitis may also be visible. Ultrasound or CT scan will show the presence of a joint effusion and assist with guided aspiration, if required. MRI may be helpful in assessing the presence of soft tissue collections or associated osteomyelitis. Radionucleotide scans have varying degrees of sensitivities and specificities in differentiating septic arthritis from other forms of inflammatory arthritides.

CLINICAL PEARL

Definitive diagnosis of acute septic arthritis relies on finding evidence of bacteria in the synovial fluid or membrane. Other diagnostic tests may provide useful additional information on severity and underlying risk factors, but are often non-diagnostic.

The same emergency doctor calls you back to say samples have been taken and asks for your advice on treatment while awaiting these results.

How Is Septic Arthritis Managed?

Septic arthritis is best treated with a combination of surgical washout and antibiotic therapy. Antibiotic therapy alone is not recommended and leads to worse outcomes than combination treatment. The orthopaedic team should be contacted to discuss surgery.

Surgical management:

* *Initial aspiration (arthrocentesis)*
    * Rationale: This serves both as a diagnostic and therapeutic function. Arthrocentesis provides a sample for cell count, Gram stain and culture and to look for crystals. Reduction of bacterial load leads to improved response to antibiotics. Reduction in neutrophils, proteins and enzymes leads to reduction in ongoing destruction of the joint.
    * When: As soon as possible and before antibiotics are started (if no evidence of severe sepsis).
    * How often: May be repeated instead of surgical washout for smaller joints. Should be repeated until joint dry.
    * How: Percutaneously. May need ultrasound or CT guidance especially for hip joints.
* *Surgical washout (arthroscopy)*
    * Rationale: This is the treatment of choice for septic arthritis of larger joints, and for any joint when there is lack of improvement after serial aspirations.
    * As above it serves both a therapeutic and diagnostic function, especially when arthrocentesis alone fails to provide a diagnostic sample.
    * How often: May be repeated every 2–3 days as required clinically.
* *Open procedure (arthrotomy)*
    * Rationale: As above it serves both a therapeutic and diagnostic function, and is the procedure of choice for any septic joint with an implant or prosthesis. It is also used when significant debridement is required for advanced disease.

CLINICAL PEARL

- Surgery is one of the mainstays of management of septic arthritis.
- Reduction of bacterial load improves the efficacy of the antibiotic.
- Early removal of inflammatory cells, proteins and enzyme mediators reduces the damage caused by these to the surrounding cartilage, thus minimizing joint destruction.
- The surgical options depend on the affected joint, severity of disease and presence of prosthetic material.

TABLE 4.57.1
Empirical Therapy Septic Arthritis

Situation	Antibiotic	Standard Dose	Comment
No risk factors for atypical organisms	Flucloxacillin	2 g IV 6-hourly	Consider adding a second oral agent, e.g. fusidic acid
Penicillin allergic	Vancomycin or Ceftriaxone	1 g IV 12-hourly 2 g once daily	
Risk of MRSA (e.g. care home resident, previous MRSA, recent hospital stay)	Vancomycin or Clindamycin	1 g IV 12-hourly 600 mg IV 6-hourly	Consider adding a second oral agent, e.g. fusidic acid; clindamycin use only based on susceptibility of MRSA
High risk for Gram-negative infection (e.g. recent GI surgery, recurrent UTIs) or *Neisseria gonorrhoea*	Ceftriaxone	2 g once daily	

ANTIBIOTIC THERAPY

Septic arthritis is an orthopaedic emergency as delayed treatment can lead to significant loss of joint function. Antimicrobial treatment of acute septic arthritis should be started immediately after joint and blood cultures have been taken. If the patient has signs of severe sepsis, blood cultures should be taken and antibiotics started urgently, before arthrocentesis.

There are no randomized controlled trials on the treatment of septic arthritis, and meta-analyses have not identified one treatment option as being superior to others. The principle of empiric antibiotic therapy therefore remains based on covering the most likely aetiology. As *S. aureus* and streptococci are the most common pathogens, empiric regimens must cover these at the very least. If a Gram stain result is available, empiric therapy can be based on the gram. Once culture and susceptibility results are available, treatment is changed to targeted therapy.

Table 4.57.1 provides example guidance on empiric IV therapy. Each hospital will have its own guideline based on local preference and local sensitivity patterns.

The duration of treatment is typically 2 weeks of IV followed by 4 weeks or oral therapy, provided there is resolution of infection. If symptoms have not resolved or inflammatory markers have not returned to normal, further investigation is recommended.

CLINICAL PEARL

- Early treatment leads to the best response and reduces the mortality rate and risk of irreversible damage to the joint.
- Initial intravenous antibiotic therapy improves rates of cure and should be based on the likelihood of the organism involved, modified by Gram stain and culture.
- Treatment duration is a minimum of 6 weeks in total, the first 2 weeks of which is IV. Oral stepdown treatment should include antibiotics with good absorption and joint penetration.

BIBLIOGRAPHY

García-Arias M, Balsa A, Mola EM. Septic arthritis. *Best Pract Res Clin Rheumatolo.* 2011;25:407–421.

Margaretten ME, Kohlwes J, Moore D, Bent S. Does this adult patient have septic arthritis? *JAMA.* 2007 April; 297(13):1478–1488.

Matthews CJ, Weston VC, Jones A, Field M, Coakley G. Bacterial septic arthritis in adults. *Lancet.* 2010 March;375:846–855.

Sharff KA, Richards EP, Townes JM. Clinical management of septic arthritis. *Curr Rheumatol Rep.* 2013 April;15:332.

Shirtliff ME, Mader JT. Acute septic arthritis. *Clin Microbiol Rev.* 2002 October;15(4):527–544.

4.58 Septic Bursitis

Caryn Rosmarin

CLINICAL CONSIDERATIONS

Bursitis is the term used to describe inflammation of a bursa. Bursae are fluid-filled sacs lined by synovial tissue and filled with synovial fluid, located at points of friction between bone and surrounding soft tissue. Their function is to cushion and decrease friction between these surfaces during movement to allow your joints to move with ease. There are over 150 such bursae in the body and they are located both superficially (in the subcutaneous tissue) and deep (below the fascia). Commonly affected superficial sites include the olecranon, prepatellar and infrapatellar bursae. Deep sites are less affected and include the iliopsoas, popliteal and subacromial as examples. When bursitis is present, the inflamed sac impairs movement and results in local pain, tenderness and swelling. Septic, or infectious, bursitis is less common than non-septic bursitis in causing this inflammation.

HOW DOES A BURSA BECOME INFECTED?

Superficial septic bursitis develops most often following local trauma to overlying skin, with direct inoculation into the bursa. It can also occur secondary to spread of overlying cellulitis. In the absence of an iatrogenic cause (e.g.. steroid injection into a non-infectious bursitis), deep septic bursitis is less likely to be due to direct inoculation and more likely to be secondary to haematogenous spread. The risk of deposition of bacteria in a bursa is increased in those with pre-existing non-septic bursitis.

WHAT ARE THE COMMON PATHOGENS CAUSING SEPTIC BURSITIS?

Most cases of septic bursitis are monomicrobial, with *Staphylococcus aureus* being the most common pathogen. Streptococci (especially *Streptococcus pyogenes*) are the next most commonly reported. Polymicrobial infection is not uncommon, especially when related to trauma.

Gram-negative organisms and anaerobes are relatively uncommon. Unusual pathogens known to be associated with particular geographic locations or epidemiologic risk factors include *Brucella* spp., *Mycobacterium* spp. and fungi.

WHO IS AT RISK OF DEVELOPING SEPTIC BURSITIS?

Superficial septic bursitis is most often associated with an underlying repetitive trauma, which can be occupational, recreational or situational. Examples include olecranon septic bursitis in carpenters, plumbers, gymnasts and weightlifters, and prepatellar septic bursitis in gardeners, carpet layers and cleaners ('housemaids knee'). Aside from the occupational and recreational, those with underlying diabetes and excess alcohol intake seem to have an increased risk of developing septic bursitis. Pre-existing inflammatory conditions such as gout and rheumatoid arthritis, as well as having had a previous episode of bursitis, are predisposed to developing septic bursitis.

CLINICAL PEARL

- Most cases of septic bursitis are secondary to local inoculation following trauma.
- Trauma to the bursae is associated with a range of occupations, recreational and situational activities.

CLINICAL APPROACH

HOW IS SEPTIC BURSITIS DIAGNOSED?

Clinically

It is difficult to distinguish septic from non-septic bursitis. Acute, painful swelling over the bursa and surrounding erythema are classic presenting signs of superficial bursitis. Mobility of the joint should be maintained unless the swelling limits it. Inflammation may be more significant in septic than non-septic bursitis, and there might be additional cellulitis of the region. Fever may be present but its absence does not exclude the diagnosis, especially if anti-inflammatory painkillers have been used. Deep bursitis is more likely to present with pain and reduced mobility. Fever is more likely to be present as deep septic bursitis is more often due to haematogenous spread and therefore associated with a bacteraemia.

Laboratory

Definitive diagnosis of septic bursitis relies on finding evidence of bacteria in the synovial fluid. Aspiration of synovial fluid from the bursa is mandatory for establishing the diagnosis and ideally should be taken before antibiotic therapy is started. The fluid should be sent for microscopy, culture and sensitivity (M,C&S) and examined for crystals.

The synovial fluid is likely to look turbid and have a raised WCC, which is predominantly neutrophils. While this is suggestive, it is not diagnostic as this is may also be present in non-septic bursitis, such as a milky looking fluid associated with tophaceous gout. Unlike septic arthritis, there is not a predictive fluid WCC to aid diagnosis. The Gram stain has been shown to be positive in 15%–100% of cases. Culture is positive in most cases if the patient has not received antibiotics before the sample is taken. Culture negative samples in the absence of antibiotics should raise the possibility of fastidious organisms or a non-septic bursitis.

Molecular-based techniques such as polymerase chain reaction (PCR) may be useful when antibiotics are taken prior to sampling, or in culture-negative bursitis with a high index of suspicion of infection.

Blood cultures are another important diagnostic sample for deep septic bursitis, as most are haematogenously spread. They should be taken even in the absence of a fever.

Routine blood inflammatory markers (WCC, CRP, ESR) and uric acid levels should be performed even though raised levels do not distinguish infective from non-infective causes.

Radiologically

Imaging is useful to determine if the bursitis is intact, communicating with the joint, or associated with underlying disease such as osteomyelitis. It is also useful to assess soft tissue infection and look for foreign bodies. Ultrasound, CT or MRI will be beneficial in different clinical scenarios and with different joints.

CLINICAL PEARL

- Definitive diagnosis relies on finding evidence of bacteria in the synovial fluid.
- Blood cultures should be taken for deep septic bursitis.

WHAT IS THE TREATMENT FOR SEPTIC BURSITIS?

Unlike septic arthritis, the treatment of septic bursitis is often antibiotic therapy alone, without surgical intervention. Surgery is usually only necessary when the infection is not responding to antibiotics and is associated with complications of its own.

Aspiration of the bursa is required for diagnosis, but regular aspiration and washout is not routinely indicated.

There are no guidelines on the treatment of septic bursitis regarding choice of antibiotic, route of delivery or duration of treatment. The principle of therapy therefore remains based on covering the most likely aetiology, *S. aureus*. Flucloxacillin is the usual empiric choice, unless penicillin allergic or having a risk for MRSA infection, when vancomycin would be treatment of choice. Additional cover should only be provided if the Gram stain is suggestive of a non-staphylococcal or mixed infection. Once culture and susceptibility results are available, treatment is changed to targeted therapy.

Initial intravenous therapy is usually recommended, especially in those with systemic symptoms or moderate to severe inflammation or cellulitis. Some authors suggest outpatient treatment with oral antibiotics may be appropriate for those with mild disease, although this should be based on culture and sensitivity results to ensure appropriate oral agents are available; otherwise, there is a risk of recurrence. These should include antibiotics that are well absorbed and have good penetration into the bursa.

The ideal duration of treatment is not established but typically 2–3 weeks of treatment is recommended, provided symptoms resolve. If symptoms have not resolved or inflammatory markers have not returned to normal, further investigation, and possibly surgical drainage, may be required.

CLINICAL PEARL

- Antibiotics form the mainstay of treatment.
- Initial antibiotic therapy should always cover for *S. aureus*.
- Antibiotics may be delivered IV or oral depending on the severity of disease and clinical response.
- Treatment duration is not established.

BIBLIOGRAPHY

Hanrahan JA. Recent developments in septic bursitis. *Curr Infect Dis Rep.* 2013 October;15(5):421–425.

Khodaee M. Common superficial bursitis. *Am Fam Physician.* 2017;95(4):224–231.

Wasserman AR, Melville LD, Birkhahn RH. Septic bursitis: A case report and primer for the emergency clinician. *J Emerg Med.* 2009 October;37(3):269–272.

Zimmerman B, Mikolich DJ, Ho G. Septic bursitis. *Semin Arthritis Rheum.* 1995 June;24(6):391–410.

4.59 Splenectomy
From Prophylaxis to Treatment

Anda Samson

CLINICAL CONSIDERATIONS

WHO IS AT RISK?

Patients can be asplenic after a splenectomy, or be functionally asplenic/hyposplenic. In the past, haematological illnesses such as immune thrombocytopenic purpura (ITP) and malignancies were the main reason for splenectomy. Currently, the need for splenectomy is prevented wherever possible, in trauma as well as in haematological patients. Splenectomy now occurs around 30%–40% as a result of surgery after a major trauma, and 60%–70% as a result of medical reasons.

Some patients still have a spleen, but the function of their spleen is decreased or absent. This can be the case, for example, in patients with sickle cell disease, but also in patients with advanced HIV, celiac disease and some other medical conditions.

WHY IS THE SPLEEN IMPORTANT?

Although the spleen has various functions, the most important function is immunological. It removes foreign material and damaged erythrocytes and acts as storage for iron erythrocytes and platelets, the marginal zone, which is home to B cells and macrophages, and white pulp, consisting of B and T lymphocytes and follicles.

Immune functions comprise antigen presentation to T helper cells, the differentiation of B cells and stimulation of production of IgM antibodies. These IgM antibodies play a big role in the opsonization, phagocytosis and destruction of bacteria, particularly capsulated bacteria. Additionally, the spleen has a function in haemostasis.

Patients without a splenic function are therefore at a much higher risk of overwhelming infection caused by capsulated bacteria. Ideally, they are therefore protected by vaccination against pneumococci, meningococci and *Haemophilus influenzae* before the spleen is removed.

CLINICAL PEARL

Vaccinations as described below are preferably given a minimum of 2 weeks prior to splenectomy. If this is not feasible, then a minimum of 2 weeks but preferably 2–3 months postsplenectomy. This is to ensure the maximum immune response possible.

CLINICAL APPROACH

The approach to splenectomized patients starts with prevention of illness and extends to a little further thinking when they present with an infection to your practice.

PREVENTION OF 'STANDARD' INFECTIONS

Patients who undergo an elective splenectomy should receive the normal vaccinations as they are advised in the national vaccination program, as well as vaccinations against:

- *Haemophilus influenza* type B
- Pneumococci: PCV-13 pneumococcal polyvalent conjugate vaccine and PPV-23 pneumococcal polysaccharide vaccine
- Meningococci type ACWY conjugated vaccine, followed by (if not already received) meningococci type B vaccine
- Annual influenza vaccination

The vaccine formulations/combinations used in various countries varies, so it is advisable to check the national guidelines for vaccination against splenectomy to avoid over-vaccination, such as 'the green book in the UK'.

Additionally to vaccinations, patients will need a minimum of 2 years of antibiotic prophylaxis. Some guidelines advise lifelong continuous antibiotic prophylaxis. The most commonly used one is feneticilline 250 mg BD or 500 mg OD (adult doses). For patients with a penicillin allergy, alternatives could be clarithromycin/azithromycin, moxifloxacin or erythromycin.

CLINICAL PEARL

The majority of serious infections occur within the first 3 months post-splenectomy.

TRAVEL PROPHYLAXIS

Splenectomized patients travelling to tropical countries may need to take extra precautions. They are more susceptible to malaria and babesiosis with overwhelming sepsis as a consequence, so they will need to be extra careful not to be bitten by mosquitos or ticks, and will need to be vigilant with their prophylaxis. Similarly, the risk of salmonellosis, often acquired through uncooked or undercooked food, is higher in this group of patients. Stand-by antibiotics with a broader spectrum may be wise when patients plan on these travels.

TREATMENT OF INFECTIONS IN SPLENECTOMIZED PATIENTS

A patient with a splenectomy who presents with fever will always need antibiotics because of the risk of overwhelming post-splenectomy infection (OPSI). Although patients may have already taken an on-demand supply of antibiotics to start prior to seeing a doctor, they should always then go on to seek medical help, since the risk of OPSI is still increased in these patients despite adequate vaccinations and prophylactic antibiotics post-splenectomy. They need to be assessed according to the local sepsis protocols and given further antibiotic treatment if this is deemed necessary.

It is important to remember that although the above-mentioned pathogens are the usual suspects for causing infection in splenectomized patients, Gram-negative infections are also quite prevalent so always taking a careful history and physical examination is key to targeted antibiotics, whilst not forgetting about covering meningococci, *Haemophilus* and pneumococci.

CLINICAL PEARL

Avoid using the same antibiotic agents for treatment as for prophylaxis.

CLINICAL VIGNETTE

A 12-year-old boy from the Congo presents to his GP with fatigue. His GP diagnoses anaemia, and subsequent testing reveals sickle cell disease. Further investigations into his blood work shows his blood film is abnormal. The haematologist discovers Howell–Jolly bodies in the erythrocytes, and an ultrasound of the boy's abdomen shows a very small spleen. He is diagnosed as functionally asplenic and receives the appropriate vaccinations, as well as prophylactic antibiotics. Upon screening, two of his siblings also have sickle cell disease.

BIBLIOGRAPHY

Di Sabatino A, Carsetti R, Corazza GR. Post-splenectomy and hyposplenic states. *Lancet.* 2011 July 2;378(9785):86–97. Epub 2011 April 5.
HM Treasry. Immunisation of individuals with underlying medical conditions. In *The Green Book*, chapter 7. 2018. https://assets.publishing.service.gov.uk/government/uploads/system/uploads/attachment_data/file/566853/Green_Book_Chapter7.pdf.
Leone G, Pizzigallo E. Bacterial infections following splenectomy for malignant and nonmalignant hematologic diseases. *Mediterr J Hematol Infect Dis.* 2015;7(1):e2015057. Published online 2015 October 13.

4.60 The Immunocompromised Patient

Anda Samson

CLINICAL APPROACH

There are many ways of being immunocompromised, and patients may be affected in various ways. One way to assess whether or not patients are immunocompromised is to look at their lines of defence 'outside-in', starting with the skin: a first line of defence against many agents which may be overlooked, especially in patients who have been in hospital for a long time. Additionally, patients with large wounds may leak protein through those wounds and be dehydrated. Through this protein loss, important building blocks for the immune system may be lost, and the dehydration puts people at risk of infections such as urinary tract infection.

Going one layer deeper, patients undergoing chemotherapy may get severe damage to mucosal membranes, leading to predisposition to mostly Gram-negative infections and anaerobes. These organisms can translocate through inflamed mucosa and end up in the bloodstream. This is not even taking into account the damage to particular cell lineages that chemotherapy can do, but a pure physical barrier that has decreased.

Then going one virtual layer deeper again, various B and T cells can be malfunctioning, either due to genetic defects, due to HIV or other viral infections, or due to medication (mostly chemotherapy). Lastly, there can be a disruption of antibodies, complement or other signalling proteins such as TNF-alpha or interleukins.

Patients may be immunocompromised in more than one way, depending on their journey through the healthcare system, and the severity of immunosuppression may vary from period to period, for example, through adaptations in medication. Table 4.60.1 shows various ways a patient can be immunocompromised and some of the specific pathogens to be aware of. Please note that this table is far from exhaustive and is meant to help you structure your thinking around immunosuppression.

> ### CLINICAL PEARL
>
> Consider whether drug or treatment reactions can cause the picture of fever and inflammation.

CLINICAL APPROACH

When dealing with an immunocompromised patient, there are three fundamental questions that will aid in determining therapy for the patient. Often it is helpful to discuss these with the physician who is treating the patient for their underlying condition.

WHAT CAUSES THE INFECTION—AND IS THERE INFECTION AT ALL?

Immunocompromised patients may be prone to similar infections as the general population is; they may just present differently. For example, patients with a pneumonia may present hypoxic, but not with a clear infiltrate on the chest X-ray; this is because there are no leukocytes to address the

TABLE 4.60.1

Examples of Immunosuppression and Likely Pathogens

Type of Immunodeficiency	Acquired vs Lifelong	Examples	Possible Pathogens
Skin and mucosal problems is an example of first-line defence	Acquired	Chemotherapy	S. aureus
		Burn wounds	Other skin organisms
	Lifelong	Eczema, other skin conditions	
		Crohn's disease	
		IgA deficiency	
B-cell dysfunction, lymphopenia and T-cell deficiency/dysfunction are all examples of lymphocytopaenia	Acquired	Splenectomy	Capsulated bacteria
		HIV	
	Lifelong	Sickle cell disease	
		CVID	
		Specific hypoglobulinaemia	
		Hyper-IgE syndrome	
	Acquired	Overwhelming viral infection (including HIV)	Viral infections
			PCP
		Malnutrition	Fungal infection
	Lifelong	SCID	CMV, EBV
			Parasitic infection
	Acquired	Steroids	Fungal infection
		Chemotherapy	TB
		HIV	Nocardia
		Lymphoma	Cryptococcus
	Lifelong	Diabetes mellitus (uncontrolled)	
Complement deficiency is an example of Innate immunity	Acquired	Endocarditis	Capsulated bacteria, particularly
		Osteomyelitis	N. meningitidis and
		Cryoglobulinaemia	S. pneumoniae
		MPGN (C3)	
		Eculizumab therapy (C5)	
	Lifelong	Lupus (C3 & C4)	
		C-1 inhibitor deficiency (C4)	
Neutropaenia	Acquired	Chemotherapy	Fungal and yeast infection
		Bone marrow transplant	
		Alcoholism	
	Lifelong	Diabetes	
		Chronic granulomatous disease	

infection. After giving G-CSF, the patient's condition can seemingly deteriorate because of the increased inflammatory response when recruiting neutrophils.

Similarly, it is important to consider which specific pathogens or groups of pathogens a patient may be at risk of judging by the type of immunosuppression. Last but not least, consider whether a non-infectious cause such as radiation pneumonitis, or a drug reaction, can cause the clinical picture.

CAN THE PATIENT'S IMMUNE FUNCTION BE IMPROVED—PERMANENTLY OR TEMPORARILY?

In patients on immunosuppressive drugs, the level of immunosuppression can sometimes be reduced; either temporarily to allow the infection to be cleared or long term dose reduction. Similarly, some patients with neutropaenia secondary to chemotherapy need G-CSF to stimulate their bone marrow to overcome the neutropaenic phase; oncologists can usually predict the duration of neutropaenia.

CAN THE INFECTION BE CLEARED?

Some infections can be cleared, just like in non-immunosuppressed patients. The duration of treatment may need to be a bit longer and the dose of the antibiotic may need to be a bit higher, because more depends on the ability of the antibiotic to kill the bacterium and less on the immune system of the patient. In patients where the infection cannot be cleared, you can opt for suppressive therapy; for example, co-trimoxazole in patients with low CD4 cells, or ciprofloxacin in patients with neutropaenia and at risk of mucositis.

CLINICAL PEARL

When assessing an immunocompromised patient, assess whether the immunosuppression can be decreased, and how long the patient will be immunosuppressed for.

CLINICAL PEARL

Although immunosuppressed patients are vulnerable to a variety of pathogens, immunosuppression does not protect from the most common infections. They can present in atypical patterns.

CLINICAL PEARL

The immune system consists of the complex humoral and cellular immune systems, but also of the more direct barriers to pathogens: skin integrity, saliva, mucosal tissue, nutritional status and hydration status.

CLINICAL VIGNETTES

Mrs Jones is an 89-year-old woman who has been in hospital for over a month. She is on a general medical ward for analysis of general deterioration but doesn't seem to get better. She is also on prednisolone for rheumatoid giant cell arteritis. You are phoned to by the FY1 to ask what antibiotic to start her on for her 'UTI' because she has a dipstick full of leucocytes and whether or not they should stop the prednisolone. After assessment of the patient by the bedside, you conclude that the patient is immunocompromised because of her pressure ulcers (lack of skin integrity), making her vulnerable to staphylococcal infections, and Gram negatives if the pressure ulcers are on the lower back. There is also her urinary catheter, which makes her vulnerable to ascending infections, and her diabetes, which makes her more vulnerable for fungal infections, especially if dysregulated. She has lost 10 kg over the duration of her stay so is likely malnourished, leading to a variety of immune deficiencies, and lastly, she is on prednisolone. After your assessment, the catheter is removed, the pressure ulcers heal with very strict position change and with adequate nutrition, the diabetes is regulated more strictly. Mrs Jones slowly improves and is able to go home after another month.

- Often elderly patients are immunocompromised by a variety of invasive and less-invasive iatrogenic factors.
- Optimizing nutrition, skin care and removal of foreign bodies can result in improvement.

You are phoned about a patient with a renal transplant who is on prednisolone, cyclosporine and mycofenolate. They have a pneumonia but the SHO that phones says that otherwise they seem quite well; they are treating as a normal CAP and have remembered that clarithromycin and erythromycin interact with the immunosuppressives. The patient is not getting better though. After probing, the patient has a mild headache too. You advise blood cultures, an LP and a cryptococcal antigen. You also advise to do cyclosporine levels and consider lowering prednisolone doses. All blood cultures, as well as the CSF, show Cryptococcus neoformans, *and the cryptococcal antigen is 1:512.*

- Non-HIV-infected, immunocompromised patients often show a lower burden of cryptococcosis and lower numbers of CNS infection; conversely, it often gets missed.
- Think about mild presentations of symptoms that may trigger further investigations.

BIBLIOGRAPHY

Bratton EW, El Husseini N, Chastain CA, Lee MS, Poole C, Stürmer T, Juliano JJ, Weber DJ, Perfect JR. Comparison and temporal trends of three groups with cryptococcosis: HIV-infected, solid organ transplant, and HIV-negative/non-transplant. *PLOS ONE.* 2012;7(8):e43582.Epub 2012 August 24.

Brizendine KD, Baddley JW, Pappas PG. Predictors of mortality and differences in clinical features among patients with cryptococcosis according to immune status. *PLOS ONE.* 2013;8(3):e60431. Epub 2013 March 26.

George MP, Masur H, Norris KA, Palmer SM, Clancy CJ, McDyer JF. Infections in the immunosuppressed host. *Ann Am Thorac Soc.* 2014 August;11(Supplement 4):S211–e4S220.

In: Bennett JE, Dolin R, Blaser MJ (eds). *Mandell, Douglas, and Bennett's Principles and Practice of Infectious Diseases.* Philadelphia, PA: Elsevier/Saunders, 2015.

Viscoli C, Varnier O, Machetti M. Infections in patients with febrile neutropenia: Epidemiology, microbiology, and risk stratification. *Clin Infect Dis.* 2005 April 1;40(Suppl 4):S240–S245.

4.61 Typhoid Fever

Julian Anthony Rycroft and Marina Basarab

CLINICAL CONSIDERATIONS

THE IMPORTANCE OF A GOOD TRAVEL HISTORY

Typhoid fever is the most likely diagnosis underlying a fever in a traveller returned from South Asia in whom malaria has been excluded. Typhoid fever, or enteric fever, is more common in children and young adults than older adults, and it is ubiquitous in Latin America, sub-Saharan Africa, South Asia and Southeast Asia. Although normally associated with poor sanitation in lower income countries, transmission from contact with an index case has been reported in the absence of travel to an endemic area. Other risk factors include consuming food from street vendors, sharing kitchen utensils and poor hand hygiene.

Although prior vaccination is recommended, the vaccine is not completely effective, and the diagnosis should not be excluded on the basis of a positive vaccination history—particularly given the vaccine is ineffective against strains lacking the Vi antigen (i.e. most Paratyphi strains). Other diagnoses to consider include malaria, dengue fever, leptospirosis, amoebiasis and Q fever.

DIAGNOSIS OF TYPHOID FEVER

Clinical features develop 5–21 days following exposure to contaminated food or water. *Salmonella* spp. invade the gut epithelium and then the lymphoid tissue in the intestinal mucosa. They are professional intracellular pathogens that are able to actively mediate entry into host cells as well as exploit phagocytic mechanisms, resulting in passive uptake. Once internalized, the pathogen manipulates host-cell function, which is associated with subsequent haematogenous dissemination of infection.

Presentation is indolent and non-specific, and is characterized by fever which gradually increases over days before presentation. Change in bowel habit is not a consistent feature—patients variably report diarrhoea, constipation or no change. Although classically typhoid fever presents with the 'rose spot' rash, these are present in less than one-third of cases and are difficult to identify on patients with dark skin.

CLINICAL PEARL

Signs and symptoms of typhoid fever:

- Fever and chills (classically no rigours)
- Dull headache
- Abdominal pain, anorexia and nausea
- Dry cough
- Myalgia
- Travel to an endemic area

TABLE 4.61.1

Practical 'In-House' Differential Serotyping of Most Common Isolates of *Salmonella enterica*

	O Antigen	H1 Antigen	H2 Antigen
S. Paratyphi A	2	a	0
S. Paratyphi B	1, 4	b	1, 2
S. Paratyphi C*	6, 7	c	1, 5
S. Typhi*	9	d	0
S. Enteritidis	1, 9	g, m	0
S. Typhimurium	1, 4	i	1, 2

* Indicates pathogenic strains carrying the capsular Vi 'K' antigen.

On assessment, the patient will be febrile with a heart rate not consistent with the temperature (relative bradycardia). While leucocytosis is common in children, leucopenia is more often the case in adults; leucocytosis in adults should raise the concern of perforation.

The cornerstone of diagnosis is blood culture. Serological testing is not useful in endemic areas where many individuals may test positive because of previous infection. Although demonstrating a fourfold increase in antibody titres can aid diagnosis, this will only make the diagnosis retrospectively—decisions regarding treatment will need to have been made ahead of this. Bacterial burden is often low in the bloodstream, so a large volume of blood will improve the sensitivity (usually 50%–70%). Stool culture has an even lower sensitivity (30%–40%) and is not helpful as a routine test in the absence of any diarrhoea. Bone marrow culture is the gold standard but is rarely necessary for diagnosis.

CLINICAL APPROACH

HANDLING THE ORGANISM

Enteric fever is most commonly associated with infection with *Salmonella enterica* serotype Typhi (*S.* Typhi), although infection with *S.* Paratyphi (A, B or C) and *S.* Choleraesuis also cause the clinical syndrome (see Table 4.61.1. for common serotypes). Typhoidal serotypes of *Salmonella* are restricted to human hosts; no animal reservoir has been found.

The identification of a Gram-negative organism in the context of this history should prompt discussion with the laboratory. *Salmonella* Typhi is a hazard-group 3 organism, which laboratory staff should suspect upon receipt of a sample which appropriately specifies the patient's travel history. Once isolated, the organism can be identified by MALDI-ToF or biochemical profile and also provisionally serotyped pending confirmation by a reference laboratory. An azithromycin MIC should be performed; an MIC ≤16 mcg/mL is considered susceptible.

MANAGEMENT

Typhoid fever usually requires single-agent therapy. Depending on local resistance patterns, oral azithromycin (5–7 days), oral ciprofloxacin (7–10 days) or intravenous ceftriaxone (10–14 days) are options. Parenteral therapy should be initially used where infection is severe or complications are present—here, corticosteroids (dexamethasone 3 mg/kg followed by 1 mg/kg every 6 hours for 48 hours) can be considered in addition to antimicrobials. The clinical diagnosis of typhoid fever should be notified to the relevant public health authority.

CLINICAL VIGNETTE

You are called in the middle of the night by the resident medical officer. The patient is on day 4 of azithromycin. He continues to spike high-grade temperatures, although does not mount a tachycardia and maintains his blood pressure. The patient reports no new symptoms, and there are no new clinical signs, although his abdomen remains somewhat tender.

It is tempting to become concerned that the patient is failing oral azithromycin. Although in house sensitivities for the isolate should have come back by now to reassure the microbiologist that this is not the case, it is possible this information might not yet be available. The most likely cause for this midnight call is the protracted time of recovery for typhoid fever—mean time to defervescence is 4–6 days and does not imply treatment failure.

Drug resistance continues to be a concern, however. Multidrug-resistant strains of *S.* Typhi and Paratyphi account for the majority of cases in Bangladesh and parts of Southeast Asia—as a result, ampicillin, cotrimoxazole and chloramphenicol are no longer recommended. While resistance to fluoroquinolones is an increasing problem, most isolates remain susceptible to azithromycin and ceftriaxone. Resistance to the latter, however, results from infection with ESBL-producing isolates. Where extensively drug-resistant (XDR) isolates emerge, carbapenems are recommended, if azithromycin cannot be used.

The following night, the same resident medical officer calls. The patient is spiking again, but this time is hypotensive (78/58 mmHg), tachycardic (110 bpm) and he is guarding his right iliac fossa.

Ileal perforation is a late complication of typhoid fever and should be suspected in the patient with a surgical abdomen and leucocytosis. The patient should be fluid resuscitated, and an urgent surgical opinion sought.

CLINICAL PEARL

Complications of typhoid fever:

- Hepatosplenomegaly
- Gastrointestinal bleeding
- Intestinal perforation (usually terminal ileum) with peritonitis
- Metastatic seeding of infection (e.g. osteomyelitis, meningitis, mycotic aneurysms)
- Typhoid encephalopathy
- Overwhelming sepsis, multiorgan failure and death
- Relapse of infection (10%)
- Chronic carriage (4%)

The patient returns to see his GP 6 weeks following completion of treatment, as he suffers a bout of watery diarrhoea. The GP sends a stool sample, from which S. *Typhi is isolated. You contact the GP, who reports that the patient's symptoms have since resolved.*

Although there is persistent shedding of the organism in this patient's stools, excretion beyond 12 months is required to be deemed chronic carriage. Chronic carriage is not associated with relapse of infection, and hosts demonstrate high antibody titres. Risk factors for chronic carriage include female sex and biliary tract abnormalities—and chronicity has been associated with malignancy, especially in the gallbladder. Treatment with ciprofloxacin 750 mg BD for 4 weeks eradicates carriage in over 90% of cases.

BIBLIOGRAPHY

Azmatullah A, Qamar FN, Thaver D, Zaidi AK, Bhutta ZA. Systematic review of the global epidemiology, clinical and laboratory profile of enteric fever. *J Glob Health*. 2015;5(2):020407.
Basnyat B et al. Enteric (typhoid) fever in travelers. *Clin Infect Dis*. 2005;41:1467–1472.
Connor BA, Schwartz E. Typhoid and paratyphoid fever in travellers. *Lancet Infect Dis*. 2005;5:623–628.
Wain J et al. Typhoid fever. *Lancet*. 2015;385:1136–1145.

4.62 Urinary Tract Infections

Firza Alexander Gronthoud

CLINICAL CONSIDERATIONS

Almost half of women will develop a urinary tract infection (UTI) at least once during their lifetime. Urinary tract infections are increasingly being caused by multidrug-resistant organisms. Increasing complex urological procedures are performed more frequently, leading to an increased rate of complicated urinary tract infections with altered urological anatomy. Advancements in molecular tools have shown that the urinary tract is not sterile and, like the gut, has its own microbiome that may potentially be influenced by antibiotic use.

Treatment of urinary tract infections has become more challenging, and misdiagnosis and inadequate antibiotic treatment are major contributors to antibiotic consumption and antimicrobial resistance. It is therefore worthwhile to consider the following.

Urinary tract infections are categorized based on:

- Upper or lower urinary tract infection (pyelonephritis versus cystitis)
- Presence of factors that influences management of the UTI (complicated versus uncomplicated UTI)

COMPLICATED URINARY TRACT INFECTION

- Complicated UTI is defined as indwelling catheter, recent urinary instrumentation, urinary stones, prostatic obstruction, diabetes, immunosuppression, pregnancy, functional or anatomical urological abnormality.
- These factors interfere with urinary flow, causing urine stasis, accumulation of bacteria and increased risk of infection.

CATHETER-ASSOCIATED URINARY TRACT INFECTION (CAUTI)

- CAUTI is the most common nosocomial infection.
- Patients with indwelling urinary catheters are a major reservoir of antimicrobial-resistant uropathogens in healthcare settings.
- Patients with indwelling urinary catheters are often exposed to antibiotics and are at risk of cross-transmission of multidrug-resistant pathogens.
- Catheterized patients are vulnerable to both symptomatic CAUTI and long-term colonization.
- After colonization, a biofilm is formed on the catheter protecting the bacteria against the immune system and antimicrobials.
- Treatment of CAUTI is only indicated if systemic signs of infection are present in the absence of other causes of infection.
- *Pseudomonas aeruginosa* and enterococci are more often seen in CAUTI.
- The presence of pyuria or malodorous urine alone is not a reason for treatment.
- Treating of CAUTI without catheter removal will result in selection of more-resistant organisms.

CLINICAL PEARL

Renal colic can mimic urosepsis:

- Very severe cramping pain resulting from distension of the ureter and pelvis above an obstruction such as a renal stone.
- Often accompanied by frequency, urgency and haematuria.
- Hypertension and tachycardia often present as a result of the severe pain.
- Presence of hypotension should raise suspicion of infection.
- Co-presence of a lower urinary tract infection increases risk of pyelonephritis and/or pyonephrosis.

SYMPTOMS

Diagnosis of a UTI is a clinical diagnosis and supported by clinical, microbiological and radiological findings:

- Symptoms compatible with cystitis: Urgency, dysuria, suprapubic pain, confusion
- Symptoms compatible with pyelonephritis: Fever, rigors, loin pain
- Lower UTI symptoms may be present or absent
- Radiological findings: Dilated ureters, hydronephrosis, stones, renal abscess
- Up to 30%–40% of patients diagnosed with a urinary tract infection may not have an UTI
- There is less likely to be an UTI if there are signs and symptoms compatible with other organ involvement (i.e. dyspnoea, cough or skin lesions)

UROPATHOGENS

- Uropathogenic *E. coli* (UPEC) cause the majority of urinary tract infections.
- After invasion of bladder epithelial cells, UPEC can persist intracellularly and evade host defences and may serve as a reservoir for persistent or recurrent infections.
- *Proteus mirabilis*, *Pseudomonas aeruginosa*, and *Enterococcus* spp. predominantly cause complicated infections and are more commonly isolated in hospitals and long-term care facilities. *Corynebacterium urealyticum* is an important nosocomial uropathogen associated with indwelling catheters. *Staphylococcus saprophyticus* tends to cause infection in young women who are sexually active.
- *Proteus* spp. hydrolyzes urea to ammonium, raising urine pH to neutral or alkaline values, potentiating crystallization of struvite (magnesium ammonium phosphate), which can lead to struvite stones.
- *Candida* spp. in urine usually represent colonization. They may cause UTIs in patients with indwelling catheters who are receiving antibiotic therapy or in immunocompromised individuals (see Chapter 4.12).

URETHRITIS

In men, urethritis is commonly caused by sexually transmitted diseases and is associated with urethral discharge. The main organisms responsible are: *Neisseria gonorrhoeae* (gonococcal urethritis), *Chlamydia trachomatis* and *Mycoplasma genitalium*.

COMPLICATIONS OF UTI

Renal abscesses are localised in the renal cortex and may occur as a result of bacteraemia. Pyuria may also be present, but urine culture is usually negative. Renal abscesses are increasingly being seen as complications of acute pyelonephritis caused by Gram-negative bacilli. The rare condition of emphysematous pyelonephritis, which results in multifocal intrarenal abscesses and gas formation within the renal parenchyma, is usually seen in diabetic patients or as a complication of renal stones. *Escherichia coli* is the commonest cause. (See Table 4.62.1.)

DIPSTICK

- In women with uncomplicated urinary infection, the highest positive predictive value for strip testing was for having nitrite alone or nitrite with either positive leucocyte esterase or blood.
- A positive urine culture or dipstick test will not differentiate between UTI and asymptomatic bacteriuria.
- Patients with asymptomatic bacteriuria may have white blood cells in the urine just as in true infection. In older patients, including those with dementia, diagnosis should be based on a full clinical assessment, including vital signs.

CLINICAL PEARL

Pyuria without apparent bacteriuria (i.e. no growth on routine culture media) may be the result of many factors: as a result of prior treatment with antimicrobial agents, catheterization, calculi (stones), bladder neoplasms, genital tract infection, sexually transmitted diseases (e.g. *C. trachomatis*) or an infection with a fastidious organism.

- Bacteriuria without apparent pyuria may be due to the lysis of the white blood cells in alkaline urine, which occurs in infection with *Proteus* spp.
- Renal tuberculosis may also be implicated in sterile pyuria but is uncommon, although should be considered if clinically indicated (e.g. in high-risk populations).

RISK FACTORS FOR UTI

- *Dehydration*: It is now well accepted that dehydration is a major risk factor. *E. coli* bacteraemias typically peak during summer months. By far, the most common source of *E. coli* bacteraemias is the urinary tract.
- *Indwelling catheter*: Intermittent catheterization is associated with a lower incidence of asymptomatic bacteriuria than long-term catheterization.

TABLE 4.62.1

Complications of Urinary Tract Infections

Chronic pyelonephritis (chronic interstitial nephritis, or reflux nephropathy): Controversy exists over the definition and cause of this syndrome. It is the second most common cause of end-stage renal failure. It is thought to be a result of renal damage caused by UTI in infants and children with vesicoureteric reflux, or by obstructive uropathy in adults. However, it is still unclear whether recurrent infection causes progressive kidney damage.

Perinephric abscess: A complication of UTI, although uncommon, that affects patients with one or more anatomical or physiological abnormalities. The abscess may be confined to the perinephric space or extend into adjacent structures. Pyuria, with or without positive culture, is seen on examination of urine, but is not always present.

Causative organisms are usually Gram-negative bacilli, but can also be staphylococci or *Candida* species. Mixed infections have also been reported.

Risk Factors for Multidrug-Resistant UTI

Risk factors include recurrent UTI, urinary catheterization, persistent urinary symptoms after an initial antibiotic, recent hospital admissions in the past 6 months, residence in a care home, recent travel and especially healthcare in a country with increased antimicrobial resistance, previously known UTI (within 1 year) caused by bacteria resistant to amoxicillin/clavulanate, cephalosporins or quinolone or recent treatment with these agents.

Cystitis in Patients with Different Urinary Anatomy

- Fistula gut to bladder
- Ileostomy

Uncommon Manifestations of UTI

- *Staphylococcus aureus* bacteraemia can lead to septic emboli to the kidneys, causing suppurative necrosis or abscess formation within the renal parenchyma. In contrast, Gram-negative bacilli rarely cause kidney infection by the hematogenous route.
- In severe cases of pyelonephritis, the affected kidney may be enlarged, with raised abscesses on the surface.

Oral Treatment for Uncomplicated Lower Urinary Tract Infection Caused by MDRO

- ESBL-producing bacteria are generally resistant to trimethoprim, ciprofloxacin, amoxicillin and cephalosporins; susceptibility to amoxicillin/clavulanate is variable.
- Resistance rates to nitrofurantoin and fosfomycin remain low.
- Regardless of ESBL production, trimethoprim resistance is common.
- Pivmecillinam (the oral form of mecillinam) can be considered alone as oral therapy for lower UTI caused by AmpC-producing *Enterobacterales*.
- Consider increasing the dose of pivmecillinam to 400 mg three times daily when treating ESBL producers as treatment failure has been documented with the standard dose (especially CTX-M-15-type ESBL).
- CTX-M-15 producers may also co-produce OXA-1, which is a penicillinase not inhibited by clavulanic acid. In this case, if no other options available, consider combination of amoxicillin/clavulanic acid 625 mg 8-hourly PO with pivmecillinam 400 mg 8-hourly PO.
- Synergy *in vitro* between cephalosporins and mecillinam because of their different target penicillin-binding proteins is likely, and synergy of cephalexin with fosfomycin is also recorded.
- For treatment of multi-drug resistant UTI including ESBLs, a seven day course is recommended as it is associated with a higher bacteriological cure rate and possibly lower rate of persistence or relapse.

Prophylaxis for Recurrent Urinary Tract Infections

- Recurrent UTI is defined as three symptomatic UTIs within 12 months or two symptomatic episodes within 6 months following clinical resolution of a previous UTI.
- Deciding whether or not to give prophylaxis is a balance between the benefits of reducing symptomatic relapse and pyelonephritis versus side effects and the risks of selecting antibiotic resistance.
- Post-coital antibiotics are equally effective as nightly prophylaxis.

- If recurrence is not too frequent: consider standby nitrofurantoin, to take as soon as symptoms occur.
- UTIs breaking through prophylaxis in recurrent infection are usually due to strains that remain susceptible, unlike the situation with trimethoprim.
- Change to a different prophylaxis based on previous urine cultures if multiple breakthroughs with a resistant strain has occurred.
- Prophylaxis with β-lactam antibiotics including cefalexin selects for resistant *Enterobacterales* in the fecal flora and is not recommended.
- Patients on prophylaxis for >6 months should be reviewed.
- Prophylaxis, if used, can usually be stopped after a year without a resumption of the recurrences, and there are now European guidelines that this review should be made at 6 months.

CLINICAL APPROACH

- Classify UTI as uncomplicated cystitis, uncomplicated pyelonephritis or complicated UTI.
- Identify the presence of a catheter, nephrostomy, stent or stones.
- Consider ultrasound urinary tract for complicated UTI.
- For uncomplicated cystitis, consider holding of antibiotics as 25%–42% of women with uncomplicated cystitis achieve clinical cure without antibiotic treatment.

Diagnosing UTI in the Elderly

- A dipstick should only be used to exclude an UTI.
- If no history can be taken, then at least three of the following symptoms should be present: dysuria, urgency, frequency, or suprapubic tenderness in combination with fever/leukocytosis AND a positive urine culture and the absence of another possible cause of infection.
- Asymptomatic bacteriuria is common in older people.

Uncomplicated Cystitis

- Nitrofurantoin 100 mg 12-hourly PO for 3 days OR
- Trimethoprim or trimethoprim/sulfamethoxazole 960 mg 12-hourly for 3 days OR
- Fosfomycin trometamol single dose 3 g OR
- Pivmecillinam 200 mg PO 8-hourly for 5 days
- Consider 7-day course for men

Oral treatment of uncomplicated cystitis caused by multidrug-resistant Gram-negative *Enterobacterales* (resistant to at least three different antibiotic classes):

- First-line options are fosfomycin trometamol 3 g PO with repeat dose on day 3 OR high dose pivmecillinam 400 mg 8-hourly for 7 days OR co-amoxiclav 625 mg 8-hourly for 7 days.
- Alternative options:
  - Oral third-generation cephalosporins: Cefixime or ceftibuten if strain is NOT producing ESBL or AmpC.
  - Oral ciprofloxacin 500 mg PO 12-hourly.
  - Consider combination of co-amoxiclav 625 mg PO 8-hourly with pivmecillinam 400 mg PO 8-hourly if significant proportion of ESBLs are CTX-M-15 type.

- Cautions:
  - If nitrofurantoin is the only oral option but the eGFR of 30–44 mL/min/1.73 m^2, a short course (3–7 days) may be used with caution.
  - Some ESBL CTX-M-15 strains co-produce OXA-1, which is not inhibited by clavulanic acid. OXA-1 has no effect on pivmecillinam, however pivmecillinam 200 mg 8-hourly PO is inadequate against CTX-M-15. Pivmecillinam at 400 mg 8-hourly PO may be more effective, in combination with amoxicillin/clavulanic acid 625 mg 8-hourly.
- Consider doxycycline 100 mg PO 12-hourly. Only CLSI has breakpoints for tetracyclines and *Enterobacterales*, with an MIC of ≤4 mg/L considered sensitive.

Oral treatment of uncomplicated cystitis caused by *Pseudomonas aeruginosa* resistant to ciprofloxacin

- If the fosfomycin MIC ≤64 mg/L: fosfomycin may be used with caution. There is no official clinical or epidemiological MIC cut-off. Most wild-type *P. aeruginosa* isolates have an MIC ≤64 mg/L.
- If the patient is to be discharged home from acute healthcare setting, then strongly consider an aminoglycoside IV stat dose.

CLINICAL PEARL

Due to toxicological properties of quinolones, risk of *C. difficile*, increasing resistance among uropathogens and risk of selecting ESBL and CPO, quinolones should no longer be a first-line treatment option for uncomplicated cystitis.

TREATMENT OF UNCOMPLICATED PYELONEPHRITIS

- Amoxicillin/clavulanic acid 625 mg PO 8-hourly 7–10 days OR
- Ciprofloxacin 500 mg PO 12-hourly 7 days

TREATMENT OF COMPLICATED UTI INCLUDING CAUTI

- Send a urine and two blood culture sets for culture and susceptibility testing before empirical treatment and review when culture results come back.
- Inpatient management:
  - Amoxicillin/clavulanic 1.2 g IV 6–8-hourly+ gentamicin 5 mg/kg IV once daily OR
  - Piperacillin/tazobactam 4.5 g 8-hourly OR
  - If risk for MDRO UTI: Either temocillin 200 mg IV 12-hourly OR meropenem 1 g IV 8-hourly
  - Consider adding vancomycin IV if CAUTI
  - Review with culture results
- Outpatient management: either amoxicillin/clavulanic acid 625 mg 8 hourly PO for 7–10 days OR ciprofloxacin 500 mg PO 12-hourly for 7 days OR trimethoprim/sulfamethoxazole 960 mg PO 12-hourly for 14 days
  - Note: Avoid trimethoprim/sulfamethoxazole if local resistance exceeds 20% or if this antibiotic has been administered to the patient in the previous 3 months.
  - Add single dose of ceftriaxone 2 g IV OD or an aminoglycoside.
  - If no signs of upper tract involvement, alternatively consider fosfomycin trometamol 3 g PO on days 1 and 3 OR pivmecillinam 200 mg PO 8-hourly for 7 days.
  - The role of fosfomycin or pivmecillinam for pyelonephritis is unclear.

- Consider ultrasound urinary tract if recurrent urinary tract infection or inadequate treatment response despite *in vitro* susceptibility.
- If urogenital abnormalities present, extend duration of treatment beyond 7 days.
- If catheter *in situ*, remove or change catheter.
- Catheters impregnated with antiseptics or antimicrobials have shown limited protection against CAUTI. Similarly, antiseptic irrigation of the catheterized bladder, antiseptic lubricants or topical therapies for meatal care have not been found to be effective.
- Discuss changing/removing nephrostomy or ureteric stents with urology.

OUTPATIENT ANTIBIOTIC TREATMENT OF COMPLICATED UTI WITH NO ORAL OPTIONS

- Ceftriaxone 2 g IV once daily.
- If lower urinary tract infection caused by ESBL producer and ceftriaxone MIC $\leq$1 mg/L: ceftriaxone 2 or 4 g IV once daily with caution. Alternative options are ertapenem 1 g IV once daily or an aminoglycoside IV once daily with therapeutic drug monitoring.
- *Pseudomonas aeruginosa* resistant to ciprofloxacin: Aminoglycoside IV once daily with therapeutic drug monitoring.

TREATMENT OF ASYMPTOMATIC BACTERIURIA

- Pregnant women and individuals soon to undergo urologic surgery, who benefit from antibiotic treatment of asymptomatic bacteriuria.
- Do not prescribe antibiotics in ASB in the elderly with or without an indwelling catheter.
- Avoid antibiotic prophylaxis for urinary catheter insertion or changes unless there is previous history of symptomatic UTI with the procedure, insertion of incontinence implant or trauma at catheterization.

PROPHYLAXIS

- Prophylactic antibiotics given at catheter change or insertion is not indicated unless:
  - History of symptomatic UTI after catheter change.
  - Traumatic catheterization (frank haematuria after catheterization or two or more attempts of catheterization).
  - Placement of an incontinence implant.
- Antibiotic choices: Nitrofurantoin 50–100 mg once daily, dose to be taken at night or trimethoprim 100 mg once daily, dose to be taken at night OR fosfomycin trometamol 3 g twice weekly.
- Long-term antibiotic prophylaxis for vesicovaginal or colovesical fistula is not indicated.

BIBLIOGRAPHY

Hawkey PM, Warren RE, Livermore DM, McNulty CAM, Enoch DA, Otter JA, Wilson APR. Treatment of infections caused by multidrug-resistant Gram-negative bacteria: Report of the British Society for Antimicrobial Chemotherapy/ Healthcare Infection Society/British Infection Association Joint Working Party. *J Antimicrob Chemother.* 2018 March 1;73(suppl_3).

Ninan S, Walton C, Barlow G. Investigation of suspected urinary tract infection in older people. *BMJ.* 2014 July 3;349:g4070.

Novelli A, Rosi E. Pharmacological properties of oral antibiotics for the treatment of uncomplicated urinary tract infections. *J Chemother.* 2017 December;29(sup1):10–18.

Zowawi HM, Harris PN, Roberts MJ, Tambyah PA, Schembri MA, Pezzani MD, Williamson DA, Paterson DL. The emerging threat of multidrug-resistant Gram-negative bacteria in urology. *Nat Rev Urol.* 2015 October;12(10):570–584.

4.63 Uveitis

Anda Samson

CLINICAL CONSIDERATIONS

Uveitis is a relatively common clinical presentation that is usually inflammatory in origin. It is an inflammation of the iris, ciliary body, choroid and retina and can be categorized anatomically (see Table 4.63.1). Overall, the aetiology is infectious only in about 20% of uveitis cases; however, the frequency of infection varies a lot depending on the location.

Granulomatous versus non-granulomatous uveitis refers to the presence or absence of clumps of white blood cells seen with slit lamp review rather than granulomas seen on pathology. The granulomatous forms of uveitis are more commonly infectious in nature, although, and the non-granulomatous forms are more often autoimmune.

CLINICAL APPROACH

DIAGNOSIS OF UVEITIS

Because uveitis is a descriptive diagnosis, the aetiology will have to be achieved through careful history taking, physical examination for other signs of (systemic) diseases and, where necessary, additional laboratory and imaging diagnostics. Collaboration with other specialists is paramount. When deciding on additional tests for infectious causes, the ophthalmic evaluation will then help to make a shift in deciding which diagnostic tests to choose.

Infection-related history will need to include travel history and exposure to TB, animal contact, sexual history and the state of the patient's immune system. If possible, a full rheumatological review needs to take place to assess for these causes as well since the majority of cases will have other causes than infection. A chest X-ray is useful to rule out any remnants of old or current TB infection and to look for signs of sarcoidosis.

LABORATORY DIAGNOSIS IN UVEITIS PATIENTS

General broad laboratory diagnostics such as inflammatory markers and kidney and liver markers, as well as possibly a serum ACE, are particularly useful in finding clues for non-infectious causes of uveitis. Syphilis serology is indicated in all patients with uveitis, and because of its frequency, *Toxoplasma* serology may be helpful.

Diagnosing ocular TB can be difficult; a diagnosis is usually made by a combination of clinical probability and the clinical pattern fitting with TB. Intra-ocular culture yield is low because of the pauci-bacillary nature of TB so a combination of history, chest X-ray and clinical symptoms and exclusion of other causes is essential.

VITREOUS/AQUEOUS SAMPLES

A vitreous sample is important if lymphoma or other malignancies are in the differential diagnosis. PCR on these samples are quite useful in case of HSV, VZV, CMV and EBV, as well as *Toxoplasma* infections. The Goldmann–Witmer coefficient is the anti-*Toxoplasma* IgG/total IgG in aqueous fluid divided by anti-*Toxoplasma* IgG/total IgG in serum.

In the case of chronic uveitis not responding, further bacterial PCR on vitrious fluid can be considered when thinking about, for example, *Mycobacterium tuberculosis*, *Tropheryma whipplei*,

TABLE 4.63.1

Classification and Aetiology of Uveitis

Anatomical Category Aetiology	Anterior Uveitis	Intermediate Uveitis	Posterior Uveitis	Panuveitis
Infectious (20%)	10%–15% herpetic, (90% of cases within the infection group) syphilis, TB, **Rare:** Lyme, Leprosy Chikungunya Brucella	Most infectious causes can also cause intermediate uveitis	50% *Toxoplasma* (25%–40%) *Toxocara* *Candida* Syphilis Acute retinal necrosis (HSV, VZV, CMV) **Rare:** Chikungunya *Brucella* Histoplasmosis West Nile virus *Bartonella henselae* Lyme	10% TB Syphilis *Candida* *Toxocara* **Rare:** Leptospirosis *Brucella* Whipple's Lyme
Autoimmune & idiopathic 80%	85% seronegative arthropathies, human leukocyte antigen (HLA)-B27-associated disease, reactive arthritis, and juvenile rheumatoid arthritis medication-related	N/A	50% lupus erythematosus, sarcoidosis, and birdshot retinochoroidopathy, (8% each) Medication-related	90% wide differential diagnosis
Malignant <1%	<1%	<1%	<1%	<1%

Bartonella henselae or *Coxiella burnettii*. These PCRs are not very sensitive, though, and a negative PCR does not rule out infection.

CLINICAL PEARL

PCR of vitreous fluid can be false negative.

TREATMENT

Treatment of uveitis depends on the underlying condition. If an infectious diagnosis is not confirmed but cannot be ruled out, empirical therapy is sometimes needed, especially in the light of immunosuppressive co-medication that is often indicated to suppress the inflammatory process and subsequent scarring.

CLINICAL PEARL

The decision to treat often needs to be made on grounds of the clinical picture; the treatment response therefore needs careful monitoring.

TREATMENT FOR SOME COMMONLY SEEN INFECTIOUS CAUSES OF UVEITIS

Herpetic uveitis is treated with oral acyclovir or valacyclovir, and topical steroids. Prophylactic acyclovir may be considered post-treatment to keep recurrence at bay. In patients with acute retinal necrosis, though, immediate intravenous acyclovir should be given, with gancyclovir if the patient is immunocompromised. Intravitreal therapy such as foscarnet is an option in severe cases.

If syphilis is the cause of the uveitis, it should be treated as a case of neurosyphilis and treated with IV benzylpenicillin or ceftriaxone for 14 days. It is important to give concurrent systemic corticosteroids to decrease the inflammation and prevent a Harisch–Herxheimer reaction. Neurosyphilis should be ruled out by lumbar puncture, and like with all cases of syphilis, further testing for presence of other sexually transmitted diseases including an HIV test is indicated.

Tuberculosis is treated the same as any other case of TB, although ethambutol should be avoided to minimize further risk of ocular damage. A short course of oral corticosteroids may be added.

In case of ocular toxoplasmosis, not every case warrants treatment, but in severe cases, pyrimethamine with sulfadiazine and leucovorin for 46 weeks is indicated.

CLINICAL PEARL

Acute retinal necrosis is an emergency and warrants immediate IV treatment for HSV/VZV, and against CMV in immunocompromised patients. Suppressive therapy should be considered post-treatment.

CLINICAL VIGNETTES

A 75-year-old man is referred from the eye hospital to your service with the request 'to rule out an infectious cause of his pan uveitis. He has served in the army as a medic for many decades and was deployed all over the world; TB exposure is likely. He has never been tested for it. A chest X-ray reveals a Gohn sign in his right upper lobe, and an interferon gamma release assay test is positive. He is not coughing, so no sputum samples can be obtained. Empirical ocular TB treatment is started with rifampicin, pyrazinamide and isoniazid, as well as steroids.

A 24-year-old man presents to the ophthalmologist with sudden loss of vision in his right eye with some concomitant pain and photophobia. Fundoscopic examination shows some areas of acute retinitis. He is admitted and a sample from the vitreous fluid is sent to the laboratory for immediate PCR for Herpes simplex. He is immediately started on high-dose steroids and IV acyclovir as well as intravitreous foscarnet. His vision then stabilizes and the pain disappears slowly. Post-discharge he is continued on oral acyclovir as suppressive therapy.

BIBLIOGRAPHY

In: Bennett JE, Dolin R, Blaser MJ (eds). *Mandell, Douglas, and Bennett's Principles and Practice of Infectious Diseases*. Philadelphia, PA: Elsevier/Saunders, 2015.

Ng KK, Nisbet M, Damato EM, Sims JL. Presumed tuberculous uveitis in non-endemic country for tuberculosis: Case series from a New Zealand tertiary uveitis clinic. *Clin Exp Ophthalmol.* 2017;45(4):357–365.

Sève P, Cacoub P, Bodaghi B et al. Uveitis: Diagnostic work-up. A literature review and recommendations from an expert committee. *Autoimmun Rev.* 2017;16(12):1254–1264.

4.64 Varicella Zoster

Firza Alexander Gronthoud

CLINICAL CONSIDERATIONS

Chickenpox occurs most commonly during childhood, and over 90% of adults are already protected. Chickenpox is less common in tropical and subtropical climates, and a significant proportion of individuals raised in these areas may be susceptible to primary infection in adulthood. In the developed world, individuals at risk for complications of chickenpox are immunocompromised individuals, pregnant women and neonates. It is therefore worthwhile to consider the following.

CHICKENPOX

Varicella zoster virus (VZV) is a DNA virus and one of the human herpes viruses. Primary infection causes varicella (chickenpox). The virus is not cleared from the body but remains latent, present in the dorsal root and/or cranial nerve ganglia. Symptoms of varicella are fever, flu-like symptoms and generalized malaise. The classic sign of chickenpox is the appearance of blisters (vesicles) on the face and scalp, which spread to the trunk and eventually limbs. Typically, the lesions seen are in different stages, as they don't all develop at the same time. After 4–7 days, the blisters dry in.

HERPES ZOSTER

Subsequent reactivation of latent virus, typically occurring decades later, causes zoster (shingles). Shingles (zoster) is due to reactivation of the virus. It is a self-limiting, localized vesicular rash occurring over one or multiple dermatomes. The rash usually resolves within 1 or 2 weeks, but pain may persist for several weeks or become chronic (post-herpetic neuralgia).

TRANSMISSION AND PERIOD OF INFECTIOUSNESS

Chickenpox infection is primarily transmitted via respiratory droplets. Respiratory droplets containing chickenpox are transmitted 2 days before, to 5 days after, onset of the rash. The lesions are infectious until they have dried in. Shingles infection is primarily transmitted by direct contact with vesicle fluid in immunocompetent individuals but can also be transmitted via respiratory droplets from immunosuppressed patients. The infectious period for shingles is from onset of rash until all of the lesions have dried in.

COMPLICATIONS OF VARICELLA ZOSTER

Chickenpox in adults may be severe, requiring hospital admission. Risk groups for complicated infection are immunosuppressed individuals, neonates in the first week of life and pregnant women. Complications of varicella zoster are bacterial superinfections (group A *Streptococcus*), pneumonia and encephalitis. Varicella acquired in the first trimester of gestation can cause serious congenital diseases in the newborn in about 1%–2% of affected pregnancies. Newborns are at risk for varicella infection if the mother develops chickenpox 5 days before delivery until 2 days after.

COMPLICATIONS OF VARICELLA ZOSTER VIRUS REACTIVATION

The most common manifestation of varicella zoster reactivation is herpes zoster. Other complications are chronic pain (post-herpetic neuralgia), cranial nerve palsies, zoster paresis, meningoencephalitis, cerebellitis, myelopathy, herpes zoster ophthalmicus (reactivation in the trigeminal nerve) and vasculopathy mimicking giant cell arteritis. These complications may develop without a rash. Herpes zoster ophthalmicus can be accompanied by keratitis, which leads to blindness.

POST-EXPOSURE PROPHYLAXIS

Contacts who are at risk of complicated infection and who have had significant exposure to varicella zoster virus should have their VZV IgG tested. If the VZV IgG is equivocal or negative, then post-exposure prophylaxis should be offered. Post-exposure prophylaxis is 60% effective in preventing chickenpox. Pregnant women with a history of chickenpox should be considered immune and do not require post-exposure prophylaxis.

Options for post-exposure prophylaxis are the live, attenuated varicella zoster vaccine and varicella zoster immunoglobulins (VZIG). The vaccine should be given within 3–5 days after exposure. Immunocompromised individuals should receive VZIG instead, to be administered within 6 days after exposure or alternatively oral acyclovir at 10 mg/kg four times a day on days 7–14 after exposure, with a maximum of 800 mg four times a day OR valaciclovir 1000 mg three times a day can be given.

PRACTICAL TIPS FOR VZIG

VZIG is to be administered via slow intramuscular injection in the upper outer quadrant of the buttock. Contacts with bleeding disorders who cannot be given an intramuscular injection should be given intravenous human normal immunoglobulin (IVIG) at a dose of 0.2 g per kg body weight (i.e. 4 mL/kg for a 5% solution) instead. This will produce serum VZV antibody levels equivalent to those achieved with VZIG. (See Table 4.64.1.)

CLINICAL PEARL

There is no evidence that VZIG is effective in the treatment of disease. Prompt treatment with appropriate drugs (i.e. acyclovir, valaciclovir, famciclovir) should be commenced at the first signs of illness in individuals with a clinical condition which increases the risk of severe varicella.

TABLE 4.64.1
VZIG Dose Recommendations

Age	VZIG Dose
0–5 years	250 mg
6–10 years	500 mg
11–14 years	750 mg
15 years and older	1000 mg

PREVENTING HERPES ZOSTER IN THE ELDERLY

Two herpes zoster vaccines have been developed: a recombinant zoster vaccine (RZV) and a live, attenuated vaccine (ZVL). ZVL was first licensed in the US by the FDA in 2006. RZV was approved by the FDA in 2017 for use in adults aged 50 or older. ZVL is, in Europe, licensed for individuals aged ≥50 years. In Canada, ZVL was approved in 2009 and RZV in 2017. Currently, the vaccination of adults aged ≥50 years with two doses of RZV is recommended, including in subjects previously vaccinated with ZVL.

CLINICAL PEARL

The World Health Organization recommends that the varicella zoster vaccine is part of national immunization programmes, whereby an 80% coverage rate should be aimed.

CLINICAL APPROACH

DIAGNOSIS AND MANAGEMENT OF COMPLICATIONS OF VARICELLA ZOSTER VIRUS REACTIVATION

Varicella zoster pneumonia is treated with intravenous acyclovir 10 mg/kg IV three times a day for 7–10 days.

Shingles does not require treatment unless in immunocompromised individuals or in pregnant women. Treatment is with intravenous acyclovir or oral valacyclovir for 7–10 days.

If a neurological complication of varicella zoster is suspected, cerebrospinal fluid (CSF), serum and/or ocular fluids should be collected and tested for VZV DNA by PCR and for anti-VZV IgG and IgM. Detection of VZV IgG antibody in CSF is more sensitive than PCR for diagnosing VZV vasculopathy, recurrent myelopathy and brainstem encephalitis. Treatment consists of intravenous acyclovir or oral valacyclovir for 10–14 days. Post-herpetic neuralgia can be managed with tricyclic antidepressants, gabapentin, pregabalin and topical lidocaine patches.

RISK ASSESSMENT FOR PATIENTS WHO HAVE BEEN IN CONTACT WITH CHICKENPOX

Risk assessment follows the following steps:

- Was there a significant exposure?
  - Contacts in the same small room for at least 15 minutes
  - Face-to-face contact
  - Immunosuppressed contacts on large open wards
- Has the contact person a history of chickenpox or vaccination?
- Is the contact (1) pregnant or (2) immunocompromised or (3) a neonate?
- Is the contact receiving regular IVIG?
  - VZIG is not required if the most recent IVIG dose was administered ≤3 weeks before exposure.
- Is the contact on long term acyclovir/valacyclovir prophylaxis?
  - Acyclovir dose should be temporarily increased to 10 mg/kg four times a day from days 7–14 following exposure for acyclovir. For patients within 12 months of a stem cell transplant, VZIG should also be considered.

CONTACTS WITH SIGNIFICANT EXPOSURE AT RISK FOR COMPLICATED CHICKENPOX

If the contact had a significant exposure during the infectious period and is either immunosuppressed, pregnant or a neonate, then urgent VZV IgG antibody testing should be done, ideally within 24 hours.

If the contact is pregnant but has a positive chickenpox history or has been vaccinated, then no further actions are needed. Patients with a negative VZV IgG require VZIG.

CONTACTS WITH SIGNIFICANT EXPOSURE WHO ARE NOT AT RISK FOR COMPLICATED CHICKENPOX

Contacts who are aged ≥12 months, not pregnant and not immunocompromised, have no history of chickenpox and who are susceptible to chickenpox are eligible for the live, attenuated varicella zoster vaccine. If the exposure was less then 5 days ago, then the vaccine should be administered. If the exposure was more than 5 days ago, then alternatively the patient can be monitored until day 21. If no symptoms have occurred by then, the vaccine can be given to prevent any future chickenpox.

CLINICAL PEARL

The risk of acquiring infection from contact with an immunocompetent individual with non-exposed shingles lesions is remote and therefore is not an indication for VZIG.

HEALTHCARE WORKERS (HCWS) WHO ARE IN CONTACT WITH CHICKENPOX

Pregnant HCWs without a positive history of chickenpox or shingles and HCWs who are immunocompromised regardless of their history of VZV infection should be tested promptly for VZ antibodies.

Those who are antibody negative require VZIG. Pregnant HCWs with a positive history of chickenpox do not require VZIG.

Immunocompetent healthcare workers do not require VZIG.

Healthcare workers who are diagnosed with localized herpes zoster on a part of the body that can be covered with a bandage and/or clothing, and who does not work with high-risk patients, should be allowed to continue working. If the HCW is in contact with high-risk patients, then an individual risk assessment should be carried out.

HCWs with localized herpes zoster lesions that cannot be covered with a bandage and/or clothing, or who are immunocompromised, and HCWs with disseminated herpes zoster, should be excluded from the workplace until there are no new lesions and all lesions have crusted over.

CLINICAL PEARL

Healthcare workers who are diagnosed with chickenpox should remain away from the workplace until there are no new lesions and all lesions are crusted and dried in.

CLINICAL VIGNETTE

You receive a call from one of the nurses working on the haematology ward. Two days ago, she spent an afternoon with her 5-year-old nephew who today is diagnosed by the GP with chickenpox. She cannot recall a history of chickenpox. She has a negative VZV IgG and has not received the chickenpox vaccine. You advise her to remain at home from day 8 until 21 days after the chickenpox contact.

- Unvaccinated HCWs without a definite history of chickenpox or zoster with a significant exposure to VZV should either be excluded from contact with high-risk patients from 8 to 21 days after exposure or should be advised to inform their occupational department before having patient contact if they feel unwell or develop a fever or rash.

- In the majority of situations, a high level of vigilance for malaise, rash or fever (including taking temperature daily) throughout the incubation period will be adequate. Decisions about redeployment away from high-risk patients need to take into account the vulnerability of the patients and whether or not skill and staffing levels will be compromised by redeploying the exposed staff member.
- Decisions about redeployment may need to be taken in conjunction with the healthcare worker, their manager and infection control.
- Irrespective of the interval since exposure, the VZV vaccine should be offered to unvaccinated HCWs without a definite history of chickenpox or zoster and who had a significant exposure to VZV, as this will also reduce the risk VZV in the future.

BIBLIOGRAPHY

Gabutti G, Bolognesi N, Sandri F, Florescu C, Stefanati A. Varicella zoster virus vaccines: An update. *Immunotargets Ther.* 2019 August 6;8:15–28.

Macartney K, Heywood A, McIntyre P. Vaccines for post-exposure prophylaxis against varicella (chickenpox) in children and adults. *Cochrane Database Syst Rev.* 2014 June 23;(6):CD001833.

Nagel MA, Gilden D. Complications of varicella zoster virus reactivation. *Curr Treat Options Neurol.* 2013 August;15(4):439–453.

Nagel MA, Gilden D. Neurological complications of varicella zoster virus reactivation. *Curr Opin Neurol.* 2014 June;27(3):356–360.

Section V

Difficult-to-Treat Organisms

5.1 AmpC, Extended-Spectrum β-Lactamase and Carbapenemase Producers

Firza Alexander Gronthoud

CLINICAL CONSIDERATIONS

The antibacterial backbone for treatment of most bacterial infections are the β-lactams. There is emerging resistance to β-lactams caused by production of β-lactamase enzymes which hydrolyse β-lactams. Clinically important β-lactamase enzymes are AmpC and extended-spectrum β-lactamase (ESBL). Carbapenems have remained the first-line drug of choice for treatment of AmpC and ESBL producers, contributing to emergence of carbapenemase-producing *Enterobacterales*, capable of hydrolyzing all β-lactams and significantly limiting treatment options (see Table 5.1.1). Compounding this, ESBL or carbapenemase genes are transmitted on plasmids, which often contain genes encoding for resistance to other classes of antibiotics like quinolones and aminoglycosides. To optimize treatment of these multidrug-resistant organisms (MDROs), it is therefore worthwhile to consider the following.

INDUCIBLE AMPC

- AmpC enzymes are Ambler class C β-lactamases, mostly produced chromosomally, and they hydrolyze penicillins and first-, second- and third-generation cephalosporins such as ceftazidime, cefotaxime, and ceftriaxone and also cephamycins including cefoxitin and cefotetan (see Chapter 2.6).
- SPACE-M is a group of organisms that produce low levels of AmpC enzymes. Upon exposure to certain β-lactams, such as amoxicillin, ampicillin, imipenem and clavulanic acid, the AmpC gene is induced and starts to produce high-level AmpC enzymes. The consequence is that these organisms then become resistant to many β-lactam agents including first-, second- and third-generation cephalosporins.
- SPACE-M organisms are *Serratia marcescens*, *Providencia* spp., *Pseudomonas aeruginosa*, *Acinetobacter baumannii*, *Citrobacter freundii*, *Enterobacter cloacae* complex and *Morganella morganii*.
- Among a population of inducible AmpC organisms, there may also exist de-repressed AmpC mutants that already produce high levels of AmpC.
- An inducible AmpC organism is producing low levels of AmpC.
- An induced AmpC organism is producing high levels of AmpC after exposure to β-lactams.
- A de-repressed AmpC mutant produces high levels of AmpC without needing exposure to β-lactams,
- *In vitro* susceptibility may not correlate with clinical efficacy as resistance can emerge by selection of mutants expressing high levels of AmpC.
- AmpC enzymes are usually chromosomally encoded but may also be present on plasmids, of which the main occurring AmpC enzyme is CMY-2.

TABLE 5.1.1

Activity of β-Lactams against β-Lactamase Enzymes

	3G Ceph	Aztreonam	Co-Amox	Pip/ Taz	Ertapenem	Imipenem	Mero	Caz/ Avi	Cef/ Taz	Temocillin
AmpC	−	−	−	+	+	+	+	+	+	+
ESBL	−	−	+/−	+	+	+	+	+	+/−	+
KPC2	−	−	−	−	−	−	+/−	+	−	+
KPC3	−	−	−	−	−	−	+/−	+/−	−	+
OXA-48	+/−	+	−	−	−	−	−	+	−	−
MBL (VIM, NDM-1)	−	+	−	−	−	−	−	−	−	−

Note: + active, − not active. +/− variable activity depending on the MIC and antimicrobial dosing.

- Clavulanic acid, sulbactam and tazobactam β-lactamase inhibitors are generally not active against AmpC enzymes, with the exception of tazobactam, which is active against AmpC-producing *M. morganii.*
- Wild-type inducible AmpC organisms are resistant to amoxicillin and ampicillin both with and without clavulanic acid or sulbactam, resistant to first-generation cephalosporins but under restricted conditions can be treated with piperacillin, third-generation cephalosporins, aztreonam, cefepime and carbapenems.
- Amoxicillin, clavulanic acid, cefoxitin and imipenem are strong inducers of AmpC.
- Although imipenem is a strong AmpC inducer, it remains stable against AmpC.
- Piperacillin, third-generation cephalosporins and tazobactam are weak inducers of AmpC.
- Third-generation cephalosporins and piperacillin/tazobactam are active against *in vitro* sensitive inducible AmpC producers, unless de-repressed mutants are selected during treatment and high levels of AmpC are being produced.
- Piperacillin seems less prone than third-generation cephalosporins to select de-repressed mutants from the induced population.
- The selection of resistant de-repressed mutants is also dependent on bacterial inoculum, antibiotic concentration at site of infection and specific species and strains.
- Cefepime does not induce AmpC and remains stable unless there is AmpC hyperproduction.
- Carbapenems and temocillin are stable against AmpC-β-lactamase enzymes.
- Piperacillin/tazobactam remains active against *M. morganii* even when expressing high levels of its AmpC enzyme. Piperacillin/tazobactam shows some degree of synergy against most de-repressed AmpC strains, although less so with *E. cloacae* and *P. aeruginosa* compared with *C. freundii* and *M. morganii.*
- Ceftazidime, in particular, is a treatment option for *S. marcescens* infections, as the frequency of selection of de-repressed mutants remains low with de-repressed mutants displaying a low ceftazidime MIC.
- Ertapenem is less stable against AmpC than meropenem, and in combination with OmpK35 porin loss, ertapenem resistance arises whilst meropenem remains active.
- Besides induction of AmpC or selection of de-repressed mutants, other risk factors for clinical failure with cephalosporins against SPACE-M are host factors, drug PK/PD parameters and the presence of other resistance determinants (e.g. ESBL production).
- *Proteus vulgaris* and *Proteus penneri* have chromosomally encoded AmpC genes, which are not active against ceftazidime.

- Many *Aeromonas* spp. express AmpC enzymes as well as a class D penicillinase and class B metallo-β-lactamase (MBL). More than 90% of isolates are susceptible to third-generation cephalosporins; however, treatment failure with cefotaxime has rarely been described. Piperacillin/tazobactam is also usually active, although rates of resistance of 10%–50% have been reported.

EXTENDED-SPECTRUM β-LACTAMASE (ESBL) PRODUCERS

- ESBLs hydrolyze penicillins, first-, third- and fourth-generation cephalosporins and aztreonam, rendering them ineffective.
- The most common ESBLs are TEM, SHV and CTX-M types.
- ESBLs are present and transmitted on plasmids, which may also contain genes conferring resistance to quinolones and aminoglycosides.
- Carbapenems are active against ESBL producers.
- Different ESBL enzymes vary in the ability to hydrolyze specific cephalosporins.
  - Producers of TEM and SHV types of ESBLs are susceptible to cefotaxime more frequently than CTX-M producers.
  - The opposite is the case for ceftazidime and cefepime.
  - CTX-M-14 has weak activity against ceftazidime compared to CTX-M-15.
- ESBL is more often found in *Escherichia coli* compared to *Klebsiella pneumoniae*.
- In contrast to AmpC enzymes, ESBL enzymes are inhibited by clavulanic acid, tazobactam and sulbactam.
- Activity of piperacillin/tazobactam against ESBL producers depends on the dose used (at least 4.5 g 8-hourly IV), source of infection and bacterial inoculum (higher inoculum is associated with lower efficacy).
- Piperacillin/tazobactam: Mortality is 0% among those with a urinary source; among those with a non-urinary source, mortality is 0% if the MIC is ≤2 mg/L, 38% if the MIC is between 4 mg/L and 8 mg/L and 44% if the MIC is ≥16 mg/L.
- Amoxicillin/clavulanic acid is not affected by inoculum effect.
- Regardless of the presence of ESBL, for third generation cephalosporins the underlying relationship between MIC, drug exposure and outcome remains the same.
- The degree of ESBL activity is dependent on the β-lactam, whether or not a β-lactamase inhibitor is used to protect the β-lactam and the particular ESBL variant.
- Increased risk of therapeutic failure in ESBL infections with β-lactam therapy is mediated by the increase in MIC.
  - From 2010 onwards, CLSI lowered its breakpoints for cephalosporins so that all clinically important resistance mechanisms are detected and recommends reporting sensitivities according to MIC.
  - EUCAST gives a similar recommendation: the presence or absence of an ESBL does not influence the categorization of susceptibility.
- β-lactamase hyperproduction and coproduction of plasmid-mediated AmpC enzymes, among other factors, can affect inhibitor activity.
- Piperacillin/tazobactam has comparable clinical outcome to carbapenem for ESBL-producing *Enterobacterales* if the MIC is less than 4 mg/L and a dose of at least 4.5 g 8-hourly IV is used.
- Piperacillin/tazobactam may be a suitable alternative to carbapenems for UTI and biliary sepsis including bacteraemias provided *in vitro* sensitivity and source control.
- Amoxicillin/clavulanic acid is active against CTX-M-14 enzyme.
- CTX-M-15 may co-exist with OXA-1, an inhibitor-resistant penicillinase, which is not inhibited by amoxicillin/clavulanic acid.

- Both ceftazidime/avibactam and ceftolozane/tazobactam are suitable last-resort options. Resistance rate among ESBL producers may be higher for ceftolozane/tazobactam than for ceftazidime/avibactam, particularly for ESBL-producing *K. pneumoniae*.

CLINICAL PEARL

- The CTX-M-15-type ESBL is the most prevalent ESBL worldwide and is associated with the epidemic *E. coli* sequence type 131 (ST131).
- ST131 strains are associated with distinct combinations of extraintestinal virulence factors and can cause persistent or recurrent urinary tract infections or higher sepsis rates.
- Within the ST131 clone, the most prevalent subclone is H30 ST131 and is associated with combined resistance to three antibiotic classes and with expressing CTX-M-15 type ESBL.
- ST131 strains account for 70%–80% of fluoroquinolone-resistant *E. coli* isolates and for nearly two-thirds of ESBL-producing isolates.
- Infections due to ESBL-positive ST131 are associated with international travel.
- Similar to *Clostridioides difficile*, use of quinolones and cephalosporins contributes to emergence and spread of ST131.

CLINICAL PEARL

- Both ESBL and AmpC producers are resistant to some or all cephalosporins, but they exhibit some differences.
- ESBLs are inhibited by β-lactam inhibitors and do not hydrolyze cephamycins, while AmpC enzymes are not inhibited by classic β-lactam inhibitors and confer resistance to cephamycins but do not efficiently hydrolyze cefepime.
- ESBLs are typically encoded by plasmid-borne genes, whereas AmpC can be encoded by plasmid genes or be produced as a result of de-repression of chromosomal genes in some *Enterobacterales*.
- Repressed AmpC producers may *in vitro* test susceptible to cephalosporins, but resistance can develop while on treatment with these drugs.
- The proportion of AmpC producers (by either plasmid-borne genes or de-repressed or hyper-expressed chromosomal genes) that are susceptible to cephalosporins (except cefepime) is lower compared to ESBL producers.

CARBAPENEMASE-PRODUCING *ENTEROBACTERALES* (CPE)

- Carbapenem resistance occurs due to carbapenemase production or a combination of loss of porins with hyperproduction of ESBL or AmpC.
- Carbapenemases belong to either the serine β-lactamases (KPC, OXA-48 like enzymes) or the zinc-dependent MBLs (IMP, VIM and NDM-1).
- Serine β-lactamases belong to Ambler class A, C or D. MBLs belong to Ambler class B.
- Although all carbapenemases have the capacity to hydrolyze carbapenems, the rate and extent of hydrolysis vary, resulting in a range of susceptibilities from a fully susceptible to a highly resistant isolate.

- There are several factors thought to contribute to this variability, including the amount of carbapenemase that is produced, the specific carbapenem tested, and the coexistence of other mechanisms of resistance, such as porin loss, efflux pumps, and the expression of other β-lactamases.
- OXA-48 carbapenemases typically have the lowest minimum inhibitory concentrations (MICs) to carbapenems and, consequently, are the hardest to identify, followed by MBLs and lastly KPCs, which have the highest MICs.
- Although *in vitro* clavulanic acid, tazobactam and sulbactam weakly inhibit KPC and OXA-48-like enzymes, they are not considered to be clinically effective against them.
- Emerging resistance to ceftazidime/avibactam has been documented both *in vitro* and *in vivo* for KPC3-producing *K. pneumoniae*.
- Only one β-lactamase inhibitor is clinically active against both KPC and OXA-48 like enzymes: avibactam, which is available in combination with ceftazidime.
- Currently, there are no clinically useful β-lactam-β-lactamase inhibitors available with activity against the class B metallo-β-lactamases. Ceftriaxone/sulbactam/EDTA and aztreonam/avibactam are new β-lactam-β-lactamase inhibitors being evaluated for treatment of MBLs and have shown promising *in vitro* results.
- Cyclic boronate 2 has been shown *in vitro* to inhibit all classes of β-lactamases, but with limited activity against VIM-2 producing *P. aeruginosa*.
- With the exception of aztreonam, MBLs hydrolyze all β-lactams including penicillins, cephalosporins, carbapenems and serine-inhibitors including clavulanic acid, sulbactam, tazobactam and avibactam.
- However, coproduction of other β-lactamases, such as AmpCs and extended-spectrum β-lactamases, often hinders the use of aztreonam.
- Carbapenemase-producing organisms (CPOs) can be either a CPE or a carbapenemase-producing *Pseudomonas aeruginosa* or *Acinetobacter baumannii*. This section will only cover CPE (see Chapters 5.2 and 5.4 for resistance mechanisms and treatment of *Acinetobacter baumannii* and *Pseudomonas aeruginosa*, respectively).
- In contrast to ESBL, carbapenemase enzymes are more prevalent in *K. pneumoniae* than in *E. coli*.
- Carbapenemase activity against carbapenems varies according to the enzyme and, probably, the expression levels of carbapenemase genes.
- Probability of reaching the target pharmacodynamic parameter is around 80% for isolates with a MIC of ≤8 mg/L if meropenem is administered at 2 g 8-hourly by extended infusion.
- KPC has a higher affinity for ertapenem than other carbapenems, which led to the hypothesis that use of ertapenem might allow the other carbapenem to survive. This seems to work *in vitro* only if the meropenem MIC is ≤128 mg/L and not for all strains.
- Most frequent antibiotics used in combination are polymyxins, tigecycline, fosfomycin and aminoglycosides. Some isolates are susceptible to minocycline, doxycycline, chloramphenicol, trimethoprim/sulfamethoxazole and temocillin.
- The new β-lactamase inhibitors, avibactam, vaborbactam and relebactam, inhibit KPC (avibactam is the only new β-lactamase inhibitors that also inhibits OXA-48) but not MBLs.
- Many CPE also produce ESBLs, and the impact of the production of both enzymes on treatment is not well established.
- The use of carbapenem for CPE infections facilitates the emergence of higher levels of carbapenem resistance due to permeability problems or increased expression of carbapenemases.
- Because of the scarcity of information, fosfomycin is not a first option against serious CRE infections when other active drugs are available, but it may be needed in some patients with scarce options. In such cases, a fosfomycin dose of 16–24 g per day as part of combination therapy is recommended.

CLINICAL APPROACH

AmpC Producers

- Carbapenems are drugs of choice for treatment of serious infection with *Enterobacterales* caused by ESBL or AmpC producers.
- Inducible AmpC
  - Both cefepime and piperacillin/tazobactam have a low risk of selecting de-repressed AmpC mutants and are therefore alternatives to carbapenem for inducible AmpC producers if *in vitro* sensitive. Use with caution in serious infections where source control is not available.
  - High-dose temocillin 2 g 8-hourly IV is a carbapenem and piperacillin/tazobactam-sparing option for UTI or pneumonia +/− bacteraemia.
  - Third-generation cephalosporins may potentially be used for *E. cloacae* complex, *S. marcescens* and *C. freundii* if *in vitro* sensitive and limited therapeutic options. Therapy failure has been documented in up to 20% of cases despite *in vitro* susceptibility. Restrict use to infections where cephalosporins reach high concentrations (i.e. UTI) and monitor closely, but preferably use alternative agent.
- De-repressed AmpC
  - Drugs of choice are carbapenems.
  - High dose temocillin 2 g 8-hourly IV is a carbapenem-sparing option for UTI or pneumonia +/− bacteraemia.
  - De-repressed *M. morganii*: Piperacillin/tazobactam is a carbapenem-sparing option if *in vitro* sensitive.
  - De-repressed *S. marcescens*: Ceftazidime is a carbapenem- and piperacillin/tazobactam-sparing option if *in vitro* sensitive.
- Chromosomal AmpC producers are generally sensitive to high-dose cefepime, unless other mechanisms of resistance are present, i.e. ESBL production. However, clinical failure with *Enterobacter* spp. and cefepime may occur if AmpC de-repressed mutants are selected, i.e. in high-inoculum infections. Clinical effectiveness of cefepime against plasmid-mediated AmpC producers is uncertain.
- Alternative agents for both inducible and de-repressed AmpC producers
  - *UTI*: Aminoglycosides in stable patients. Serum trough levels should be closely monitored using therapeutic drug monitoring.
  - *Intra-abdominal infection*: Tigecycline, consider high dose 200 mg loading dose, thereafter 100 mg 12-hourly.
  - Quinolones and trimethoprim/sulfamethoxazole may be used for oral stepdown. Quinolones are high risk for causing *C. difficile infection* in *C. difficile* carriers. Trimethoprim/sulfamethoxazole may carry increased risk of therapy failure for bloodstream infections.

Extended-Spectrum β-Lactamase Producers

- Carbapenems are drugs of choice for treatment of serious infections with *Enterobacterales* caused by ESBL or AmpC producers.
- Ertapenem can be considered with susceptible isolates for outpatient parenteral antimicrobial therapy (OPAT).
- High-dose temocillin 2 g 8-hourly IV is a carbapenem- and piperacillin/tazobactam-sparing option for UTI or pneumonia +/− bacteraemia.
- Piperacillin/tazobactam may be considered for urinary tract infection and biliary sepsis +/− associated bacteraemia. Piperacillin/tazobactam should be dosed at 4.5 gram 8-hourly or 6-hourly and MIC should be less than 4 mg/L.

- Oral amoxicillin/clavulanic acid may be considered for lower urinary tract infections, provided *in vitro* fully sensitive. Based on *in vitro* sensitivities, preferred options are nitrofurantoin, fosfomycin, pivmecillinam, trimethoprim and ciprofloxacin.
- It is not recommended to use third-generation cephalosporins for treatment of ESBL infections. Third-generation cephalosporins may be considered on the following grounds: (1) alternative options are not available, (2) MIC *in vitro* is equal to or lower than the MIC breakpoint, (3) high dose is used and (4) used for treatment of stable patients with nonobstructive UTI or if the source of infection has been removed as high inoculum increases risk of selection of ESBL hyperproducers.
- Cefepime may be considered if MIC $\leq$2 mg/L.
- Aminoglycosides are alternative options for treatment of urosepsis in stable patients. Serum trough levels should be closely monitored using therapeutic drug monitoring.
- Tigecycline is an alternative option for intra-abdominal infections.

CLINICAL PEARL

If the bacteria responsible for the infection are subsequently shown to produce neither ESBLs nor AmpC β-lactamase, carbapenem use should reasonably be stepped down to narrower-spectrum agents.

CARBAPENEMASE-PRODUCING ENTEROBACTERIACEAE

- MBL producers are susceptible to aztreonam if they are not ESBL or AmpC producers.
- OXA-48 producers are susceptible to ceftazidime and ceftolozane/tazobactam if they do not coproduce ESBL, AmpC or other carbapenemase enzymes.
- OXA-48 producers that co-produce ESBL but not AmpC, or other carbapenemase enzymes, are susceptible to ceftolozane/tazobactam.
- Isolates with MBLs or OXA-48 and no ESBL or AmpC production may be susceptible to aztreonam (those with OXA-48 alone are likely also to be susceptible to ceftazidime and ceftolozane/tazobactam).
- OXA-48 producers are frequently susceptible to ceftazidime/avibactam.
- KPC producers are frequently susceptible to ceftazidima/avibactam, meropenem/vaborbactam and imipenem-relebactam.
- Overall, combinations including tigecycline, colistin and meropenem are associated with the lowest mortality, and combination therapy with new β-lactam/β-lactamase inhibitors is promising.
- Among the various antibiotic combinations, lower mortality is seen with a meropenem-containing combination if the meropenem MIC is between 2 and 8 mg/L and high-dose meropenem extended infusion: 2 g 8-hourly over 3 hours.
- Colistin resistance is associated with increased mortality.
- Carbapenem monotherapy may be an option for UTI caused by carbapenem-susceptible CPE.
- If combination therapy is used, the inclusion of tigecycline for complicated UTI and tigecycline or aminoglycosides for ventilator-associated pneumonia should be avoided.
- Temocillin may be potentially used in infections caused by KPC producers.

CLINICAL PEARL

Selection for de-repressed AmpC mutants can occur in high-inoculum infections, where there is a non-eradicated focus or in sites where adequate drug levels are harder to achieve.

CURRENT β-LACTAM AGENTS WITH ACTIVITY AGAINST KPC AND OXA-48, BUT NOT MBL

- Ceftazidime/avibactam (active against both KPC and OXA-48)
- Meropenem/vaborbactam (no activity against OXA-48)
- Imipenem/cilastatin/relebactam (weak and variable activity against OXA-48-producing *Enterobacterales*)
- Cefiderocol (FDA recommendation for approval for treatment of complicated UTI)

AGENTS IN DEVELOPMENT WITH ACTIVITY AGAINST METALLO-β-LACTAMASE ENZYMES

- Aztreonam/avibactam
- Ceftriaxone/sulbactam/EDTA/tazobactam

BIBLIOGRAPHY

Banerjee R, Johnson JR. A New Clone Sweeps Clean: The Enigmatic Emergence of *Escherichia coli* Sequence Type 131. *Antimicrob Agents Chemother.* 2014 September;58(9):4997–5004.

Cahill ST, Cain R, Wang DY et al. Cyclic Boronates Inhibit All Classes of β-Lactamases. *Antimicrob Agents Chemother.* 2017 March 24;61(4).

Harris PN, Ferguson JK. Antibiotic Therapy for Inducible AmpC -Lactamase-Producing Gram-Negative Bacilli: What Are the Alternatives to Carbapenems, Quinolones and Aminoglycosides? *Int J Antimicrob Agents.* 2012 October;40(4):297–305.

Hawkey PM, Warren RE, Livermore DM, McNulty CAM, Enoch DA, Otter JA, Wilson APR. Treatment of Infections Caused by Multidrug-Resistant Gram-Negative Bacteria: Report of the British Society for Antimicrobial Chemotherapy/Healthcare Infection Society/British Infection Association Joint Working Party. *J Antimicrob Chemother.* 2018 March 1;73(suppl_3).

Rodríguez-Baño J, Gutiérrez-Gutiérrez B, Machuca I, Pascual A. Treatment of Infections Caused by Extended-Spectrum-β- Lactamase-, AmpC-, and Carbapenemase-Producing Enterobacteriaceae. *Clin Microbiol Rev.* 2018 February 14;31(2).

5.2 *Acinetobacter baumannii*

Firza Alexander Gronthoud

CLINICAL CONSIDERATIONS

Acinetobacter baumannii is a Gram-negative, aerobic, oxidase-negative, non-fermenting coccobacillus. Its natural habitat is soil and water. *Acinetobacter baumannii* is difficult to decolourize with Gram stain and may be misidentified for a Gram-positive bacterium. As it is catalase positive, it may initially be misidentified for a *Staphylococcus aureus*. Although usually *Acinetobacter baumannii* may represent colonization when cultured from non-sterile samples, it has the potential to cause difficult-to-treat opportunistic infections. In fact, in some regions of the world, it is one of the most common causes of hospital-acquired infections. It can persist in the environment for a prolonged time and has multiple resistance mechanisms by which it causes prolonged outbreaks and severe, difficult-to-treat infections. It is therefore worthwhile to consider the following.

RISK FACTORS FOR *ACINETOBACTER BAUMANNII* INFECTIONS

Infections with *A. baumannii* are more common in southern Europe, North America, South America and Asia. It is less common in northern European countries and Australia, where it more often represents colonization in clinical cultures. Prolonged hospitalization and multiple antibiotic courses are significant risk factors in these countries, and *A. baumannii* has caused numerous outbreaks in intensive care units in these countries.

Population at risk for *Acinetobacter baumannii* infections are immunosuppressed individuals and patients with underlying pulmonary conditions.

Factors promoting infections are colonization pressure, broad-spectrum antibiotic treatment, especially prolonged or multiple courses, indwelling catheters or intravascular catheters, mechanical ventilation, multiple invasive procedures and burns.

PROPERTIES OF *ACINETOBACTER BAUMANNII*

- Survives for prolonged periods on dry surfaces (months to years) and has been found in disinfectants.
- Transmission through contaminated hands of healthcare workers and contaminated equipment and environment.
- More worryingly, airborne transmission has been described although this requires further investigation.
- Similar to *Pseudomonas aeruginosa*, *A. baumannii* possesses multiple antibiotic-resistance mechanisms: enzymatic inactivation of antibiotics, alteration of bacterial targets, permeability barriers to uptake of antimicrobials or active efflux pumps.
- Carbapenem resistance is predominantly caused by class D OXA-like β-lactamases.
- OXA-23, OXA-24, OXA-40, OXA-51, OXA-58 and OXA-143 are the major carbapenemases.
- OXA-23 producers may also co-produce ArmA-encoded 16S ribosomal methyltransferases, conferring resistance to all aminoglycosides.
- In addition, *A. baumannii* can also produce certain class B metallo-β-lactamases (IMP, VIM, SIM and NDM), further contributing to resistance to all β-lactams.

CLINICAL MANIFESTATIONS

Acinetobacter baumannii is mainly associated with hospital-acquired pneumonia and bloodstream infections which may be reflected by its high colonization rate of the respiratory tract and intravascular devices in ICU patients. Other clinical presentations are catheter-associated urinary tract infections, burn infections and neurosurgical infections including ventriculitis.

CLINICAL PEARL

Multidrug-resistant (MDR) *A. baumannii* mainly causes outbreaks in ICU settings.

In contrast, ESBL and carbapenemase-producing *Escherichia coli* and *Klebsiella* spp. cause infection in a wider group of patients, both in the community and in the healthcare setting and thus have far greater potential to spread rapidly.

ANTIMICROBIAL SUSCEPTIBILITY TESTING

There are two main issues with antimicrobial susceptibility testing. Firstly, EUCAST has clinical breakpoints for few antibiotics: imipenem, meropenem, ciprofloxacin, levofloxacin, gentamicin, tobramycin, amikacin, colistin and trimethoprim/sulfamethoxazole. In contrast, CLSI has a wider selection of clinical breakpoints including: ampicillin/sulbactam, piperacillin/tazobactam, third- and fourth-generation cephalosporins, imipenem, meropenem, ciprofloxacin, levofloxacin, gentamicin, tobramycin, amikacin, colistin, tetracyclines and trimethoprim/sulfamethoxazole (see CLSI M100 29th edition supplement for a full overview of all antimicrobials).

Secondly, the presence of colistin heteroresistance may be missed by standard phenotypic antimicrobial susceptibility testing. Heteroresistance is the presence of a subpopulations of resistant organisms in an isolate.

CLINICAL APPROACH

DIFFERENTIATING COLONIZATION FROM INFECTION

The presence of *A. baumannii* in the respiratory tract, urinary tract, surgical wounds and other fluids may represent infection or colonization. *A. baumannii* forms biofilms on foreign bodies such as an endotracheal tube, explaining the high rate of colonization in some countries. *A. baumannii* usually represents colonization at first, but prolonged antibiotic courses select out *A. baumannii*, promoting infection.

If *A. baumannii* has been identified in cultures, it is essential to prevent unnecessary antibiotic courses and keep antibiotic course duration as short as possible. It is also be beneficial to remove or change urinary catheters or intravascular devices.

TREATMENT OPTIONS

Wild-type *A. baumannii* (non MDR): Sulbactam, fluoroquinolones, trimethoprim/sulfamethoxazole, minocycline, tigecycline, doxycycline, meropenem, aminoglycosides and polymyxins are the agents most often used.

MDR *A. baumannii*: Sulbactam used to be a treatment option but is less effective now due to widespread resistance. The antibiotics with the highest *in vitro* activity against MDR *A. baumannii* are colistin and minocycline. Ertapenem is not active against *A. baumannii*, and minocycline is more potent than doxycycline. Based on *in vitro* data, the suggested first-line treatment option is intravenous colistin + intravenous or oral minocycline. Other agents that could be used depending on *in vitro* antimicrobial susceptibility results are carbapenems and aminoglycosides.

Although a clinical breakpoint has been defined by neither CLSI nor EUCAST, tigecycline should be avoided even as part of combination therapy if the MIC is ≥ 2 μg/mL, as it is associated with higher mortality rates.

ERADICATION OF *ACINETOBACTER BAUMANNII*

The combination of colistin and rifampicin could be an option for eradication in persistent colonized individuals or recurrent infections, as the addition of rifampicin demonstrated an excellent microbial eradication rate in a multicentre randomized trial, but no impact on mortality rate was observed.

AEROSOLIZED COLISTIN

Aerosolized colistin could be considered in addition to systemic antibiotic therapy for respiratory tract infections. Bronchospasm could occur.

BIBLIOGRAPHY

CLSI. *Performance Standards for Antimicrobial Susceptibility Testing*, 29th ed., CLSI supplement M100. Wayne, PA: Clinical and Laboratory Standards Institute, 2014.

Garnacho-Montero J, Timsit JF. Managing *Acinetobacter baumannii* infections. *Curr Opin Infect Dis.* 2019 February;32(1):69–76.

Vila J, Pachón J. Therapeutic options for *Acinetobacter baumannii* infections: An update. *Expert Opin Pharmacother.* 2012 November;13(16):2319–2336.

Wong D, Nielsen TB, Bonomo RA, Pantapalangkoor P, Luna B, Spellberg B. Clinical and pathophysiological overview of *Acinetobacter* infections: A century of challenges. *Clin Microbiol Rev.* 2017 January;30(1):409–447.

5.3 *Achromobacter xylosoxidans*

Firza Alexander Gronthoud

CLINICAL CONSIDERATIONS

- *Achromobacter* species (formerly known as *Alcaligenes*) is an aerobic, motile, oxidase- and catalase-positive, non-fermenting Gram-negative bacillus.
- Although strictly an aerobe, it can survive and proliferate in hypoxic and even anoxic environments.
- It has been found in fresh and brackish water, soil and municipal and hospital water supplies.
- *Achromobacter xylosoxidans* and *Achromobacter denitrificans* are the two most reported clinical species.
- Belongs to the Burkholderiales order, within the Alcaligenaceae family.
- They grow well on simple media, and on nutrient agar colonies, they are flat or slightly convex with smooth margins and range from white to light grey.
- Opportunistic pathogen in immunosuppressed patients, cystic fibrosis, haematologic and solid organ malignancies and renal failure.
- Causes a wide range of infections: bacteraemia, pneumonia, meningitis, urinary tract infections and nosocomial infections from contaminated medications, nebulizers, dialysis fluids, saline solution, disinfectants (chlorhexidine) and contact lens fluid.
- It is an environmental organism, can be found on plants and in soil and may be wise to keep plants from high-risk patient groups within hospitals.
- Antimicrobial agents with the highest *in vitro* activity are imipenem, meropenem, piperacillin/tazobactam, ticarcillin/clavulanic acid and ceftazidime.
- May also be susceptible to trimethoprim/sulfamethoxazole, colistin, chloramphenicol and minocycline/tigecycline.
- Resistant to amoxicillin/clavulanic acid, aztreonam, ertapenem, aminoglycosides, expanded spectrum cephalosporins other than ceftazidime, quinolones.
- Intrinsic resistance through multiple efflux pumps, aminoglycoside modifying enzymes and narrow-spectrum class D β-lactamases.
- *Achromobacter* species can acquire antimicrobial resistance through mobile genetic elements such as integrons containing extended-spectrum β-lactamase and metallo-β-lactamase enzymes have been reported.
- Despite *in vitro* resistance, aerosolized tobramycin or colistin may be effective owing to high local concentrations.
- Neither EUCAST nor CLSI provide *Achromobacter* spp.-specific breakpoints. CLSI does provide clinical breakpoints for non-*Enterobacterales* which in clinical practice has been cautiously applied to *Achromobacter* species.

CLINICAL PEARL

Biofilm production is associated with resistance to environmental factors by promoting intimate attachment to surfaces, resistance to phagocytic activity and other host immune factors, shielding from antimicrobial activity and enhanced spread across surfaces via bacterial motility. In polymicrobial infections, interspecies interactions have been demonstrated such that different species within the same biofilm can respond to each other's signalling systems and provide survival advantages to the entire polymicrobial community.

CLINICAL APPROACH

ESTABLISH CLINICAL SIGNIFICANCE

- If either alone or with other organisms from non-sterile sites (e.g. sputum, wound swabs, and urine cultures), their role in disease may be difficult to ascertain.
- Antimicrobial treatment is indicated if
  - isolated from sterile sites (e.g. cerebrospinal fluid, blood and joint aspiration), but always correlate with clinical symptoms.
  - Repeated isolation of inpatients with clinical symptoms of infection.

ANTIBIOTIC OPTIONS

- The optimal treatment is unknown.
- Treatment options are piperacillin/tazobactam, meropenem, trimethoprim/sulfamethoxazole, ceftazidime, minocycline and chloramphenicol.
- Aminoglycosides, fluoroquinolones, fosfomycin and aztreonam have poor activity.
- Consider combination therapy for the treatment of *Achromobacter* spp. pulmonary exacerbations in CF, with or without inhaled colistin or tobramycin in patients with cystic fibrosis.

BIBLIOGRAPHY

Abbott IJ, Peleg AY. Stenotrophomonas, Achromobacter, and Nonmelioid Burkholderia Species: Antimicrobial Resistance and Therapeutic Strategies. *Semin Respir Crit Care Med.* 2015 February;36(1):99–110.

Hu Y, Zhu Y, Ma Y, Liu F, Lu N, Yang X, Luan C, Yi Y, Zhu B. Genomic Insights into Intrinsic and Acquired Drug Resistance Mechanisms in *Achromobacter xylosoxidans. Antimicrob Agents Chemother.* 2015 February;59(2):1152–1161.

Swenson CE, Sadikot RT. Achromobacter respiratory infections. *Ann Am Thorac Soc.* 2015 February;12(2):252–258.

5.4 *Pseudomonas aeruginosa*

Firza Alexander Gronthoud

CLINICAL CONSIDERATIONS

Pseudomonas aeruginosa is an environmental organism and an important opportunistic pathogen causing nosocomial infections and infections in critically ill and immunocompromised individuals. Although initially it can be susceptible to a wide range of antimicrobials, it has the ability to rapidly become resistant owing to multiple intrinsic resistance mechanisms, and cause severe morbidity and mortality. It is therefore worthwhile to consider the following:

Important risk factors for *Pseudomonas aeruginosa* colonization and infection:

- Prior antimicrobial treatment
- Urinary catheter, intravascular catheter, mechanical ventilation
- Critically ill
- Immunocompromised (i.e. neutropaenia)
- Underlying chronic lung disease

MUCOID *PSEUDOMONAS AERUGINOSA*

Mucoid *Pseudomonas aeruginosa* is seen in cystic fibrosis. These *P. aeruginosa* variants produce an alginate-containing matrix providing protection from opsonization, phagocytosis and antibiotics.

ECTHYMA GANGRENOSUM

- Necrotic skin lesions caused by mini septic emboli and can be seen in *P. aeruginosa* bloodstream infections in immunocompromised individuals
- Initially painless erythematous areas with papules and/or bullae which rapidly progress to painful gangrenous ulcers
- Single or multiple and preferentially found in the gluteal and perineal areas
- Biopsies of these lesions grow *P. aeruginosa*
- Not specific to *P. aeruginosa*, as also described in *Staphylococcus aureus* and *Fusarium* spp.

RESISTANCE MECHANISMS

- Antibiotic resistance mechanisms include decreased cell wall permeability, efflux pumps, antibiotic inactivation enzymes, production of AmpC and metallo-β-lactamase enzymes and antibiotic target modifications.
- These resistance mechanisms are chromosomally encoded (intrinsic), through mutations or acquired through mobile genetic elements (plasmids and integrons). These mobile genetic elements often carry multiple resistance genes.
- Aminoglycoside-modifying enzymes (AME)
  - Acetyltransferases (AAC), phosphotransferases (APH) and nucleotidyltransferases (ANT).
  - Among aminoglycoside resistance, resistance to gentamicin develops first followed by tobramycin and later on amikacin.
  - Tobramycin is more potent against *P. aeruginosa* than gentamicin.

- Efflux pumps
  - *Pseudomonas aeruginosa* has three groups of proteins that work together to confer resistance to virtually all antibiotics except polymyxins.
  - Group 1: Efflux pumps which are located in the cytoplasmic membrane: MexB, MexD, MexF and MexY.
  - Group 2: Membrane porins OprM, OprJ and OprN.
  - Group 3: Efflux pumps and membrane porins are connected through proteins in the periplasmic space: MexA, MexC, MexE and MexX.
  - The main antibiotic resistance combinations are MexAB-OprM, MexCD-OprJ, MexEF-OprN and MexXY-OprM.
  - Quinolones are substrates of all efflux systems and, as such, can trigger resistance to other classes of antibiotics.
- Reduced permeability
  - Reduced permeability is caused by several mechanisms, which affect all classes of antibiotics including polymyxins.
  - Of note, porin oprD mutations affect imipenem. This mutation is often associated with overexpression of efflux system. Imipenem can thus trigger resistance to other classes of antibiotics.
- β-lactamase enzymes
  - AmpC, ESBL, carbapenemase enzymes and OXA-type enzymes.
  - *Pseudomonas aeruginosa* is resistant to penicillins, first- and second-generation cephalosporins and third generation cephalosporins with exception of ceftazidime, due to a combination of low-level AmpC expression, efflux pumps and reduced permeability.
  - Metallo-β-lactamase (MBL): VIM and IMP, although KPC has been reported as well.
  - Nevertheless, AmpC overexpression is associated with quinolone resistance, which, with aminoglycoside resistance, is already known to be associated with efflux pumps.
  - Enhanced AmpC production and depressed oprD causes resistance to meropenem.
- Drug target modifications
  - β-lactams resistance: Modification of the penicillin binding protein 4 (PBP4) or overexpression of PBP3.
  - Quinolone resistance: Alterations in DNA gyrase and topoisomerase which are enzymes involved in DNA replication. These alterations are a result of point mutations in GyrA and GyrB which are subunits of DNA gyrase and mutations in parC and parE which are subunits of topoisomerase IV.
  - Polymyxin resistance: Structural modifications of lipopolysaccharides (LPs).

CARBAPENEMS SHOULD NOT BE A FIRST-LINE CHOICE FOR *PSEUDOMONAS AERUGINOSA* TREATMENT

- Meropenem resistance is associated with efflux pumps and AmpC overexpression.
- In contrast, piperacillin/tazobactam and ceftazidime resistance is more commonly associated with AmpC overexpression alone, making non-carbapenems preferable agents for avoidance of MDR strains.
- As mentioned previously, imipenem can trigger multidrug resistance.
- In contrast to *Enterobacterales*, rates of resistance to carbapenems are generally higher than those to ceftazidime, piperacillin/tazobactam or aminoglycosides.

LABORATORY DETECTION OF RESISTANCE MECHANISMS

- Disk diffusion and Etest are not reliable because colistin diffuses poorly into agar diffusion.
- Automated systems such ViTeK are also less reliable.
- Gold standard remains microbroth dilution.
- Carbapenemase production can be detected with various phenotypic tests, with MALDI-TOF MS or with molecular tests.

TREATMENT

- Multidrug resistance, defined as resistance to an antipseudomonal β-lactam AND an aminoglycosides AND fluoroquinolones is frequent and isolates resistant to all antipseudomonal antibiotics, is increasingly common.
- Combination therapy has been more controversial in treating fully susceptible *P. aeruginosa*, failing to improve survival in bacteraemia or affect outcome in VAP.
- Most common sources of *P. aeruginosa* bloodstream infections are respiratory tract, urinary tract and central venous catheter. Less commonly, skin and soft tissue (mainly seen in neutropenic patients, surgical site infections, burns and infected chronic ulcers).
- To lower the bacterial burden, bacterial burden and reduce risk of drug resistance, source control is essential: removal of catheters, drainage of abscess or even tracheostomy change.
- The nature of the resistance mechanism may undermine the use of combination therapy in *P. aeruginosa* infections, such as single efflux mutations affecting both β-lactams and fluoroquinolones. When resistance is mutational, meropenem and tobramycin are most likely to retain activity for the β-lactam and aminoglycoside classes compared to other β-lactam and aminoglycoside agents.
- For multidrug-resistant strains, combination therapy is the cornerstone of therapy on the basis that singularly resistant, and inactive antibiotics can obtain a synergistic or additive effect.
- Therapy for multidrug-resistant and pan-resistant strains of *P. aeruginosa* depends on the mechanism of resistance but largely encompasses colistin or an aminoglycoside in combination with an antipseudomonal β-lactam.

CLINICAL APPROACH

ANTIBIOTICS WITH ANTIPSEUDOMONAL ACTIVITY

- Oral/intravenous: ciprofloxacin or levofloxacin.
- Intravenous: aztreonam, piperacillin/tazobactam, ceftazidime, cefepime, meropenem, imipenem, gentamicin, tobramycin, amikacin, colistin and the newer cephalosporins ceftolozane/tazobactam and ceftazidime/avibactam.
- Inhaled: colistin, tobramycin.
- *Pseudomonas aeruginosa* has lower MICs for ciprofloxacin compared to levofloxacin. Levofloxacin on the other hand has better lung penetration.
- *Pseudomonas aeruginosa* is intrinsic resistant to tetracyclines, tigecycline, ertapenem. It is *in vitro* resistant to trimethoprim/sulfamethoxazole and chloramphenicol, but clinical success has been seen in patients with cystic fibrosis.
- Quinolones should be reserved for uncomplicated non-severe infections as *P. aeruginosa* rapidly develops resistance.

CLINICAL PEARL

Fosfomycin has *in vitro* activity against *P. aeruginosa* and is a potential oral alternative to quinolones for treatment of a urinary tract infection. However, no CLSI or EUCAST breakpoints exist.

TREATMENT APPROACH

- *First-line IV options*: Ceftazidime or piperacillin tazobactam
- *Oral stepdown*: Ciprofloxacin
- *For pneumonia and if second agent is needed*: Preferred options are tobramycin or amikacin

COMBINATION TREATMENT

Although the evidence for using combination therapy instead of monotherapy is conflicting, combination therapy may be preferred if:

- High bacterial burden
- Uncontrollable source
- Empirical treatment in setting of high antimicrobial resistance
- Major risk factors for drug resistance—recent antibiotic courses in past 3 months, recent hospital admissions (especially intensive care)

IF ON MONOTHERAPY

- If clinically and biochemically improving, continue monotherapy
- Only start second agent if the patient starts to deteriorate
- If the patient is stable but there is no clinical response to monotherapy, review original diagnosis, perform MIC testing if possible, investigate source control and carefully consider adding a second agent

SOURCE CONTROL

- Debridement of necrotic lesions
- Drainage of collections/abscesses
- Removal of urinary catheters or intravascular catheters
- Tracheostomy changes

TOPICAL TREATMENT

Superficial wound infections have a yellow or green colour with a malodorous smell. Superficial wound infections generally do not require systemic antibiotic treatment. Alternatively, dressings containing 1% acetic acid are highly effective against *P. aeruginosa* wound infections.

DURATION OF TREATMENT

- Hospital-acquired pneumonia including VAP and UTI: 7 days
- Intra-abdominal source: up to 7 days after source control
- Exacerbation bronchiectasis: 14 days

AEROSOLIZED TREATMENT

Aerosolized treatment is often used in patients with chronic lung disease such as cystic fibrosis. Main indications are eradication of *Pseudomonas aeruginosa* and suppression of chronic infection. Aerosolized treatment has also been used as an adjunct to systemic infection in severe respiratory infections in other populations such as critically ill patients. Main agents used for aerosolized treatment are colistin, tobramycin and aztreonam. Bronchospasm can occur as a side effect.

DETECTION OF ECTHYMA GANGRENOSUM

Collection of blood cultures, culture of exudates from an aspirate or skin biopsy should be performed and sent to the microbiology laboratory for culture.

BIBLIOGRAPHY

Bassetti M, Vena A, Croxatto A, Righi E, Guery B. How to manage *Pseudomonas aeruginosa* infections. *Drugs in Context*. 2018;7:212527.

Lister PD, Wolter DJ, Hanson ND. Antibacterial-Resistant *Pseudomonas aeruginosa*: Clinical Impact and Complex Regulation of Chromosomally Encoded Resistance Mechanisms. *Clin Microbiol Rev*. 2009 October;22(4):582–610.

Mesaros N, Nordmann P, Plésiat P et al. *Pseudomonas aeruginosa*: Resistance and therapeutic options at the turn of the new millennium. *Clin Microbiol Infect*. 2007 June;13(6):560–578. Epub 2007 January 31.

Nagoba BS, Selkar SP, Wadher BJ, Gandhi RC. Acetic acid treatment of pseudomonal wound infections—A review. *J Infect Public Health*. 2013 December;6(6):410–415.

Strateva T, Yordanov D. *Pseudomonas aeruginosa* – A phenomenon of bacterial resistance. *J Med Microbiol*. 2009 September;58(Pt 9):1133–1148.

5.5 *Stenotrophomonas maltophilia*

Firza Alexander Gronthoud

CLINICAL CONSIDERATIONS

Stenotrophomonas maltophilia is a low-virulent, non-fermenting Gram-negative rod. It is found in the environment, mainly in water and soil. When found in screening and clinical cultures, it often represents colonization. Particularly in immunocompromised patients and patients with underlying lung disease including cystic fibrosis, the presence in a culture may indicate infection. Because there are limited data on effective antimicrobial treatment of *S. maltophilia* and antimicrobial susceptibility testing is challenging, it is worthwhile to consider the following.

DIAGNOSIS IN THE LABORATORY

- Aerobic, glucose non-fermentative, weak oxidase-positive, Gram-negative bacillus.
- When isolated in clinical specimens, it often represents colonization initially.
- Like other non-fermenters (*Pseudomonas aeruginosa* and *Acinetobacter baumannii*), it is a low-virulent, opportunistic organism causing infection when host defence is compromised.

RISK FACTORS

- Hospitalized patients with indwelling intravascular catheters
- Ventilated patients in the ICU
- Immunocompromised patients
- Individuals with underlying pulmonary diseases
- Repeated and prolonged antibiotic courses

CLINICAL MANIFESTATIONS

It most commonly causes respiratory tract infections and bloodstream infections, but has also been isolated from patients with wound infections, soft tissue infections, urinary tract infections and even meningitis.

ANTIMICROBIAL RESISTANCE

Stenotrophomonas maltophilia has multiple resistance mechanisms conferring widespread antibiotic resistance: efflux pumps, altered membrane protein, chromosomal β-lactamase production, antibiotic modifying enzymes, point mutations in antibiotic target sites and changes in lipopolysaccharide (LPS). *Stenotrophomonas maltophilia* can also acquire resistance to trimethoprim/sulfamethoxazole through mobile genetic elements (integrons). *Stenotrophomonas maltophilia* can also undergo changes in penicillin binding protein 1 (PBP1), which coincides with hyperproduction of β-lactamase L1 and L2.

ANTIMICROBIAL AGENTS

Antimicrobials commonly used for treatment of *S. maltophilia* infections are trimethoprim/ sulfamethoxazole, minocycline, tigecycline, fluoroquinolones and ceftazidime.

The preferred treatment is trimethoprim/sulfamethoxazole. Fluoroquinolones may have similar activity compared to trimethoprim/sulfamethoxazole, with levofloxacin and moxifloxacin more active than ciprofloxacin. *In vitro*, synergy between quinolones and β-lactams has been demonstrated.

Other antimicrobials that have been used in various combinations include ticarcillin/clavulanate, piperacillin/tazobactam, minocycline, tigecycline, colistin, chloramphenicol and ceftazidime. Minocycline is *in vitro* more potent than doxycycline. No clinical breakpoints exist for tigecycline.

ANTIMICROBIAL SUSCEPTIBILITY TESTING

Susceptibility test results for agents other than trimethoprim/sulfamethoxazole should be treated with caution as there are no data to support a relationship between susceptibility testing results and clinical outcome with *S. maltophilia* infection. Susceptibility testing of trimethoprim/sulfamethoxazole is more reproducible than antibiotics. When interpreting trimethoprim/sulfamethoxazole disk diffusion, faint growth within the zone of inhibitions should be ignored and only the clear edge of inhibition should be measured. EUCAST has only clinical breakpoints for trimethoprim/sulfamethoxazole, whereas CLSI has additional clinical breakpoints for commonly used antibiotics including ceftazidime, minocycline, fluoroquinolones, piperacillin/tazobactam, ticarcillin/clavulanate, aztreonam, imipenem and meropenem (see CLSI M100 29th edition supplement for a full overview of all antimicrobials).

CLINICAL APPROACH

Stenotrophomonas maltophilia usually initially represents colonization and should not be treated in the first instance, unless it is isolated from a sterile culture such as a blood culture.

Antibiotic courses in patients colonized with *S. maltophilia* should be as short as possible to avoid selection of *S. maltophilia* and increasing likelihood of subsequent infection.

The main treatment option is trimethoprim/sulfamethoxazole 960 mg 12-hourly or increased to 1440 mg 12-hourly if necessary. The main side effects are hyperkalaemia, nephrotoxicity, myelosuppression, rash and on rare occasions Stevens–Johnson syndrome.

Second-line treatment consists of combinations of levofloxacin, minocycline or tigecycline, ceftazidime and meropenem if *in vitro* sensitive. Colistin and aztreonam have also been used.

BIBLIOGRAPHY

Abbott IJ, Peleg AY. Stenotrophomonas, Achromobacter, and Nonmelioid Burkholderia Species: Antimicrobial Resistance and Therapeutic Strategies. *Semin Respir Crit Care Med*. 2015 February;36(1):99–110.

Adegoke AA, Stenström TA, Okoh AI. Stenotrophomonas maltophilia as an Emerging Ubiquitous Pathogen: Looking Beyond Contemporary Antibiotic Therapy. *Front Microbiol*. 2017 November 30;8:2276.

Chang YT, Lin CY, Chen YH, Hsueh PR. Update on infections caused by *Stenotrophomonas maltophilia* with particular attention to resistance mechanisms and therapeutic options. *Front Microbiol*. 2015 September 2;6:893.

CLSI. *Performance Standards for Antimicrobial Susceptibility Testing*, 29th ed. CLSI supplement M100. Wayne, PA: Clinical and Laboratory Standards Institute, 2019.

5.6 *Staphylococcus aureus*

Firza Alexander Gronthoud

CLINICAL CONSIDERATIONS

Staphylococcus aureus is one of the most common causes of community-acquired and hospital-acquired infections. *Staphylococcus aureus* infections can be caused by a methicillin-sensitive *S. aureus* (MSSA) or a methicillin-resistant *S. aureus* (MRSA). Methicillin-sensitive *Staphylococcus aureus* is a commensal organism on the skin, and one-third of the population carries MSSA in the nose. Shortly after introduction of penicillin in the 1950s, MRSA emerged, which is causing more than half of all hospital-acquired *S. aureus* infections in some countries. MRSA is often multi-resistant, limiting treatment options. Both MSSA and MRSA can cause significant morbidity and mortality. It is therefore worthwhile to consider the following.

RESISTANCE MECHANISMS

More than 80% of all *Staphylococcus aureus* isolates produce a penicillinase that is active against penicillin and amoxicillin. Semisynthetic penicillin like methicillin, oxacillin, nafcillin and flucloxacillin are not affected by this β-lactamase enzyme. Semisynthetic penicillins like flucloxacillin are the drug of choice for treatment of MSSA infections. Amoxicillin/clavulanic acid, cephalosporins (except ceftazidime) and carbapenem are other β-lactams active against penicillinase producing MSSA.

Methicillin-resistant *S. aureus* has a PBP2a instead of a PBP2 in its cell wall. This confers resistance to almost all β-lactams including the semisynthetic penicillins, cephalosporins and carbapenems. PBP2a is encoded by the *mecA* gene. The *mecA* gene is located in mobile genetic element called staphylococcal cassette chromosome *mec* (SCC*mec*). SCC*mec* also frequently contains resistance genes to other antibiotics including macrolides, clindamycin and tetracycline. MRSA can spread SCC*mec* to MSSA through horizontal gene transfer.

CLINICAL PEARL

Penicillin binding protein (PBP) is an enzyme which catalyzes the cross-linking of the peptidoglycan layer, which makes up the bacterial cell wall and is the target of β-lactam agents. Most β-lactams can only bind to PBP2 but not PBP2a. In recent years, two fifth-generation cephalosporins have been developed with activity against MRSA by binding to PBP2a: ceftaroline fosamil and ceftobiprole.

Some MSSA strains are penicillinase hyperproducers and have a reduced *in vitro* susceptibility to semisynthetic penicillins. These strains are called borderline oxacillin-resistant *Staphylococcus aureus*, or BORSA. Oxacillin is used in the microbiology laboratory as a marker for susceptibility to semisynthetic penicillin. Clinically, however, semisynthetic penicillins remain effective against BORSA infections.

Finally, penicillin-tolerant *S. aureus* strains have been isolated. Due to a missing autolytic enzyme, they are reduced susceptible to penicillins.

CLINICAL PEARL

Staphylococcus lugdunensis, is a *Staphylococcus* with virulence properties similar to *S. aureus* and causes similar infections. Most *S. lugdunensis* are susceptible to penicillin G. *Staphylococcus lugdunensis* has bound coagulase enzyme but not unbound. It may therefore cause false-positive results with coagulase latex agglutinations tests but not with plasma coagulase tube tests.

VIRULENCE FACTORS

Staphylococcus aureus produces bound or free coagulase, which converts fibrinogen to fibrin, providing protection from phagocytes and enables *S. aureus* to form septic emboli and disseminate to other organs. It further prevents phagocytosis. *Staphylococcus aureus* can also produce several toxins which are associated with specific clinical syndromes. Examples are:

- Toxic shock syndrome toxin-1 (TSST-1) causing toxic shock syndrome characterized by fever, diarrhoea, shock, multiorgan failure and a scarlatiniform rash which desquamates. Blood cultures are almost always negative.
- Exfoliative toxin damages the epidermis, causing generalized skin desquamation, also known as scalded skin syndrome.
- Panton–Valentine leucocidin lyses white blood cells; is associated with recurrent skin boils and abscesses and necrotizing pneumonia.
- Enterotoxin causes food poisoning.

LABORATORY TESTING

Staphylococcus aureus grows aerobically and anaerobically and produces β-haemolytic colonies with a yellow pigment. Mannitol salt agar is a selective medium for *S. aureus* containing a high salt concentration. Coagulase testing used to be the main test to differentiate between *S. aureus* and coagulase-negative staphylococci, but nowadays MALDI-TOF MS is increasingly being used as it provides a rapid and accurate identification within 5 minutes.

A *Staphylococcus aureus* resistant to cefoxitin and oxacillin is highly indicative of MRSA. This can be confirmed with a rapid PBP2a agglutination test or using molecular techniques.

Several other methods exist for detection of MRSA:

- Chromogenic MRSA agar plates can be used where potential MRSA colonies have a green colour. This should be followed up by a confirmatory identification test, i.e. MALDI-ToF and antimicrobial sensitivity testing. In addition, a PBP2a agglutination test can be performed as well.
- Alternatively, PCR can be performed on nose, throat, axilla and groin swabs. PCR can provide a same day result and is highly sensitive. Limitations are that it is more expensive, it does not provide any antimicrobial sensitivities and some MRSA strains are missed with PCR.

CLINICAL PEARL

Staphylococcus aureus is very rarely a blood culture contaminant and all patients with a positive blood culture should be assumed to have a true bacteraemia.

CLINICAL MANIFESTATIONS

- Parotitis
- *Heart:* Pericarditis, endocarditis
- *Soft tissue:* Furuncles, carbuncles, abscesses, cellulitis
- *Respiratory tract:* Pneumonia which may be complicated by empyema; necrotizing pneumonia associated with PVL-producing *S. aureus*
- *Bone and joint:* Spondylodiscitis, epidural abscess, osteomyelitis, septic arthritis, septic bursitis
- *Central nervous system:* Brain abscess, neurosurgical CNS infections
- *Urinary tract:* In the absence of a bladder catheter or ureteric stents, *S. aureus* rarely causes a urinary tract infection

CLINICAL APPROACH

SIGNIFICANCE OF POSITIVE URINE SAMPLES

Urine cultures may grow *S. aureus* in bloodstream infections owing to the high bacterial load. *S. aureus* rarely causes UTI in the absence of a catheter. An MSU growing *S. aureus* should therefore raise suspicion of a systemic infection.

DIAGNOSTIC WORK-UP BLOODSTREAM INFECTION

Because of the high risk of septic emboli, systemic dissemination to other organs should be excluded in patients with a bloodstream infection with *S. aureus*. The following work-up should be routinely performed in *S. aureus* bloodstream infections.

Thorough physical examination to look for signs of endocarditis (skin and nails should be inspected for presence of splinter haemorrhages, Janeway lesions or Osler's node and fundoscopy to look for Roth spots) and back pain which may be indicative of spondylodiscitis. Back pain can be elicited by pressing on both shoulders thereby compressing any infected discs.

Painful, swollen and tender joints are compatible with septic arthritis and pain in extremities indicative of osteomyelitis. As *S. aureus* is a skin colonizer, a thorough examination of the skin is indicated. Headache or any other neurological symptoms should prompt for a CT with contrast or MRI to rule out brain involvement. An echocardiography should be performed to rule out endocarditis. A negative transthoracic echocardiography does not rule out endocarditis.

Blood cultures should be collected after 72 hours of therapy. Positive blood cultures at 72 hours are associated with a worse prognosis. Retention of intravascular devices is associated with increased mortality, and removal is indicated.

Uncomplicated bloodstream infection is defined as a negative-result blood culture and afebrile after 72 hours, no signs and symptoms of metastatic infection and no other foreign bodies involved.

Complicated bloodstream infection is defined as persistent positive blood cultures or fever after 72 hours, persistent source of infection or signs of systemic dissemination, for example septic emboli to skin or other organs.

Community-acquired bloodstream infection could also be regarded as a complicated *S. aureus* infection because of a longer duration of bacteraemia until presentation in the hospital and therefore increased likelihood of systemic dissemination.

MANAGEMENT OF BLOODSTREAM INFECTION

Management of uncomplicated bloodstream infections consists of intravenous therapy for 14 days from the first negative blood culture. There is emerging literature that suggests, for uncomplicated

MSSA bloodstream infections, an oral stepdown with clindamycin or linezolid may be considered after 7 days of intravenous antibiotics; however, this should be decided on an individual case-by-case basis. Duration of complicated bloodstream infection is 4–6 weeks of intravenous therapy. The first-line option for MSSA is IV flucloxacillin. In case of penicillin allergy, ceftriaxone, vancomycin or daptomycin may be considered. It should be noted that vancomycin is inferior to β-lactams for MSSA bloodstream infections. First-line options for MRSA are vancomycin or daptomycin.

Source Control

In the presence of bloodstream infections, retention of infected foreign bodies is associated with increased mortality rate and removal is indicated. Soft tissue infections with abscesses require drainage, and similarly, the mainstay of treatment of pleural empyema and iliopsoas abscess is drainage.

General Antibiotic Options for Staphylococcus aureus Infections

Benzylpenicillin is more active than flucloxacillin against penicillin-sensitive MSSA strains. However, most MSSA strains are penicillin resistant, and especially in soft tissue infections, multiple MSSA strains may be involved, some of which are penicillin resistant and may be missed in the laboratory. Flucloxacillin therefore remains the first-line option for MSSA infections. It must be noted that the oral absorption of flucloxacillin varies per individual and higher doses or switching to another agent may be advised.

Cephalosporins are also active against MSSA and are used in case of penicillin allergy. Ceftriaxone is often used for intravenous outpatient or ambulatory therapy of MSSA infections. Cefotaxime is preferred over ceftriaxone for CNS infections owing to lower MICs and better CNS penetration. A limitation of cefotaxime is it is administered 6 times a day.

Alternative intravenous options are glycopeptides, but they are inferior to β-lactams for bloodstream infections. For non-severe infections, a vancomycin pre-dose level between 10 and 15 mg/L may be sufficient. For severe infections or if the vancomycin MIC is between 1 and 2 mg/L, then a higher pre-dose level of 15–20 mg/L should be used. Teicoplanin is another glycopeptide which initially needs three loading doses, after which it is administered once a day intravenously and is used as an alternative to ceftriaxone for outpatient therapy. Although teicoplanin less often causes adverse events compared to vancomycin, it is still recommended to perform trough levels, especially in severe infections. For severe infections, a trough level between 20 and 40 mg/L should be the goal. Teicoplanin should not be used as initial treatment for severe infections including bloodstream infections because of the loading time.

Alternative intravenous options are daptomycin and linezolid.

General oral treatment options for MSSA and MRSA are clarithromycin, clindamycin, doxycycline and linezolid. Ciprofloxacin, rifampicin and fusidic acid should never be given as monotherapy because resistance develops quickly.

All patients with a spondylodiscitis, epidural abscess, septic arthritis, osteomyelitis or brain abscess should have multiple sets of blood cultures collected and undergo a full bloodstream infection work-up.

CLINICAL PEARL

Flucloxacillin has poor penetration in necrotic tissue. There is some concern that subtherapeutic flucloxacillin concentration drives up PVL production. Therefore, for necrotizing pneumonia, alternative agents should be used, preferably in combination: vancomycin, linezolid, clindamycin and rifampicin.

DECOLONIZATION TREATMENT

Decolonization treatment for MRSA carriers is a method commonly used to eradicate MRSA. Countries have different indications for MRSA-decolonization treatment. This may also depend on local MRSA carrier rates. Decolonization treatment actually suppresses the MRSA bacterial load to undetectable levels rather than eradicate MRSA and recurrences do occur. This may also depend on adherence to decolonization protocols as well as pets and household members who may be colonized as well.

Decolonization treatment consists of nasal mupirocin or chlorhexidine (for nasal carriers) for 5–7 days, in combination with a body wash containing either chlorhexidine or octenidine and daily changes of bedsheets and towels.

Wounds and eczema significantly reduce the success rate and, in these instances, systemic treatment with a combination of two oral antibiotics may be attempted. These antibiotics are usually any combination of doxycycline, clindamycin, rifampicin, trimethoprim/sulfamethoxazole and fusidic acid.

BIBLIOGRAPHY

Corey GR. *Staphylococcus aureus* bloodstream infections: Definitions and treatment. *Clin Infect Dis.* 2009 May 15;48(Suppl 4):S254–S259.

del Rio A, Cervera C, Moreno A, Moreillon P, Miró JM. Patients at risk of complications of *Staphylococcus aureus* bloodstream infection. *Clin Infect Dis.* 2009 May 15;48(Suppl 4):S246–S253.

Dijkmans AC, Hartigh Jd, van Dissel JT, Burggraaf J. A simplified oral flucloxacillin absorption test for patients requiring long-term treatment. *Ther Drug Monit.* 2012 June;34(3):356–358.

Holland TL, Arnold C, Fowler VG Jr. Clinical management of *Staphylococcus aureus* bacteremia: A review. *JAMA.* 2014 October 1;312(13):1330–1341.

Itoh N, Hadano Y, Saito S, Myokai M, Nakamura Y, Kurai H. Intravenous to oral switch therapy in cancer patients with catheter-related bloodstream infection due to methicillin-sensitive *Staphylococcus aureus*: A single-center retrospective observational study. *PLOS ONE.* 2018 November 29;13(11):e0207413.

Mitchell DH, Howden BP. Diagnosis and management of *Staphylococcus aureus* bacteraemia. *Intern Med J.* 2005 December;35(Suppl 2):S17–S24.

Thwaites GE, Edgeworth JD, Gkrania-Klotsas E, Kirby A, Tilley R, Török ME, Walker S, Wertheim HF, Wilson P, Llewelyn MJ. UK Clinical Infection Research Group. Clinical management of *Staphylococcus aureus* bacteraemia. *Lancet Infect Dis.* 2011 March;11(3):208–222.

Willekens R, Puig-Asensio M, Ruiz-Camps I et al. Early oral switch to linezolid for low-risk patients with staphylococcus aureus bloodstream infections: A propensity-matched cohort study. *Clin Infect Dis.* 2019;69(3):381–387.

5.7 Vancomycin-Resistant Enterococci

Firza Alexander Gronthoud

CLINICAL CONSIDERATIONS

Enterococci are part of the commensal gut flora. The clinically relevant enterococci which may cause infections are *Enterococcus faecium* and *Enterococcus faecalis* (see Chapter 2.1 for how commensal flora may cause disease). Commensal *Enterococcus faecium* and *E. faecalis* are sensitive to glycopeptides. Since the 1980s, vancomycin resistance is increasingly found in hospital-acquired infections caused by *E. faecium* and *E. faecalis*. They are referred to as vancomycin-resistant enterococci (VRE). Because the predominant VREs are also resistant to teicoplanin, another term used is glycopeptide-resistant enterococci. Although enterococci are low-virulent organisms, VRE infections have been associated with complicated treatment courses and increased mortality. Although this may in part be attributable to underlying medical conditions of patients who are at risk of VRE infections, it is worthwhile to consider the following.

POPULATION AT RISK FOR VRE COLONIZATION AND INFECTION

Frequent and prolonged hospital admission increases the likelihood that patients become colonized with VRE. VRE are low-virulent organisms, so it is not unsurprising that patients with breaches in physiological barriers or compromised immunity are at increased risk of progression from colonization to infection: for example, VRE infections have been well documented in liver transplant recipients, haematopoietic stem cell transplant recipients and surgical patients. Factors that further promote infection are chemotherapy-induced mucositis, neutropenia, intravascular devices, surgery and broad-spectrum antibiotics that can reduce the colonization resistance of the gut flora (see Chapter 1.1). It is important to realize that these risk factors are general infection risk factors, not specific to enterococci, and patients more often develop infections caused by Gram-negative bacteria.

TRANSMISSION AND COLONIZATION

Like commensal enterococci, VRE mainly colonize the gastrointestinal tract, but can also be found on the skin. Perhaps the latter is, in part, attributable to hygienic factors. It is therefore unsurprising that direct transmission occurs through contaminated hands of healthcare workers. VRE are indirectly transmitted by contaminated medical equipment and contaminated environment. In fact, VRE can be found in the environment for weeks to months. Finally, diarrhoea further increases transmission. Duration of carriage can be anywhere between weeks and years, with 3 years or longer described.

MECHANISM OF RESISTANCE

The two clinically most relevant glycopeptide resistance genes in VRE are *vanA* and *vanB*. These genes encode for structural changes in the cell wall preventing vancomycin and teicoplanin from binding to the cell wall. *VanA* is the dominant phenotype and confers high level resistance to vancomycin and teicoplanin whilst *vanB* is less prevalent and confers moderate to high level resistance to vancomycin but remains susceptible to teicoplanin. *VanB* is also found in other gut commensals such as some *Clostridium* species.

Enterococcus gallinarum and *Enterococcus casseliflavus* are normal inhabitants of the gut, and they are intrinsically resistant to vancomycin owing to *vanC*. They remain susceptible to teicoplanin. They are very-low-virulent organisms and will not be discussed in this chapter.

CLINICAL MANIFESTATIONS

Vancomycin-resistant enterococci are mainly associated with bloodstream infections and urinary tract infections, especially in the presence of intravascular devices or urinary catheters. Other infections that have been described are surgical site infections, intra-abdominal infections and neurosurgical infections. As applies to all enterococci, they very rarely cause respiratory tract infections, and their presence in respiratory samples should be regarded as colonization.

ANTIBIOTIC SUSCEPTIBILITY PATTERN OF VRE

- *Enterococcus faecalis*: Sensitive to nitrofurantoin, amoxicillin, piperacillin/tazobactam, tigecycline, daptomycin, linezolid
- *Enterococcus faecium*: Sensitive to nitrofurantoin, tigecycline, daptomycin, linezolid

LABORATORY DIAGNOSIS

VRE can be detected phenotypically with culture techniques or with PCR. Although PCR can provide a same-day result and has a higher sensitivity, it has a lower specificity for detecting *vanB* isolates because *vanB* is also present in other gut flora such as *Clostridium* spp. Chromogenic agar plates for VRE are commonly used in laboratories. Rectal swabs are the specimens used for surveillance, and visible stool on the swab increases culture sensitivity.

EUCAST does not have MIC breakpoint for enterococci and daptomycin. For *Enterococcus faecium*, CLSI has defined susceptible as an MIC of ≤4 mg/L, based on daptomycin 8–12 mg/kg once daily for serious infections. For *Enterococcus faecalis*, susceptible is defined by CLSI as an MIC of ≤2 mg/L, based on daptomycin 6 mg/kg once daily. *Enterococcus faecium* and *Enterococcus faecalis* isolates with a daptomycin MIC of ≥8 mg/L are considered resistant.

CLINICAL APPROACH

Enterococci are low-virulent organisms, and only a low proportion of patients colonized with VRE develop a VRE infection. For instance, in haematopoietic stem cell recipients, the VRE bloodstream infection rate in VRE-colonized patients is around 10%. Initial empirical treatment should therefore not differ between VRE and non-VRE colonized individuals, and local hospital antibiotic guidelines should be followed. Overuse of daptomycin and linezolid may also lead to increased antibiotic resistance rates in not only enterococci, but also staphylococci.

VRE BLOODSTREAM INFECTIONS

Main treatment options are daptomycin or linezolid. There are data that suggest that a daptomycin MIC of 3–4 mg/L is a risk factor for selection of resistant mutants. Therefore, for isolates with an MIC of 3–4 mg/kg, invasive infections such as endocarditis or high bacterial burden, a daptomycin dose of 10–12 mg/kg IV should be used to reduce risk of recurrence or emergence of resistance.

Linezolid is a bacteriostatic oxazolidinone antibiotic and may cause myelosuppression after 2–3 weeks of therapy. However, in haematopoietic stem cell transplant recipients, linezolid seems to show similar effectiveness as daptomycin and no significant myelosuppressive toxicity either. Linezolid can be administered intravenously and orally, whereas daptomycin is only available as an intravenous formulation.

Tigecycline should not be used for bloodstream infections or urinary tract infections because of the subtherapeutic concentration. Vancomycin-resistant *E. faecalis* can be treated with amoxicillin.

Uncomplicated cystitis can be treated with nitrofurantoin. Trimethoprim/sulfamethoxazole for treatment of UTI is less reliable, as recurrences have been described.

THE ROLE OF NEWER ANTIBIOTICS

Tedizolid is a newer oxazolidinone with a lower potential for development of resistance, but clinical data for VRE is lacking. Telavancin and dalbavancin are newer glycopeptides with activity against *vanB* isolates but not against the dominant *vanA* isolates. Similar to dalbavancin, oritavancin is another newer glycopeptide with a prolonged half-life allowing weekly doses. It has *in vitro* activity against *vanA* and *vanB* isolates, but clinical data are lacking.

SYNERGISM

Synergism between daptomycin and amoxicillin, rifampicin or fusidic acid has been described whereby a combination of daptomycin with amoxicillin may potentially decrease daptomycin MIC.

PREVENTING VRE TRANSMISSION AND INFECTION

The most effective methods are hand hygiene and antimicrobial stewardship. Restricting broad-spectrum antibiotics and metronidazole preserves the colonization resistance of the gut flora against multidrug-resistant organisms such as VRE, extended-spectrum β-lactamase producers and carbapenemase-producing organisms. Vancomycin, metronidazole and cephalosporins are commonly being associated with increasing risk of VRE colonization.

Patients with diarrhoea should be moved to a single room, not only to minimize environmental contamination but also because the diarrhoea could be attributable to *Clostridioides difficile* or norovirus, for example. Although there is increasing evidence that contact precautions do not reduce colonization and infection rates of VRE in endemic settings, local hospital policies should be followed and annually reviewed based on local epidemiology and literature studies. There is insufficient evidence to suggest that antibiotic prophylaxis with daptomycin or linezolid or fecal transplant reduces the infection rate in VRE-colonized patients.

SCREENING FOR VRE

Enterococci species, including VRE, are low-virulent organisms. Despite resistance to glycopeptides, several effective treatment options exist. Similar to a lack of evidence for contact precautions, the beneficial effect of rectal screening on carriage rate or infection rate is unclear. Institutions should perform a risk assessment for their setting to ascertain whether or not it is still cost-effective to continue VRE surveillance.

BIBLIOGRAPHY

Benamu E, Deresinski S. Vancomycin-Resistant *Enterococcus* Infection in the Hematopoietic Stem Cell Transplant Recipient: An Overview of Epidemiology, Management, and Prevention. Version 1. *F1000Res.* 2018;7:3. Published online 2018 January 2.
Britt NS, Potter EM, Patel N, Steed ME. Comparative Effectiveness and Safety of Standard-, Medium-, and High-Dose Daptomycin Strategies for the Treatment of Vancomycin-Resistant Enterococcal Bacteremia Among Veterans Affairs Patients. *Clin Infect Dis.* 2017 March 1;64(5):605–613.
Faron ML, Ledeboer NA, Buchan BW. Resistance Mechanisms, Epidemiology, and Approaches to Screening for Vancomycin- Resistant Enterococcus in the Health Care Setting. *J Clin Microbiol.* 2016 October; 54(10): 2436–2447. Prepublished online 2016 May 4. Published online 2016 September 23.
Martin EM, Bryant B, Grogan TR, Rubin ZA, Russell DL, Elashoff D, Uslan DZ. Noninfectious Hospital Adverse Events Decline After Elimination of Contact Precautions for MRSA and VRE. *Infect Control Hosp Epidemiol.* 2018 July;39(7):788–796.

5.8 *Helicobacter pylori*

Firza Alexander Gronthoud

CLINICAL CONSIDERATIONS

CLINICAL MANIFESTATIONS

Helicobacter pylori is a Gram-negative, microaerophilic bacterium, transmitted human to human and often acquired in childhood. Infection is chronic. Initially, the infection is asymptomatic but later on progresses to gastritis with development of a peptic ulcer disease, gastric cancer, mucosa-associated lymphoid tissue (MALT) lymphoma. *Helicobacter pylori* eradication cures gastritis and can alter the progression to long-term complications, or recurrence of disease.

OESOPHAGOGASTRODUODENOSCOPY

Oesophagogastroduodenoscopy (OGD) is indicated to rule out gastric cancer if the following alarm symptoms are present: weight loss, dysphagia, gastrointestinal bleeding, abdominal mass or iron-deficiency anaemia.

CLINICAL PEARL

Patients with thrombocytopaenia of unknown origin should be investigated for *Helicobacter pylori*, hepatitis B and hepatitis C.

MALTOMA

- Localized-stage gastric MALToma is strongly associated with *H. pylori* infection.
- In the early (Lugano I/II) stage, low-grade MALT lymphoma can be cured by *H. pylori* eradication in 60%–80% of cases.
- *H. pylori* eradication treatment is ineffective.
- Chemotherapy or radiotherapy is indicated if lymphoma t(11;18)/API2-MALT1 translocation is present or if no response or progression despite *H. pylori* eradication treatment.

INDICATION FOR TESTING

- In young patients with dyspepsia, it is recommended to test for *H. pylori* using a non-invasive strategy.
- In individuals at risk for gastric cancer, i.e. older adults, an OGD should be considered.

DIAGNOSIS

- UBT (urea breath test) is the most investigated and best recommended non-invasive test in the context of a 'test-and-treat strategy'.
- Monoclonal SAT (Stool Antigen Test) can also be used.
- Serology does not discriminate between past and active infection.
- UBT and SAT for confirmation of *H. pylori* eradication should be performed at least 4 weeks after completion of therapy.

- Proton-pump inhibitor (PPI) should be discontinued at least 2 weeks before testing for *H. pylori* infection.
- Antibiotics and bismuth compounds should be discontinued at least 4 weeks before performing UBT or SAT.
- H2 receptor antagonists have minimal effect on the sensitivity of UBT and SAT.
- If endoscopy is performed, a rapid urease test (RUT) on tissue sample can be performed.
- RUT should be performed 4 weeks after cessation of antibiotics or bismuth, and PPIs should be stopped at least 2 weeks prior to RUT.
- A negative result does not rule out *H. pylori* because of occurrence of false-negative results.
- False-positive results are rare and may be due to the presence of other urease-containing bacteria such as *Proteus mirabilis, Citrobacter freundii, Klebsiella pneumoniae, Enterobacter cloacae* and *Staphylococcus aureus*.
- Most cases of *H. pylori* infection can be diagnosed from gastric biopsies using histochemical staining.

MICROBIOLOGY TESTING

- After a first failure, if an endoscopy is carried out, antimicrobial susceptibility testing (AST) should be considered in all regions before giving a second-line treatment, because the chance of having a resistant organism is high, in the range of 60%–70% for clarithromycin.
- A gastric biopsy allows culture and AST of clarithromycin, levofloxacin, metronidazole, rifamycin and eventually amoxicillin and tetracycline.
- The correlation between AST performed by culture and antibiogram versus a molecular test, essentially real-time PCR, is not perfect.
- If bismuth-based quadruple therapy is used as second-line treatment, AST does not necessarily need to be performed because of low tetracycline resistance, and metronidazole resistance can be overcome by using higher doses.
- *H. pylori* eradication results in significant improvement of gastritis and gastric atrophy but not of intestinal metaplasia.
- Factors affecting treatment effectiveness:
  - Development of resistance during treatment.
  - Inoculum effect.
  - Protective effect gastric mucus layer.
  - Intracellular location bacteria.
  - Subpopulation of resistant strains.
  - Compliance to treatment.
  - Age <60 years, type of gastritis, presence of non-ulcer dyspepsia, CYP 2C19 polymorphisms (affecting proton pump inhibitor [PPI] metabolism), smoking and increased body mass index.
  - But most importantly, compliance, high gastric acidity, high bacterial load and bacterial strains, but the most important is the increase in *H. pylori* resistance to clarithromycin.
- There is increased resistance to clarithromycin and metronidazole. Resistance to amoxicillin is rare.

TREATMENT

- Clarithromycin should not be used if local resistance rate is higher than 15%.
- It may take 6 months or longer before symptoms improve.
- *H. pylori* can resist antibiotic therapy through
  - Shelter from antibiotics through biofilm formation and invasion of gastric cells.
  - High bacterial load increases likelihood of subpopulations of resistant strains.

- Most antibiotics are less active in the acid environment of the stomache, and the use of PPI increases antibiotic activity.
- *In vitro* susceptibility therefore does not correlate directly with *in vivo* effectiveness.
- Antibiotics used are clarithromycin, amoxicillin, metronidazole, tetracycline, levofloxacin, furazolidone and bismuth.
- Worldwide resistance is often a problem with metronidazole, macrolides (e.g. clarithromycin) and fluoroquinolones (e.g. levofloxacin).
- Metronidazole resistance can be overcome by increasing the dose to 1500 mg or more and increasing duration of therapy from 10 to 14 days.
- Increasing the pH to approximately 6 will trigger the bacteria to enter in a replicative state and become phenotypically susceptible to antibiotics effective with replicating organisms.

CLINICAL APPROACH

- PPI treatment should be continued after successful eradication in patients who receive NSAIDs, coxibs or even low-dose aspirin after a peptic ulcer bleeding event.
- Testing for *H. pylori* should be performed in aspirin and NSAID users with a history of peptic ulcer.

FIRST-LINE EMPIRICAL THERAPY

- Clarithromycin 500 mg 12-hourly PLUS amoxicillin 1 g 12-hourly PLUS a PPI (40 mg esomeprazole equivalent per dose) for 14 days.
- Clarithromycin 500 mg 12-hourly PLUS a nitroimidazole (tinidazole 500 mg 12-hourly or metronidazole 500 mg 8-hourly) plus a PPI (40 mg esomeprazole equivalent per dose) for 14 days.

If first-line treatment fails, preferably an OGD should be performed for culture and antimicrobial susceptibility testing, after which targeted treatment can be started.

If either local clarithromycin resistance rate >15% or first-line treatment fails and OGD is not performed, then second-line empirical therapy options are:

- *First option: Bismuth quadruple therapy*—Bismuth subsalicylate or bismuth subcitrate two tablets and tetracycline hydrochloride (500 mg) both 4 times daily with meals and at bedtime plus metronidazole/tinidazole (500 mg) 3 times daily with meals and a PPI twice daily for 14 days.
- *Second option: Quinolone-based therapy*—Standard dose PPI, levofloxacin 500 mg and amoxicillin 1 g, all 12-hourly for 10 days.
- *Alternative options:*
  - Quadruple regimen (PPI, amoxicillin, quinolone and bismuth).
  - Concomitant therapy amoxicillin, clarithromycin and metronidazole) PLUS a PPI, all twice daily for 10–14 days.
  - *Sequential therapy:* PPI plus amoxicillin for the first 5 days followed by a triple regimen including a PPI, clarithromycin and a nitroimidazole (metronidazole or tinidazole) for the following 5 days.
  - *Hybrid therapy (efficacy unclear):* A 7-day dual therapy with a PPI (standard dose 12-hourly) and amoxicillin (1 g 12-hourly) followed by a 7-day quadruple therapy with a PPI (standard dose BID), amoxicillin (1 g 12-hourly), clarithromycin (500 mg 12-hourly) and metronidazole (500 mg 12-hourly).

An advantage of concomitant therapy versus sequential therapy is efficacy against dual-resistant (clarithromycin and metronidazole) strains where the sequential therapy is reportedly more likely to fail.

TARGETED TREATMENT (IF ANTIMICROBIAL SUSCEPTIBILITIES ARE KNOWN)

- *Clarithromycin sensitive:* Amoxicillin (1 g) and clarithromycin (500 mg) plus a PPI all given twice daily for 14 days (40 mg esomeprazole equivalent per dose).
- *Metronidazole sensitive:* Amoxicillin (1 g) and tinidazole (500 mg) or metronidazole (500 mg) plus a PPI all given twice daily for 14 days (40 mg esomeprazole equivalent per dose).
- *Fluoroquinolone sensitive:* Fluoroquinolone (e.g. levofloxacin 500 mg once daily), plus a PPI and amoxicillin 1 g twice daily for 14 days (40 mg esomeprazole equivalent per dose).
- *If allergic to penicillin:* Clarithromycin (500 mg), and tinidazole (500 mg) or metronidazole (500 mg) plus a PPI (40 mg esomeprazole equivalent per dose) all given twice daily for 14 days.

CLINICAL PEARL

Antibiotic-susceptibility testing should be carried out after two consecutive treatment failures to determine optimal combination treatment.

SALVAGE THERAPY (EMPIRIC SALVAGE THERAPY AFTER TWO OR MORE FAILURES WITH DIFFERENT DRUGS)

- Furazolidone quadruple therapy with tetracycline
  - Bismuth subsalicylate or bismuth subcitrate two tablets and tetracycline hydrochloride (500 mg) both 4 times daily with meals and at bedtime plus furazolidone 100 mg 8-hourly with meals and PPI twice daily for 14 days.
  - Furazolidone quadruple therapy with amoxicillin Bismuth subsalicylate or bismuth subcitrate two tablets 4 times daily with meals and at bedtime plus furazolidone 100 mg and amoxicillin 1 g 8-hourly, with meals plus a PPI twice daily for 14 days.
- Rifabutin therapies
  - Rifabutin (150 mg once or twice daily), amoxicillin (1.5 g), and esomeprazole 40 mg (or an equivalent PPI) every 8 h for 14 days.
  - Rifabutin 150 mg, amoxicillin 1 g, bismuth subcitrate or subsalicylate two tablets, a PPI all twice daily for 14 days.
- High-dose PPI–amoxicillin dual therapy
  - PPI (e.g. rabeprazole 20 mg, esomeprazole 40 mg) plus amoxicillin (500–750 mg) all 4 times daily at approximately 6 h intervals for 14 days (can use 8-h interval at night) (effective for CYP2C19 poor metabolizers).

CONFIRMATION OF SUCCESSFUL ERADICATION

Eradication can be confirmed via UBT or SAT at least 4 weeks after completion of therapy.

BIBLIOGRAPHY

Georgopoulos SD, Papastergiou V, Karatapanis S. Current options for the treatment of *Helicobacter pylori*. *Expert Opin Pharmacother.* 2013 February;14(2):211–223.

Graham DY, Dore MP. *Helicobacter pylori* therapy: A paradigm shift. *Expert Rev Anti Infect Ther.* 2016 June;14(6):577–585.

Malfertheiner P, Megraud F, O'Morain CA et al. El-Omar EM; European *Helicobacter* and Microbiota Study Group and Consensus panel. Management of *Helicobacter pylori* infection—the Maastricht V/Florence Consensus Report. *Gut.* 2017 January;66(1):6–30.

5.9 *Clostridioides difficile*

Firza Alexander Gronthoud

CLINICAL CONSIDERATIONS

Clostridium difficile, or now classified as *Clostridioides difficile*, is the most common cause of hospital-acquired diarrhoea, has high relapse rates of 20% and differentiation between colonization and disease can be challenging. It is therefore worthwhile to consider the following.

DIAGNOSIS

Diagnosing *Clostridium difficile* infection (CDI) is challenging as the presence of toxins or a toxin-producing strain does not necessarily indicate infection. The diagnosis is based on a combination of clinical picture, presence of *C. difficile* and free toxins in the stool in the absence of other causes of diarrhoea OR evidence of pseudomembranous colitis. Diarrhoea is often defined as three or more stools per day, taking the shape of their container OR Bristol stool chart types 5–7.

LABORATORY TESTS

Diagnostic tests for *C. difficile* include detection of glutamate dehydrogenase (GDH), which is an enzyme produced by *C. difficile*, detection of toxin A and B (Tox A/B) or a nucleic acid amplification test (NAAT) for detection of the toxin gene. Reference tests are toxigenic culture or cytotoxin assay. These tests require specialized laboratories and are time consuming. A positive GDH EIA alone will only tell you that the patient is colonized with *C. difficile*.

The GDH and PCR are the most sensitive tests with the toxin A/B EIAs being less sensitive but more specific, as they will only detect those samples with free toxin present.

PCR, on the other hand, is less specific as detection of the toxin genes does not necessarily mean the strain is producing toxins. Finally, it is important to be aware of the local prevalence, as this has an impact on the predictive value and thus clinical utility of the assays.

C. DIFFICILE IN INFANTS

Asymptomatic *C. difficile* carriage in children 1–2 years old is common and the presence of toxin-producing strains in the stools of children aged 1–2 years represents colonization.

Children up to 1–2 years do not have toxin receptors in their immature gut mucosa.

SEVERE DISEASE AND COMPLICATIONS OF C. DIFFICILE

There are no official definitions for severe disease. Parameters used to asses increased risk of developing severe disease include leucocytosis >15,000 cells/mm³, serum creatinine >1.5 times the premorbid level or decreased albumin <30 g/L, age ≥65 years, severe underlying comorbidity (DM, cardiovascular, respiratory and kidney disease, malignancy), immunodeficiency and admission to the ICU. Infection with ribotypes 027 and 079 are associated with severe disease. Individuals with an inability to mount an adequate humoral immune response (e.g. patients on rituximab) or individuals with low levels of anti-toxin antibodies (e.g. elderly patients) may also be at risk of severe disease or a more protracted course. Complications of CDI are hypotension, shock, ileus or megacolon.

Recurrence

A first episode of CDI is complicated by a recurrence in 30% of the cases. Recurrence is defined as recurrent symptoms within 8 weeks after the onset of a previous successfully treated episode, caused by either a relapse or reinfection with a new isolate. Prognostic markers for increased risk of recurrence include age ≥65 years, use of antibacterial agents after diagnosis of CDI and/or after CDI treatment, history of previous CDI and severe comorbidities.

Antibiotic Treatment

Antibiotic treatment is successful if there is no diarrhoea for two consecutive days. The three main drugs used are oral metronidazole, oral vancomycin and oral fidaxomicin. Metronidazole is cheap and was the drug of choice for non-severe CDI. However, because it reaches low luminal concentrations and has been shown to be inferior to vancomycin, it is no longer first-line treatment for non-severe CDI. Oral vancomycin reaches high luminal concentrations and induces rapid suppression of *C. difficile* to undetectable levels during therapy and faster resolution of diarrhoea compared to metronidazole. Vancomycin orally and metronidazole are both broad-spectrum agents that may lead to significant disruption of the commensal colonic microbiota and reducing colonization resistance (see Chapter 1.1).

Fidaxomicin is a newer narrow-spectrum macrocyclic antibacterial that is only active against Gram-positive bacteria, in particular *C. difficile*. It is poorly absorbed from the gastrointestinal tract and is licensed for the treatment of CDI with a treatment duration of 10 days. It has a significant lower recurrence rate compared to metronidazole and vancomycin. Its effectiveness for treatment of severe CDI needs further research.

Treatment Response

A daily stool chart should be kept to document stool frequency and stool consistency. In addition, clinical parameters such as temperature, WBC and albumin and, if indicated, an abdominal X-ray.

Treatment response should be observed daily and evaluated after at least 3 days as it can take 3–5 days before clinical response occurs (in particular with metronidazole). Even with successful treatment, it can take weeks for stool consistency and frequency to normalize.

Sustained cure is defined as initial clinical cure of the baseline episode of CDI and no recurrent infection through 12 weeks of follow-up.

CLINICAL PEARL

The detection of either *C. difficile tcdB* gene or GDH in combination with a negative toxin test likely indicates asymptomatic colonization.

CLINICAL APPROACH

Diagnostic Algorithm

Preferably a two- or three-stage algorithm is performed to diagnose *C. difficile disease*, in which a positive first test is confirmed with one or two confirmatory tests. No single test is suitable to be used as a stand-alone test. This first test should have a high negative predictive value.

Antibiotic Treatment of a First Episode

For non-severe CDI cases in non-epidemic situations where CDI likely is induced by antibiotics, withdrawal of the initiating antibiotic can be tried first. If antibiotic treatment is still needed after

48 hours monitoring, vancomycin 125 mg 6-hourly PO for 10 days can be started. In patients with high risk factors for relapse, fidaxomicin 200 mg 12-hourly PO for 10 days can be used as first-line option.

For severe CDI cases, first-line treatment is vancomycin 125 mg 6-hourly PO for 10 days. In case of ileus, higher doses up to 500 mg 6-hourly PO can be tried.

ANTIBIOTIC TREATMENT OF RECURRENT INFECTION

For a first recurrent infection, vancomycin 125 mg 6-hourly PO for 10 days can be used again or fidaxomicin 200 mg 12-hourly for 10 days. In case of multiple recurrences, use either vancomycin 125 mg 6-hourly PO for 10 days followed by a pulsed regimen (125–500 mg/day every 2–3 days for at least 3 weeks) or followed by tapered regimen (gradually decreasing the dose to 125 mg per day). Alternatively, fidaxomicin 200 mg 12-hourly for 10 days may be used.

ALTERNATIVE REGIMENS

Bezlotoxumab is a monoclonal antibody which blocks toxin B. In combination with standard antibiotic treatment, it has been shown to significantly reduce the rate of recurrence. Currently more studies are needed to investigate the optimal role and indication for use. Bezlotoxumab may increase risk of congestive heart failure.

Fecal transplant has been shown to be effective in treating multiple recurrent CDI.

Metronidazole remains the only parenteral antibiotic therapy supported by case series. Intravenous metronidazole (500 mg intravenous three times daily) may be added to oral vancomycin, if the patient has ileus or significant abdominal distension.

Intracolonic instillation of vancomycin could be cautiously tried but its effectiveness is unknown. When oral treatment is not possible, intravenous metronidazole should be used and can be combined with intracolonic (vancomycin retention enema 500 mg in 100 mL normal saline four times daily intracolonic) or nasogastric administration of vancomycin.

CLINICAL PEARL

In limited case studies, oral teicoplanin showed significantly better bacteriological cure compared to vancomycin and was borderline superior in terms of symptomatic cure, but the quality of the evidence is very low and further research is needed.

ROLE OF SURGERY

Surgical intervention is indicated in patients in whom there is no response to antibiotic treatment, septic shock, toxic megacolon or bowel perforation. Early colectomy is associated with improved survival with septic shock, increased serum lactate ($\geq$5 mM), mental status changes, end organ failure and renal failure, and the need for preoperative intubation and ventilation are independent risk factors for mortality.

PREVENTION

Patients should be isolated in a side room with strict precautions (gloves and gowns) until 48 hours after diarrhoea has settled. Hand hygiene should be performed with water and soap instead of alcohol. Environmental cleaning of hospital inpatient rooms or bed spaces of *C. difficile* patients should be carried out daily with at least 1000 ppm of chlorine. During periods of increased incidence, it may be necessary to temporarily increase to 5000 ppm of chlorine, but it has a strong smell and is corrosive to the fabric of the environment. In addition, it may be beneficial to use sporicidal wipes to further enhance cleaning. Rapid environmental tests exist to confirm environmental elimination of *C. difficile* spores. Antimicrobial stewardship is important to decrease gut colonization rate and reduce colonization pressure and prevent progression from *C. difficile* colonization to CDI.

CLINICAL VIGNETTE

An 87-year-old male is admitted generally unwell, with dehydration, AKI and constipation. He receives fluids and laxatives. During admission, he develops a hospital-acquired pneumonia for which he receives piperacillin/tazobactam. The following day he develops diarrhoea and a stool sample is sent for CDI which comes back negative. Because of persistent diarrhoea, a second stool sample is sent 4 days later, which again is negative for CDI.

The diagnostic benefit of repeat testing within a 7-day period with both toxin A/B EIA and PCR is low and should be discouraged.

Repeat testing for CDI within 28 days post-treatment is not useful as *C. difficile* can still be found in the stool and not necessarily mean infection. It is a clinical judgement to decide whether to start CDI treatment again. It is important to rule out other causes of diarrhoea.

BIBLIOGRAPHY

Beinortas T, Burr NE, Wilcox MH, Subramanian V. Comparative efficacy of treatments for Clostridium difficile infection: A systematic review and network meta-analysis. *Lancet Infect Dis.* 2018;18(9):1035–44.
Debast SB, Bauer MP, Kuijper EJ. European Society of Clinical Microbiology and Infectious Diseases. European Society of Clinical Microbiology and Infectious Diseases: Update of the treatment guidance document for *Clostridium difficile* infection. *Clin Microbiol Infect.* 2014 March;20(Suppl 2):1–26.
Nelson RL, Suda KJ, Evans CT. Antibiotic treatment for *Clostridium difficile*-associated diarrhoea in adults. *Cochrane Database Syst Rev.* 2017 March 3;3:CD004610.

5.10 Actinomycosis

Firza Alexander Gronthoud

CLINICAL CONSIDERATIONS

Actinomycosis is an endogenous chronic, granulomatous infectious disease with an indolent disease course. *Actinomyces* species are part of the commensal flora in the gastrointestinal and genital tracts. After trauma, surgical procedures or foreign bodies, which disrupt the mucosal barrier, they can invade deeper tissues and cause significant disease which may go unrecognized for a prolonged time. It is therefore worthwhile to consider the following:

- *Actinomyces* species cause indolent, slowly progressing granulomatous disease mostly involving the orocervicofacial, thoracic and abdominopelvic sites.
- Other presentations are localized cutaneous actinomycosis, central nervous system (CNS) infection or disseminated disease.
- Species commonly found in clinical cultures are *A. israelii*, *A. gerencseriae*, *A. naeslundii*, *A. odontolyticus*, *A. meyeri*, *A. georgiae* and *A. neuii* subsp. *neuii*.
- Normal habitat: oral cavity (*A. odontolyticus* predominant *Actinomyces* species), pharynx, distal oesophagus and urogenital tract.
- Diagnosis is often late due to nonspecific signs and symptoms of the disease.
- Characteristic features of actinomycosis include chronic manifestations, abscess formation with sinus tracts and purulent discharge.
- Hard macroscopic grains, 'sulfur granules,' in pus is a classical finding although not always present.
- When crushed and viewed under a microscope, these granules reveal Gram-positive branching, filamentous rods surrounded by neutrophils.
- Some actinomycosis cases have been linked to specific conditions, such as osteoradionecrosis or bisphosphonate-related osteonecrosis of the jaws.
- The disease can appear in both immunocompetent and immunocompromised individuals.
- Often cultures remain negative if a patient has received prior antimicrobial treatment in the past.
- *Actinomyces* are very susceptible to β-lactam agents but intrinsically resistant to metronidazole.
- *Actinomyces* species have different susceptibilities to antibiotics with *A. europaeus* and *A. turicensis* being the most resistant.
- *Actinomyces* may present as polymicrobial infections.

OROCERVICOFACIAL ACTINOMYCOSIS

- Most common presentation of actinomycosis.
- Poor oral hygiene, smoking and alcohol use are significant risk factors, facilitated by dental procedures.

THORACIC ACTINOMYCOSIS

- The main source of thoracic actinomycosis is considered to be the aspiration of oropharyngeal secretions, although haematogenous spread or direct spread from local infections can result in actinomycotic lesions at pulmonary sites.
- Alternative causes to be considered in differential diagnoses include lung cancer, pneumonia and tuberculosis.

- Since the spread of an actinomycotic lesion occurs despite anatomic barriers, invasion into the pleura or the chest wall can result in empyema or actinomycosis in the chest wall and surrounding bone structures.
- Multiple lung abscesses mimicking coccidioidomycosis and organizing pneumonia with microabscesses.
- Rarely, a progressing thoracic lesion extends to extra-thoracic tissues, with abscess formation on the thoracic wall and pus eroding through the chest wall, causing 'empyema necessitatis'.

ABDOMINAL AND PELVIC ACTINOMYCOSIS

- Abdominal actinomycosis is mainly a consequence of invasive procedures or abdominal infection such as appendicitis.
- Laparoscopic cholecystectomy with a lost gallstone(s) has been reported to be a potential complication leading to actinomycosis; *A. naeslundii* and an unspecified *Actinomyces* spp. were detected in two cases of abdominal abscesses, while *A. meyeri* was found in a case of abdominal actinomycosis extending from the kidney up to the thorax and in an actinomycotic subphrenic abscess.
- *A. israelii* and *A. meyeri* have been identified in pus specimens from periappendical abscesses.
- In some abdominal actinomycosis cases arising from an abdominal source or even from the mouth, *Actinomyces* can result in pericarditis or the involvement of the liver.
- Pelvic actinomycosis has usually been connected to *Actinomyces* present on an intra-uterine contraceptive device (IUCD) after its prolonged use.
- Risk of pelvic actinomycosis in relation to the use of IUCDs is very low.

Cutaneous actinomycosis is usually a secondary infectious process, with an underlying focus at deeper tissues, or it appears as a result of hematogenous spread from actinomycotic lesion elsewhere in the body. Manifestations with a single or with multiple draining sinuses can occur at various body sites, including the face, chest, midriff and hip, as well as upper and lower extremities.

CLINICAL APPROACH

In the case of actinomycosis, it has been considered that a long duration of antimicrobial therapy with high doses is necessary, with treatment extending up to 1 year (or even longer). This concept is changing, and medications are now adjusted on the basis of individual treatment needs. The same is valid for surgery, which was previously used routinely for treatment of actinomycotic lesions; however, the current trend is to limit invasive procedures and to rely on a targeted antibiotic regimen instead. Treatment of abscesses usually requires drainage, whereas surgical resection may be indicated only in cases with extensive necrotic lesions or when antimicrobial therapy fails. Actinomycosis is often a polymicrobial infection. for severe infections an initial intravenous course of two weeks is recommended, followed by an oral stepdown. Intravenous options are amoxicillin/clavulanic acid or ceftriaxone with or without metronidazole. Oral options include amoxicillin/clavulanic acid, doxycycline or a macrolide with or without metronidazole. Clindamycin or quinolones should be avoided unless in vitro susceptible.

BIBLIOGRAPHY

Könönen E, Wade WG. *Actinomyces* and related organisms in human infections. *Clin Microbiol Rev.* 2015 April; 28(2):419–442. Published online 2015 March 18.
Song JU, Park HY, Jeon K, Um SW, Kwon OJ, Koh WJ. Treatment of thoracic actinomycosis: A retrospective analysis of 40 patients. *Ann Thorac Med.* 2010 April;5(2):80–85
Valour F, Sénéchal A, Dupieux C et al. Actinomycosis: Etiology, clinical features, diagnosis, treatment, and management. *Infect Drug Resist.* 2014;7:183–197. Published 2014 July 5.
Wong VK, Turmezei TD, Weston VC. Actinomycosis. *BMJ.* 2011 October 11;343:d6099.

5.11 Nocardia

Firza Alexander Gronthoud

CLINICAL CONSIDERATIONS

Nocardia causes opportunistic infections in immunocompromised individuals. *Nocardia* spp. can be found in soil and decomposing vegetation, as well as in fresh and salt water. Although trimethoprim/sulfamethoxazole is considered as one of the first-line treatment options, depending on the *Nocardia* species, resistance occurs, and prolonged courses of up to 12 months or longer is often needed. It is therefore worthwhile to consider the following.

MICROBIOLOGY

Nocardia spp. are Gram-positive, aerobic, branching rods, commonly found in dust, soil and water. *Nocardia* belong to the order of Actinomycetales, suborder Corynebacteriaceae and family Nocardiaceae. Common *Nocardia* species are *N. asteroides sensu stricto, N. farcinica, N. nova, N. cyriacigeorgica* and *N. brasiliensis*.

POPULATION AT RISK

Nocardia spp. are opportunistic pathogens and are mainly associated with pulmonary infections and brain infections in immunosuppressed individuals, especially in the presence of cell-mediated immune deficiencies including lymphoma, human immunodeficiency virus infection and solid organ or hematopoietic stem cell transplant recipients, as well as long-term treatment with steroids or other drugs that suppress cell-mediated immunity. Graft-versus-host disease and subsequent additional immunosuppressive treatments may possibly contribute to a higher incidence of nocardiosis in allogeneic stem cell transplant recipients compared to those receiving an autologous haematopoietic stem cell transplant. Finally, up to one-third of patients with nocardiosis are immunocompetent.

CLINICAL PEARL

Nocardia classically causes a granulomatous inflammation most commonly affecting the lungs, brain and soft tissue. A classical feature of extrapulmonary nocardiosis is abscess formation and can resemble a pyogenic bacterial infection

PULMONARY INFECTION

Pulmonary nocardiosis is the most common clinical presentation of infection because inhalation is the primary route of bacterial exposure. The onset of symptoms ranges from subacute to chronic. Symptoms and radiological findings are similar to tuberculosis, aspergillosis, actinomycosis and malignancy and include productive or non-productive cough, shortness of breath, chest pain, haemoptysis, fever, night sweats, weight loss and progressive fatigue.

Thoracic imaging can show focal or multifocal disease with nodules, consolidation, pleural effusion and cavitary lesions. Pulmonary nocardiosis can spread to other body sites including the brain through haematogenous dissemination or a contiguous spread of necrotizing pneumonitis into the pleura, pericardium, mediastinum and vena cava.

Brain Abscess

Brain abscess is the most common extrapulmonary location for nocardiosis. A solitary lesion or multiple brain lesions may be present. Brain lesions may resemble a malignancy or vascular infarct. Associated symptoms are headache, nausea, vomiting, seizures or altered mental status. Neurologic symptoms typically have a slow onset but may rapidly progress.

Cutaneous Nocardiosis

Soil containing *Nocardia* can inoculate wounds after a traumatic injury and cause a primary cutaneous infection. This presentation is usually seen in immunocompetent individuals. Cutaneous nocardiosis can present as cellulitis, skin abscesses, nodules, ulcers, abscesses and fistulas, and also spread to lymph nodes. *Nocardia brasiliensis* and *N. asteroides* may be involved. Mycetoma may also develop, resembling a fungal infection (sporotrichosis and coccidioidomycosis), actinomycosis or a tumour. Mycetoma usually develops on feet and legs and is predominantly seen in men working on farms where skin abrasions are more likely to occur. Mycetoma contains nodules and fistula, and abscesses may drain granules containing *Nocardia*.

CLINICAL APPROACH

Diagnosis

The modified Ziehl–Neelsen stain on clinical samples shows beaded acid-fast rods on microscopy. Gram stain shows branching filamentous Gram-positive rods. *Nocardia* spp. grows aerobic and buffered charcoal yeast extract (BCYE) agar is a selective agar used for *Nocardia* spp. as well as for *Legionella* spp.

CLINICAL PEARL

Pulmonary nocardiosis may be complicated by central nervous system involvement, and neuroimaging is recommended in pulmonary cases.

Treatment

Trimethoprim/sulfamethoxazole (TMP-SMX) or imipenem/cilastatin in combination with amikacin are the two most used and effective treatment options. The combination of imipenem/cilastatin with amikacin is synergistic against *Nocardia* species and is frequently used in patients with cerebral abscesses.

For localized disease such as cutaneous nocardiosis, the recommended treatment dose is 5–15 mg/kg per day of the trimethoprim component. The TMP/SMX ratio is usually 1:5. For severe, extensive or disseminated disease, 15 mg/kg TMP and 75 mg/kg SMX intravenously or by mouth should be used. Alternatively, imipenem 500 mg–1 g 6-hourly in combination with amikacin 15 mg/kg/day may be used.

Trimethoprim/sulfamethoxazole is active against most *Nocardia* species. Resistance to TMP-SMX and other antibiotics is more commonly seen in *N. farcinica*, *N. brasiliensis* and *N. otitidiscaviarum*.

In general, *Nocardia* species have different antimicrobial susceptibility patterns, emphasizing the importance of specimen collection and phenotypic antimicrobial susceptibility testing.

Alternative antimicrobial agents with activity against *Nocardia* spp. include meropenem, ceftriaxone, cefotaxime, minocycline, moxifloxacin, levofloxacin, linezolid, tigecycline and amoxicillin/clavulanic acid. Although imipenem is more potent than meropenem against

Gram-positive organisms, *Nocardia* spp. display variable *in vitro* susceptibilities to meropenem and imipenem, and *in vitro* antimicrobial susceptibility testing is recommended to choose the agent with the lowest MIC.

Linezolid is *in vitro* active against all *Nocardia* species and has successfully been used in clinical practice. Linezolid has excellent brain penetration, but long-term treatment may cause myelosuppression and rarely optic neuritis and peripheral neuropathy. Another adverse event which requires discontinuation is lactic acidosis. Tedizolid is a newer generation oxazolidinone and may be associated with a lower incidence of myelosuppression, but more clinical data is needed for prolonged treatment.

Amoxicillin/clavulanic acid is moderately active against many strains of *N. asteroides*, *N farcinica* and *N. brasiliensis*. Moxifloxacin has also been used with success.

Combination therapy with imipenem and cefotaxime, amikacin and TMP-SMX, imipenem and TMP-SMX, amikacin and cefotaxime or amikacin and imipenem may provide enhanced activity.

For brain abscess, the combination of imipenem/cilastatin with amikacin is less suitable because amikacin has poor CNS penetration and high-dose imipenem can increase risk of seizures, especially in patients with renal impairment, disrupted blood–brain barrier and brain lesions such as brain abscess. It may be better to use either a combination of TMP-SMX with ceftriaxone or, alternatively, linezolid.

DURATION OF TREATMENT

Duration of treatment is generally prolonged to minimize risk of disease relapse. Immunocompetent patients with pulmonary with or without extrapulmonary involvement may be successfully treated with 6–12 months of antimicrobial therapy. Immunocompromised individuals and all patients with a brain abscess, however, should be treated for at least 12 months. A duration of up to 3 months may be sufficient for soft tissue infections.

PREVENTING *NOCARDIA* IN IMMUNOCOMPROMISED PATIENTS

TMP-SMX 960 mg thrice weekly or 480 mg once daily is used in allogeneic stem cell transplant recipients and immunocompromised individuals receiving high-dose steroids for ≥4 weeks to prevent *Pneumocystis jirovecii* infection, and reactivation of toxoplasma in HSCT recipients. This regimen coincidentally also prevents nocardiosis; however, breakthrough infection has been reported. Interestingly, these *Nocardia* isolates may still be susceptible to TMP-SMX.

BIBLIOGRAPHY

Welsh O, Vera-Cabrera L, Salinas-Carmona MC. Current treatment for *Nocardia* infections. *Expert Opin Pharmacother.* 2013 December;14(17):2387–2398.
Wilson JW. Nocardiosis: Updates and Clinical Overview. *Mayo Clin Proc.* 2012 April;87(4):403–407.
Yildiz O, Doganay M. Actinomycoses and *Nocardia* pulmonary infections. *Curr Opin Pulm Med.* 2006 May;12(3):228–234.

Section VI

Appendix

6.1 Syndromic Approach to Infections

Firza Alexander Gronthoud

Bacterial and Viral Infections

(Continued)

Location	Clinical Syndrome	Clinical Specimen	Organism	Examples
Central nervous system	Meningitis	CSF and blood cultures	Bacteria	*Streptococcus pneumoniae, Neisseria meningitidis, Haemophilus influenzae*
			Viruses	Enterovirus, herpes simplex, Varicella zoster, Cytomegalovirus, Epstein–Barr virus, Adenovirus
			Fungi	*Cryptococcus neoformans*
	Encephalitis	CSF and EDTA Blood for PCR	Viruses	Herpes simplex, Varicella zoster, Cytomegalovirus, Epstein–Barr virus, adenovirus, HHV6, JC virus
	Brain abscess	Blood cultures, abscess fluid	Bacteria	*Staphylococcus aureus* (*Streptococcus anginosus* group, *Bacteroides* spp., *Prevotella* spp.)
	Spondylodiscitis	Blood cultures, tissue biopsy	Bacteria	*Staphylococcus aureus*, Streptococci, Enterobactericeae
Eye	Conjunctivitis	Eye swab	Bacteria	*Staphylococcus* spp., *Streptococcus pneumoniae, Haemophilus* spp., *Moraxella* spp.
		Eye swab	Viruses	Herpes simplex, Enterovirus, Adenovirus
	Endophthalmitis	Blood culture	Bacteria	Acute post-cataract: Coagulase-negative staphylococci (CoNS) Bleb-related: Viridans streptococci, *Streptococcus pneumoniae, Haemophilus influenzae* Post-traumatic: *Bacillus cereus* Endogenous: Staphylococcus
		Blood culture	Fungi	*Candida* spp., *Aspergillus* spp., *Fusarium* spp.
Upper respiratory tract	Rhinosinusitis	Washout	Bacteria	*Streptococcus pneumoniae, Haemophilus influenzae*, less common *P. aeruginosa*
		Nasopharyngeal aspirate, washout	Viruses	Adenovirus, Parainfluenza, Rhinovirus
		Washout, serum galactomannan	Fungi	*Aspergillus* spp., Zygomycetes
	Pharyngitis	Pharyngeal swab	Bacteria	Streptococcus group A, C & G, *Fusobacterium necrophorum*
		Pharyngeal swab	Viruses	Adenovirus, Herpes simplex, HIV

Bacterial and Viral Infections

Location	Clinical Syndrome	Clinical Specimen	Organism	Examples
Lower respiratory tract	Bronchiolitis	Nasopharyngeal aspirate, Nose/Throat swab	Viruses	Respiratory syncytial virus, Human metapneumovirus, Influenza, Rhinovirus, Human coronavirus HCoV-NL63
	Pneumonia	Sputum, BAL	Bacteria	CAP *Streptococcus pneumoniae, Haemophilus influenzae* HAP *Enterobacterales, Staphylococcus aureus, Pseudomonas aeruginosa*
		Sputum, BAL, NPA, Nose/Throat swab. Point-of-care test	Viruses	Influenza A, Influenza B, Respiratory syncytial virus, Human metapneumovirus SARS-CoV-1, SARS-COV-2, MERS-CoV
		Sputum, BAL, galactomannan	Fungi	*Aspergillus* spp., Zygomycetes
Ear, nose & throat	External otitis	Ear swab	Bacteria	*Streptococcus pneumoniae, Haemophilus influenzae, Moraxella catarrhalis, Pseudomonas aeruginosa*
		Ear swab	Fungi	*Aspergillus niger, Candida* spp.
	Otitis media	Ear discharge	Bacteria	*Streptococcus pneumoniae, Haemophilus influenzae, Moraxella catarrhalis*
Cardiovascular	Endocarditis	Blood culture, valve culture	Bacteria	Viridans streptococci, Enterococci, *Staphylococcus aureus*, Coagulase-negative staphylococci
		Blood culture, valve culture	Fungi	*Candida* spp., *Aspergillus* spp.
	Pericarditis	Pericardial fluid, blood culture	Bacteria	*Staphylococcus aureus*, β-Haemolytic streptococci
	Myocarditis	EDTA blood, serology	Viruses	Enterovirus, Adenovirus, Parvovirus B19, Cytomegalovirus, Epstein–Barr virus, HIV, Influenza
		EDTA blood, serology	Bacteria	*Mycoplasma pneumoniae*

(Continued)

Bacterial and Viral Infections

Location	Clinical Syndrome	Clinical Specimen	Organism	Examples
Intra-abdominal	Hepatitis	Clotted blood for serology, EDTA blood for PCR, stool for PCR (HEV only)	Viruses	Hepatitis B virus Hepatitis D virus Hepatitis C virus Hepatitis E virus Herpes simplex Adenovirus
	Cholangitis	Blood culture, bile fluid	Bacteria	*Enterobacterales*, Streptococci, Enterococci, *Bacteroides* spp., *Clostridium* spp.
Gastrointestinal tract	Peptic ulcer	Stool for antigen or gastric biopsy for culture	Bacteria	*Helicobacter pylori*
	Diarrhoea	Stool for PCR or rapid point-of-care test (lower sensitivity)	Viruses	Norovirus Enterovirus Rotavirus
			Bacteria	Cytomegalovirus (immunocompromised) *Salmonella* spp. *Shigella* spp., *Yersinia enterocolitica.*, *Campylobacter spp.*, *Clostridioides difficile*
Urinary tract	Cystitis	Urine, blood culture	Bacteria	*Enterobacterales* (mostly *Escherichia coli*), *Pseudomonas aeruginosa*
	Pyelonephritis	Urine, blood culture	Fungi	*Candida* spp.
Skin and soft tissue	Vesicles + rash	Vesicle scrape and fluid	Viruses	Herpes simplex Varicella zoster Enterovirus
	Cellulitis/erysipelas	Tissue biopsy, abscess fluid	Bacteria	β-Haemolytic streptococci, *Staphylococcus aureus*, *Enterobacterales*
Bone & joint	Osteomyelitis & septic arthritis	Bone, tissue, aspirate	Bacteria	*Staphylococcus aureus*, Streptococci, *Enterobacterales*, *Neisseria gonorrhoea*
		Bone, tissue, aspirate	Fungi	*Candida* spp.

(Continued)

Bacterial and Viral Infections

Location	Clinical Syndrome	Clinical Specimen	Organism	Examples
Reproductive organs	Chancre		Bacteria	*Treponema pallidum* (syphillis, lues), *Haemophilus ducreyi*
	Warts		Viruses	Human papilloma virus (HPV)
	Vesicles		Viruses	Herpes simplex virus
	Urethritis		Bacteria	*Neisseria gonorrhoea, Chlamydia trachomatis*
	Bacterial vaginosis		Bacteria	Decrease in lactobacilli, increae in *Gardnerella vaginalis, Prevotella* spp., *Porphyromonas* spp., *Bacteroides* spp., *Peptostreptococcus* spp., *Mycoplasma hominis, Ureaplasma urealyticum* and *Mobiluncus* spp.
	Genital thrush		Fungi	*Candida* spp.
	Pelvic inflammatory disease		Bacteria	*Neisseria gonorrhoeae, Chlamydia trachomatis, Actinomyces* spp. and other vaginal bacterial flora
	Endometritis		Bacteria	Polymicrobial (group B streptococci, enterococci, other aerobic streptococci, *G. vaginalis, E. coli, P. bivia, Bacteroides* spp. and peptostreptococci)

Parasitic Infections

Group	Disease	Organism	Clinical Syndrome
		Protozoa	
Lumen-dwelling protozoa	Amebiasis	*Entamoeba histolytica*	Diarrhoea, dysentery, liver abscess, lung abscess
	Giardiasis	*Giardia lamblia*	Diarrhoea, steatorrhea, malabsorption
		Dientamoeba fragilis	Diarrhoea, abdominal pain
	Balantidiasis	*Balantidium coli*	Dysentery, colitis
	Cystoisosporiasis	*Cystoisospora belli*	Diarrhoea, anorexia, weight loss
	Cryptosporidiosis	*Cryptosporidium parvum*	Diarrhoea, anorexia, weight loss, abdominal pain
	Cyclosporiasis	*Cyclospora cayetanensis*	Diarrhoea, anorexia, weight loss, abdominal pain
	Microsporidiosis	*Enterocytozoon bieneusi, Encephalitozoon intestinalis*	Chronic diarrhoea and wasting (primarily disease of HIV a patients)
Blood- and tissue-dwelling protozoa	Malaria	*Plasmodium falciparum, P. vivax, P. ovale, P. malariae, P. knowlesi*	Fever, rigors, headache, back pain, anaemia, thrombocytopenia, splenomegaly
	African trypanosomiasis (sleeping sickness)	*Trypanosoma brucei gambiense, T. b. rhodesiense*	Winterbottom's sign (lymphadenopathy along the back of the neck), fever, headache, 'sleeping sickness'
	Chagas	*Trypanosoma cruzi*	Romaña's sign (also known as chagoma, refers to periorbital swelling, palpebral oedema and conjunctivitis seen 1-2 weeks following infection), fever, hepatosplenomegaly, myocarditis
	Babesiosis	*Babesia microti, Babesia divergens*	Chills and fever, headache, fatigue, anaemia
	Leishmaniasis	*Leishmania* spp.	Cutaneous Skin ulcer
			Mucocutaneous Ulcers of skin, and oral and nasal mucosa
			Visceral (Kala-azar) Hepatosplenomegaly, anaemia, fever, weight loss
	Toxoplasmosis	*Toxoplasma gondii*	Usually asymptomatic. Otherwise, mononucleosis-like syndrome with fever, headache, myalgia, lymphadenitis, and extreme fatigue. Intrauterine infection can lead to retinochoroiditis, encephalomyelitis, and hydrocephalus or microcephaly
		Sarcocystis spp.	Myositis, dyspnoea, and wheezing, associated with eosinophilia
	Primary amoebic meningoencephalitis (PAM)	*Naegleria fowleri*	Severe frontal headache, fever, nausea, vomiting, stiff neck (associated with swimming)
	Granulomatous amoebic encephalitis (GAE)	*Acanthamoeba* spp. *Balamuthia mandrillaris*	Altered mental state, headache, seizures, stiff neck (*Acanthamoeba* spp. can also cause keratitis, associated with mainly soft contact lenses)

(Continued)

Parasitic Infections

Group	Disease	Organism	Clinical Syndrome
Helminths			
Trematodes	Fasciolopsiasis	*Fasciolopsis buski*	Abdominal pain, diarrhoea, oedema, ascites, eosinophilia
	Fascioliasis	*Fasciola hepatica*	Hepatomegaly, eosinophilia, jaundice, portal cirrhosis
	Schistosomiasis (bilharziasis)	*Schistosoma* spp.	Hepatosplenomegaly, diarrhoea, portal fibrosis, haematuria, hypertension, bladder carcinoma
	Paragonimiasis	*Paragonimus westermani*	Haemoptysis, cough, fever, eosinophilia
Cestodes	Diphyllobothriasis	*Diphyllobothrium latum* (fish tapeworm)	Majority asymptomatic; can cause vitamin B12 deficiency, anaemia
	Taeniasis	*Taenia saginata* (beef tapeworm), *T. solium* (pork tapeworm)	Vague digestive disturbances, anorexia; majority asymptomatic
	Cysticercosis	*Cysticercus cellulosae* (larva of *T. solium*)	Asymptomatic to Jacksonian seizures, hydrocephalus, visual problems
	Echinococcosis (hydatid disease)	*Echinococcus granulosus*, *E. multilocularis*, *E. multilocularis*	Chronic space-occupying lesions of involved organs
	Hymenolepiasis	*Hymenolepis nana*, (dwarf tapeworm), *H. diminuta* (rat tapeworm)	Enteritis, diarrhoea, abdominal pain, anorexia; majority asymptomatic
Intestinal nematodes	Ascariasis	*Ascaris lumbricoides*	Cough, pneumonitis, vague GI symptoms
	Enterobiasis	*Enterobium vermicularis*	Anal pruritus, restless sleep
	Ancylostomiasis (necatoriasis)	*Ancylostoma duodenale, Nector americanus* (Hookworms)	Dermatitis, cough, diarrhoea, abdominal pain, anaemia, eosinophilia
	Strongyloidiasis	*Strongyloides stercoralis*	Cough, epigastric pain, diarrhoea, eosinophilia
	Trichuriasis	*Trichuris trichiura* (Whipworm)	Abdominal pain, mucous diarrhoea, eosinophilia
	Anisakiasis	*Anisakis* spp.	Epigastric pain, nausea, vomiting, diarrhoea, variable eosinophilia

(Continued)

Parasitic Infections

Group	Disease	Organism	Clinical Syndrome
Blood- and tissue-dwelling nematodes	Lymphatic filariasis	*Wuchereria bancrofti, Brugia malayi, B. timori*	Lymphangitis, lymphadenitis, oedema, fever, eosinophilia, (hydrocele, elephantiasis)
	Loiasis	*Loa loa* (eye worm)	Calabar (fugative), swellings, pruritus, eosinophilia, worm migrates across eye
	Onchocerciasis (river blindness)	*Onchocerca volvulus* (blinding worm)	Subcutaneous nodules, pruritic dermatitis, hyperpigmentation, visual disturbances, blindness
	Dracunculiasis	*Dracunculus medinensis,* (Guinea worm)	Pruritus, blister, ulcer, eosinophilia, secondary infection
	Trichinellosis	*Trichinella spiralis*	Fever, eosinophilia, muscle pain, orbital oedema
	Visceral larva migrans	*Toxocara canis, T. cati*	Hepatomegaly, hypereosinophilia, hyperglobulinemia
Arthropods	Scabies, Norwegian scabies	*Sarcoptes scabiei*	Very small vesicles, intense itching
	Lice (head, pubic)	*Pediculus humanus*	Itchiness, lymphadenopathy
	Myiasis	*Dermatobia hominis, Cordylobia anthropophaga* (tumbu fly)	Painful, indolent ulcers or furuncle-like sores of long-standing

The Returning Traveller

Incubation period <21 days	Undifferentiated fever	*Rickettsia* spp., *Leptospira* spp., *Salmonella* spp., typhoid fever	Dengue, Chikungunya, Zika virus	Malaria, Babesia, amoebic liver abscess. *Schistosoma* spp.
	Fever with rash	*Rickettsia* spp., typhoid fever	Dengue, Chikungunya, HIV, CMV, EBV, Rare: Viral haemorrhagic fever (Ebola, Marburg)	*Schistosoma* spp.
	Fever with jaundice	*Leptospira* spp. *Borrelia recurrentis* (relapsing fever)	Yellow fever. Rare: Viral haemorrhagic fever (Ebola, Marburg)	
	Fever with hepatosplenomegaly	*Leptospira* spp. *Borrelia recurrentis* (relapsing fever)		Amoebic liver abscess, malaria
	Meningoencephalitis	*Neisseria meningitidis*	Japanese encephalitis, tick-borne encephalitis, dengue, West Nile virus	Malaria
	Lower respiratory tract infection	*Burkholderia pseudomallei* (melioidosis)	Influenza, Middle East respiratory syndrome, corona virus	
	Diarrhoea	*Shigella* spp., *Salmonella* spp., *Yersinia enterocolitica*, *Campylobacter* spp., *Vibrio* spp., *Escherichia coli* O157:H7		*Entamoeba histolytica, Isospora belli, Cyclospora cayetanensis*
	Skin		*Herpes simplex, herpes zoster*	Hookworm larvae, myiasis, tungiasis, filariasis, scabies
Incubation period >21 days	Undifferentiated fever	*Leptospira* spp., *Brucella* spp., typhoid fever	HIV	Malaria, Babesia, amoebic liver abscess
	Fever with rash			*Fasiocla hepatica*
	Fever with jaundice	*Leptospira* spp.	Hepatitis viruses	*Fasiocla hepatica*
	Fever with hepatosplenomegaly	*Brucella* spp. *Leptospira* spp.,		Amoebic liver abscess, African trypanosomiasis, malaria
	Meningoencephalitis	*Borrelia burgdorferi, Listeria monocytogenes,* syphilis	HIV	African trypanosomiasis, malaria
	Lower respiratory tract infection	*Mycobacterium tuberculosis* (tuberculosis), *Burkholderia pseudomallei* (melioidosis)		
	Diarrhoea			*Entamoeba histolytica*
	Skin			*Leishmania* spp.

BIBLIOGRAPHY

Bennett JE, Dolin R, Blaser MJ, Mandell GL, Douglas RG. *Mandell, Douglas, and Bennett's Principles and Practice of Infectious Diseases*, Philadelphia, PA: Elsevier/Saunders, 2015.
John DT, Markell EK, Petri WA, Voge M, Markell EK. *Markell and Voge's Medical Parasitology*, Elsevier, 2013.

6.2 Specimen Collection

Firza Alexander Gronthoud

- Bloodstream infection
  - *Clinical symptoms*: Fever, rigors, tachycardia, hypotension.
  - *Specimen*: Two blood culture sets, each set containing an aerobic and anaerobic bottle. Volume is more important than timing. Collect 20–30 mL per blood culture set.
- Central line bloodstream infection
  - *Clinical symptoms*: Fever, rigors, tachycardia, hypotension. Exit site may be red swollen, tender and discharging pus.
  - *Specimen*: Blood culture sets from each lumen and a peripheral blood culture set. If the catheter is to be removed, also send tip for culture. If discharge from exit site, send a swab.
- Urinary Tract Infection
  - *Clinical symptoms*: Dysuria, frequency, and urgency.
  - *Specimen*: Midstream urine in a sterile container.
- Catheter-Associated Urinary Tract Infection
  - *Clinical symptoms*: Fever and systemic signs of infection not explained by other conditions.
  - *Specimen*: Remove or change catheter, then collect a fresh urine culture to avoid diagnosing catheter colonization.
- Lower respiratory tract infection
  - *Clinical symptoms:* Diverse but may include cough, fever, sputum production, pleuritic chest pain.
  - *Specimen*: Sputum culture, endotracheal aspirate, bronchoalveolar lavage. For respiratory viruses, the following samples are also suitable: dacron, rayon swab or Nylon flocked swabs (Viral swabs) for nose/throat swab or send a nasopharyngeal aspirate. Nasopharyngeal swabs have a higher yield than oropharyngeal swabs.
- Skin and soft tissue infection
  - *Clinical manifestations*: Cellulitis, erysipelas, abscesses, necrotizing fasciitis (NF).
  - *Specimen*: Pus should be collected from abscesses and carbuncles through incision and drainage. NF requires urgent debridement with tissue samples sent. Blood cultures are positive in around 10% of the cases. Indications for blood cultures are immunosuppression, malignancy, animal bites and/or immersion injuries.
- Bone and joint infection
  - *Clinical symptoms*: Fever, painful and swollen joints, tenderness and decreased range of motion.
  - *Specimen*: Aspiration of synovial fluid cultures, bone biopsy, two sets of blood cultures. Gram stain on synovial fluid has a low sensitivity for the diagnosis of joint infections.
- Prosthetic joints infection
  - *Clinical symptoms*:
    - *Early onset*: Acute joint pain, warmth, erythema, edema, wound drainage or dehiscence, joint effusion, and fever.
    - *Late onset*: Persistent joint pain, with or without early implant loosening, fever
  - *Specimen*: Two sets of blood cultures, joint aspiration and 5–7 intraoperative pus and tissue samples. If X-ray is negative, consider MRI. Superficial swab culture from

draining wounds is useful in identifying the etiologic microorganism of acute prosthetic joint infections, especially when *S. aureus* or Gram-negative bacilli were identified. Poor concordance between superficial swab and intraoperative tissue cultures in chronic prosthetic joint infections.

- Endocarditis
  - *Clinical symptoms*: Fever, rigors, flu-like symptoms, malaise, dyspnoea, chest pain, arthropathy, anaemia, weight loss.
  - *Specimen*: Collect three sets of blood cultures within 24 hours. If a transthoracic echo is negative, consider a transoesophageal echo.
- Secondary peritonitis
  - *Clinical symptoms:* Fever, abdominal pain, rigid abdomen, rebound tenderness.
  - *Specimen:* Drain fluid in collection bag for hours may be less reliable as colonizing agents may overgrowth and misrepresent the pathogenic flora and lead to inappropriate antibiotic treatment. The absence of anaerobic bacteria does not rule out their involvement as they require specific transport medium and culture environments, often not present on routine laboratories. Factors that increase likelihood of a positive drain culture are leucocytosis (sens. 62%, spec. 53%), gas in the collection on CT (sens. 59%, spec. 77%), purulent material aspiration (sens. 76%, spec. 76%) and presence of polymorphonuclear cells in the specimen. Air-only intra-abdominal collections with signs of infection should be considered for percutaneous management similar to that of conventional infected fluid collections. Although fluid is not visible on CT, these collections can produce fluid that contains organisms.
- Meningitis
  - *Clinical symptoms*: Classical symptoms including fever, altered mental status, neck stiffness and photophobia may be absent.
  - *Specimen*: Cerebrospinal fluid (CSF) for cell count and culture. If Gram stain and culture negative, consider polymerase chain reaction (16 s PCR, meningococcal or pneumococcal PCR).
- Gastroenteritis
  - *Clinical symptoms*: Stool may be watery, bloody or greenish colour, fever, abdominal pain or cramps, nausea, malaise, weight loss.
  - *Specimen*: Stool cultures may be considered in patients who present with persistent diarrhoea or bloody diarrhoea, or who have recently travelled to areas with poor public sanitation systems. Stool samples from patients who developed diarrhoea >3 days after admission will only be tested for *Clostridioides difficile*. Chronic diarrhoea + weight loss indicates parasitic infection such as *Giardia lamblia*. Always document on request form if patient is immunocompromised, bloody diarrhoea, foreign travel, animal exposure and if consumption of shellfish, unpasteurized dairy products or uncooked or raw meat. Stool samples are not routinely tested for viruses in most laboratories.

6.3 Spectrum of Activity of Antibiotics

Firza Alexander Gronthoud

	Gram negative										Anaerobes			Gram positive						
	Moraxella catarrhalis	*Neisseria* spp.	*Stenotrophomonas maltophilia*	*Acinetobacter baumanii*	*Pseudomonas aeruginosa*	Carbapenemase-Producing Enterobacterales	ESBL-producing Enterobacterales	*Citrobacter freundii, Serratia marcescens, Enterobacter cloacae*	*Proteus mirabilis, Klebsiella pneumoniae, Escherichia coli*	*Haemophilus influenzae*	*Bacteroides fragilis*	*Clostridioides difficile*	*Clostridium perfringens*	*Streptococcus pneumoniae*	*Enterococcus faecium*	*Enterococcus faecalis*	Haemolytic streptococci (Strep. A,C,G & Strep B)	Staphylococcus Coagulase negative	MRSA *Staphylococcus aureus*	MSSA *Staphylococcus aureus*
Penicillins																				
Benzylpenicillin	–	✓								–	–	–	✓	✓	–	–	✓	–	–	?
Ampicillin/Amoxicillin	–	✓							✓	✓	–	–	✓	✓	–	✓	✓	–	–	?
Co-amoxiclav	✓	✓							✓	✓	✓	–	✓	✓	–	✓	✓	?	–	✓
Piperacillin/Tazobactam	✓	✓	?	?	✓		?	✓	✓	✓	✓	–	✓	✓	–	✓	✓	✓	–	✓
Flucloxacillin														?	–	–	✓	?	–	✓
Temocillin	✓						✓	✓	✓	✓		–	–	–	–	–	–	–	–	–
Aztreonam	✓	✓		?	✓		–	?	✓	✓	–	–	–	–	–	–	–	–	–	–
Cephalosporins																				
Cefalexin (Cephalexin)									✓	✓	–		–	?	–	–	✓	✓	–	✓
Cefuroxime	✓	✓						✓	✓	✓	–		–	✓	–	✓	✓	✓	–	✓
Ceftriaxone	✓	✓	?	?			?	?	✓	✓	–		–	✓	–	–	✓	?	–	?
Ceftazidime				?	✓		?	✓	✓	✓	–		–	?	–	–	✓	?	–	✓
Cefepime					✓		✓	✓	✓	✓	–		–	✓	–	–	✓	?	–	–
Ceftazidime/Avibactam				?	✓	✓	✓	✓	✓	✓	–		–	?	–	–	–	–	–	–
Ceftolozane/Tazobactam			?		✓		✓	✓	✓	✓	–		–	–	–	–	✓	–	–	–
Ceftobiprole	✓	✓			✓			?	✓	✓	–		✓	✓	–	✓	✓	✓	✓	✓
Ceftaroline fosamil	✓	✓					✓	✓	✓	✓	–		✓	✓	–	✓	✓	✓	✓	✓
Carbapenem																				
Meropenem	✓	✓		✓	✓		✓	✓	✓	✓	✓	–	✓	✓	–	✓	✓	✓	–	✓
Imipenem-cilastatin	✓	✓		?	?		✓	✓	✓	✓	✓	–	✓	✓	–	✓	✓	✓	–	✓
Ertapenem	✓	✓					✓	✓	✓	✓	✓	–	✓	✓	–	?	?	✓	–	✓
Macrolides/Linocosamides																				
Erythromycin	✓	–										–	–	✓	–	–	✓	?	?	✓
Clarithromycin	✓	–										–	–	✓	–	–	✓	?	?	✓
Clindamycin	–	–									?	–	✓	–	–	–	–	?	?	✓

	Gram positive							Anaerobes			Gram negative									
	Staphylococcus aureus MSSA	Staphylococcus aureus MRSA	Coagulase negative Staphylococci	Haemolytic streptococci (Strep. A, C, G & Strep B)	Enterococcus faecalis	Enterococcus faecium	Streptococcus pneumoniae	Clostridium perfringens	Clostridioides difficile	Bacteroides fragilis	Haemophilus influenzae	Escherichia coli, Klebsiella pneumoniae, Proteus mirabilis	Enterobacter cloacae, Serratia marcescens, Citrobacter freundii	ESBL-producing Enterobacterales	Carbapenemase-Producing Enterobacterales	Pseudomonas aeruginosa	Acinetobacter baumannii	Stenotrophomonas maltophilia	Neisseria spp.	Moraxella catarrhalis
Aminoglycosides																				
Gentamicin	?	?	?	-	-	-	-	-	-	-	-	✓	✓	✓	?	✓	?	-	-	-
Tobramycin	?	?	?	-	-	-	-	-	-	-	-	✓	✓	✓	?	✓	✓	-	-	-
Amikacin	?	?	?	-	-	-	-	-	-	-	-	✓	✓	✓	?	✓	✓	-	-	-
Diaminopyrimidines																				
Trimethoprim	✓	✓	-	-	?	?	-	-	-	-	✓	✓	✓	✓	?	-	-	-	-	-
Trimethoprim/sulfamethoxazole	✓	✓	-	-	?	?	-	-	-	✓	✓	✓	✓	✓	?	-	✓	✓	?	✓
Quinolones																				
Ciprofloxacin	✓	✓	-	-	✓	✓	-	-	-	-	✓	✓	✓	✓	?	✓	✓	?	✓	✓
Levofloxacin	✓	✓	✓	✓	✓	✓	✓	-	-	✓	✓	✓	✓	✓	?	✓	✓	?	✓	✓
Moxifloxacin	✓	✓	✓	-	-	-	✓	-	✓	✓	✓	✓	✓	✓	?	-	✓	?	✓	✓
Glycopeptides																				
Vancomycin IV	✓	✓	✓	✓	✓	✓	✓	✓	-	-	-	-	-	-	-	-	-	-	-	-
Teicoplanin	✓	✓	✓	✓	✓	✓	✓	?	-	-	-	-	-	-	-	-	-	-	-	-
Vancomycin PO	-	-	-	-	-	-	-	-	✓	-	-	-	-	-	-	-	-	-	-	-
Nitromidazoles																				
Metronidazole	-	-	-	-	-	-	-	✓	✓	✓	-	-	-	-	-	-	-	-	-	-
Tetracyclines																				
Doxycycline	✓	✓	✓	?	?	?	✓	?	-	-	✓	?	?	-	-	-	✓	✓	?	✓
Tigecycline	✓	✓	✓	✓	✓	✓	✓	✓	✓	✓	✓	✓	✓	✓	✓	-	✓	✓	✓	✓
Other agents																				
Rifampicin	✓	✓	✓	✓	-	-	✓	-	-	-	?	-	-	-	-	-	✓	-	✓	-
Fosfomycin	✓	✓	✓	-	✓	-	✓	-	-	✓	-	✓	✓	✓	?	-	-	-	-	-
Linezolid	✓	✓	✓	✓	✓	✓	✓	✓	✓	-	-	-	-	-	-	-	-	-	-	-
Daptomycin	✓	✓	✓	✓	✓	✓	✓	✓	✓	-	-	-	-	-	-	-	-	-	-	-

✓ Clinical activity
- Inappropriate therapy or usually resistant
? Variable activity

6.4 Doses of Common Antimicrobials

Firza Alexander Gronthoud

Oral Antibiotics	Standard Dose	High Dose	Important Side Effects
		β-LACTAMS	
Phenoxymethylpenicillin (Penicillin V)	500 mg 6-hourly	2 g 6-hourly	Allergic reaction
Amoxicillin	500 mg 8-hourly	750 mg to 1 g 8-hourly (2 g 8-hourly for typhoid fever or late disseminated Lyme disease)	Allergic reaction
Amoxicillin/clavulanic acid	625 (500/125) mg 8-hourly 1 g (875/125) tablets are available in US and Australia	1 g (875/125) 8-hourly Amoxicillin 1000 mg with clavulanate 62.5 mg extended release tablets is licensed for CAP; dose is 2 tablets twice daily 7–10 days	Allergic reaction, hepatotoxicity
Flucloxacillin	500 mg 8-hourly	1 g 6-hourly	Allergic reaction, hepatotoxicity
Mecillinam	200 mg 6- or 8-hourly	400 mg 6- or 8-hourly	Allergic reaction
Ceftibuten	400 mg once daily		
		TETRACYCLINES	
Doxycycline	100 mg 12-hourly day 1 followed by 100 mg once daily	100 mg 12-hourly Neurosyphilis: 200 mg 12-hourly for 28 days	GI upset, bone discolouration, teeth discolouration (children <8 years and tetra>doxy), photosensitivity
Minocycline	Initial loading dose of 200 mg followed by maintenance dose 100 mg 12-hourly		
Tetracycline	250 mg 6-hourly	500 mg 6-hourly	
		MACROLIDES	
Erythromycin	250–500 mg 6-hourly	1 g 6-hourly	Erythromycin infusion associated with thrombophlebitis, Ery+clari strong CYP450 inhibitor, prolonged QT interval ery>clari>azithro, exacerbation myasthenia gravis, infrequently rash. Azithromycin not CYP450 inhibitor. Rate of side effects lowest with azithromycin
Clarithromycin	250 mg 12-hourly	500 mg 12-hourly	
Azithromycin	500 mg once daily	1 g once daily. Gonorrhoea: 2 g once	

(Continued)

Oral Antibiotics	Standard Dose	High Dose	Important Side Effects
		LINCOSAMIDE	
Clindamycin	600 mg 8-hourly or 150–300 mg 4-hourly	900 mg 8-hourly or 450 mg 6-hourly	Diarrhoea, rashes, fever, erythema multiforme, transient hepatitis, neutropaenia, thrombocytopenia, prolonged QT interval
		OXAZOLIDINONE	
Linezolid	600 mg 12-hourly	600 mg 8-hourly may be necessary i.e. when in combination with rifampicin	Myelosuppression after 2–3 weeks, deranged LFTs, peripheral neuropathy, optic neuropathy, in combination with SSRIs: serotonin syndrome, lactic acidosis
Tedizolid	200 mg once daily	–	
		QUINOLONES	
Ciprofloxacin	500 mg 12-hourly	750 mg 12-hourly	Ciprofloxacin lowers seizure threshold. All quinolones: prolonged QT interval, peripheral neuropathy, mild deranged LFTs, Achilles tendinitis/ ruptured tendon, neuromuscular blockade
Levofloxacin	500 mg once daily or 500 mg twice daily	500 mg twice daily	
Moxifloxacin	400 mg once daily	400 mg once daily	
Ofloxacin	200 mg once daily	400 mg twice daily	
Nitrofurantoin	50 mg 6-hourly	100 mg 6-hourly	Allergic reaction, pneumonitis
		OTHER	
Fosfomycin tromethamine suspension	3 g for one dose		Diarrhoea, headache
Fosfomycin calcium monohydrate capsule	500 mg 8-hourly	1 g 8-hourly	
Trimethoprim	200 mg 12-hourly		Trimethoprim: hyperkalaemia, sulfamethoxazole: nephrotoxicity, rash. Other side effects: myelosuppression, rarely Stevens–Johnson syndrome
Trimethoprim/sulfamethoxazole	960 mg 12-hourly	1440 mg 12-hourly for *S. maltophilia*. 12 mg/kg/ day in 2–4 doses for PJP	
Rifampicin (only to be used as part of combination therapy)	450 mg 12-hourly	600 mg 12-hourly	Strong CYP450 inducer
Metronidazole	400–500 mg 8-hourly		Peripheral neuropathy, encephalopathy
Fidaxomicin	200 mg 12-hourly for 10 days		
Fusidic acid (only use as part of combination therapy)	500 mg 8-hourly	1 g 8-hourly	
Chloramphenicol	50 mg/kg 6-hourly OR 1 g 6-hourly. Max dose 4 g/day	For meningococcal meningitis: 2 g 6-hourly	Myelosuppression

Intravenous Antibiotics	Standard Dose	Critically Ill or Invasive Disease	Side Effects
		B-LACTAMS	
Benzylpenicillin	0.6–1.2 g 6-hourly OR 1 million units 6-hourly	1.2–2.4 g 4 hourly OR 2–4 million units 4- or 6-hourly	Allergic reaction, seizures
Amoxicillin	1 g 6- or 8-hourly	2 g 4-hourly for Endocarditis or Brain abscess	Allergic reaction, GI symptoms
Amoxicillin/clavulanic acid	1.2 g 8-hourly	1.2 g 6-hourly. 4-hourly dose may be necessary for Gram-negative infection with increased MIC	Allergic reaction, GI symptoms, hepatotoxicity
Piperacillin/tazobactam	4.5 g 8-hourly	4.5 g 6-hourly OR Continuous infusion. Use local guidance as various in continuous infusion regimens exist. Example 4.5 g loading dose followed by maintenance dose 13.5 g/day	Allergic reaction, drug fever
Ampicillin/sulbactam	3 g 8-hourly	3 g 8-hourly	Allergic reaction
Flucloxacillin	2 g 6-hourly OR 1 g 4-hourly	2 g 4–6-hourly	Allergic reaction, hepatotoxicity
Temocillin	2 g 12-hourly	2 g 8-hourly	Allergic reaction
Cefazolin	500 mg 8-hourly	1 g 4-hourly	Allergic reaction, encephalopathy
Cefuroxime	750 mg 8-hourly	1.5–3 g 8-hourly	
Ceftriaxone	2 g once daily	4 g/day in 1 or 2 doses	
Cefotaxime	1 g 8-hourly	2 g 8-hourly If meningitis: 2 g 4-hourly	
Ceftazidime	1 g 8-hourly	2 g 8-hourly	Allergic reaction, seizures
Ceftazidime/avibactam	2.5 g 8-hourly		
Cefepime	1 g 8-hourly	2 g 8-hourly	
Ceftolozane/tazobactam	1.5 g 8-hourly	2.1 g 8-hourly (HAP & VAP)	
Ceftaroline	600 mg 12-hourly	600 mg 8-hourly (S. aureus MIC > 1 mg/L)	
Ceftobiprole	500 mg 8-hourly		
Ertapenem	1 g daily		Allergic reaction, encephalopathy
Imipenem/cilastatin	500 mg 6-hourly	1 g 6-hourly	Allergic reaction, seizures, encephalopathy
Meropenem	1 g 8-hourly OR 500 mg 6-hourly	2 g 8-hourly OR Continuous infusion 2 g loading dose followed by 4 g/24 hours	Allergic reaction, encephalopathy
		TETRACYCLINES	
Doxycycline	100 mg 12-hourly	Use alternative agent. Otherwise 100 mg 12-hourly	
Eravacycline	1 mg/kg × 2 IV		

(Continued)

Practical Clinical Microbiology and Infectious Diseases

428

Intravenous Antibiotics	Standard Dose	Critically Ill or Invasive Disease	Side Effects
GLYCYLCYCLINE			
Tigecycline	100 mg loading dose followed by 50 mg 12-hourly	200 mg loading dose followed by 100 mg 12-hourly	Prolonged QT interval, mild CYP450 inhibitor. Exacerbation myasthenia gravis
MACROLIDE			
Clarithromycin	500 mg 12-hourly	500 mg 12-hourly	
LINCOSAMIDE			
Clindamycin	600 mg to 900 mg 8-hourly	1.2 g 6-hourly	Diarrhoea, rashes, fever, erythema multiforme, transient hepatitis, neutropaenia, thrombocytopenia, prolonged QT interval
OXAZOLIDINONE			
Linezolid	600 mg 12-hourly. 600 mg 8-hourly may be necessary, i.e. when in combination with rifampicin	600 mg 12-hourly. 600 mg 8-hourly may be necessary, i.e. when in combination with rifampicin	Myelosuppression after 2–3 weeks, deranged LFTs, peripheral neuropathy, optic neuropathy, in combination with SSRIs: serotonin syndrome, lactic acidosis
Tedizolid	200 mg once daily	200 mg once daily	Similar side effects as linezolid, possibly lower frequency
GLYCOPEPTIDE			
Vancomycin	Based on body weight. Different vancomycin nomograms exist, follow own hospital policy but usually loading dose 15–20 mg/kg followed by maintenance dose 15–20 mg/kg 8- to 12-hourly. Aim for pre-dose level 10–15 mg/L	Continuous infusion 30 mg/kg with loading dose 15 mg/kg, aim for pre-dose level 20–25 mg/L. If intermittent dosing, aim for pre-dose level 15–20 mg/L (also indicated if S. aureus MIC ≥1 and ≤4 mg/L)	Red Man syndrome, nephrotoxicity, rash, myelosuppression
Teicoplanin	Three loading doses 6 mg/kg at an 12-hour interval followed by once daily 6 mg/kg	Increase loading dose and maintenance dose to 10–12 mg/kg	Rash, drug fever. Less common than vancomycin: nephrotoxicity, myelosuppression
Dalbavancin	1.5 g for 1 dose, alternatively 1 g on day 1, and 500 mg on day 8	Do not use	
Oritavancin	1.2 g over 3 hours for 1 dose	Do not use	

(Continued)

Intravenous Antibiotics	Standard Dose	Critically Ill or Invasive Disease	Side Effects
DAPTOMYCIN			
Daptomycin	6–8 mg/kg once daily	10–12 mg/kg once daily	Myalgia, muscle weakness with increased CK levels, peripheral neuropathy, eosinophilic pneumonia
QUINOLONES			
Ciprofloxacin	400 mg 12-hourly	400 mg 8-hourly	Lowered seizure threshold Cipro > Levoflox. All quinolones: neuromuscular blockade, prolonged QT interval, peripheral neuropathy, mild deranged LFTs, Achilles tendinitis/ruptured tendon. Hyperglycaemia Cipro > Levoflox
Levofloxacin	500 mg once daily or 500 mg twice daily	500 mg twice daily	
Moxifloxacin	400 mg once daily	400 mg once daily	
AMINOGLYCOSIDES			
Gentamicin	5 mg/kg/day IV	7 mg/kg IV	Ototoxicity, nephrotoxicity, neuromuscular blockade, encephalopathy
Tobramycin	5 mg/kg/day IV	7 mg/kg IV	
Amikacin	15–20 mg/kg/day IV	20–30 mg/kg IV	
POLYMYXINS			
Polymyxin B sulfate	15,000–25,000 units/kg/day OR 0.75–1.25 mg/kg q12 h OR 1.5–2.5 mg/kg/day	30,000 units/kg/day OR 3 mg/kg/day	Nephrotoxicity, neuromuscular blockade, hypokalaemia, hyponatraemia, hypochloraemia and a negative anion gap, paraesthesia
Colistin methanesulfonate (also called colistin or CMS)	Loading dose 9 million units	9 million units per day in 2 or 3 divided doses. Daily dose 12 million units per day may be required in critically ill, but insufficient data exist	
OTHER			
Trimethoprim/sulfamethoxazole	960 mg 12-hourly	1440 mg 12-hourly for *S. maltophilia*. 120 mg/kg/day in 2–4 doses for PJP	
Rifampicin (only to be used as part of combination therapy)	450 mg 12-hourly	600 mg 12-hourly	
Fosfomycin	4 g 8-hourly	8 g 8- to 12-hourly	
Metronidazole	500 mg 8-hourly		
Chloramphenicol	50 mg/kg 6-hourly OR 1 g 6-hourly. Max dose 4 g/day	For meningococcal meningitis: 2 g 6-hourly	Encephalopathy, peripheral neuropathy

Antiviral Agents

	Oral	Intravenous	Side Effects
Aciclovir	800 mg 5 times a day (valacyclovir preferred)	5–10 mg/kg 8-hourly	
Valacyclovir	1000 g 8-hourly		Nephrotoxicity, myelosuppression
Ganciclovir		5 mg/kg 12-hourly	Nephrotoxicity, myelosuppression
Valganciclovir	900 mg 12-hourly		
Foscarnet		60 mg/kg 8-hourly or 90 mg/kg 12-hourly	Nephrotoxicity
Cidofovir (in combination with hyperhydration and oral probenecid		5 mg/kg/week for 2–3 weeks, thereafter at 2-week intervals. Alternatively, 1 mg/kg three times per week	Nephrotoxicity
Ribavirin off license dose for hepatitis E and measles	600 mg 12-hourly		Haemolytic anaemia
Ribavirin for respiratory syncytial virus	Aerosolized 2 g for 1–4 hours 8-hourly by small particle generator	Ribavirin 6 mg/kg 8-hourly	Haemolytic anaemia
Oseltamivir	75 mg 12-hourly		
Zanamivir	Inhalation 10 mg twice daily	Intravenous 600 mg 12-hourly	

Antifungal Agents

	Dose	Side Effects
Fluconazole	100–200 mg once daily. Invasive disease: 800 mg loading dose followed by 400 mg once daily	Azoles inhibit CYP450, fluconazole weaker CP450 inhibitor. Polyneuropathy occurs in 10% of patients receiving triazole therapy for more than 4 months with risk highest in itraconazole > voriconazole > posaconazole. Other side effects are hepatotoxicity (more commonly with voriconazole and posaconazole), encephalopathy (mostly voriconazole) and prolonged QT interval. Isavuconazole has a lower rate of side effects compared to voriconazole compared to voriconazole. Cyclodextrin in infusion fluid voriconazole and itraconazole accumulates in renal impairment and can cause renal obstruction and necrosis. Posaconazole has lower rate of side effects. Voriconazole: visual disturbances + photosensitivity
Voriconazole	Oral 400 mg 12-hourly for 2 doses thereafter 200–300 mg 12-hourly; Intravenous 6 mg/kg 12-hourly for 2 doses thereafter 3–4 mg/kg 12-hourly	
Isavuconazole	Oral and IV loading dose 200 mg 8-hourly for 48 hours (6 doses), thereafter 200 mg once daily	
Itraconazole	Oral and IV 100–200 mg 12-hourly	
Posaconazole	Suspension 400 mg 12-hourly with food, alternatively 200 mg 6-hourly (without food); Tablet and IV loading dose 300 mg 12-hourly thereafter 300 mg once daily	
Caspofungin	70 mg loading dose. Daily maintenance dose: >81 kg: 70 mg, <81 kg 50 mg	Low rate of side effects. Hepatotoxicity and infusion-related reactions have been documented.
Anidulafungin	200 mg 'loading dose', then 100 mg/day	
Micafungin	100 mg/day	
Amphotericin B deoxycholate 'conventional amphotericin B' or Fungizone	0.5–1.5 mg/kg/day	Side effects more common with conventional amphotericin B. Infusion related reaction, nephrotoxicity, hypokalaemia, hypomagnesemia, hepatotoxicity
Liposomal amphotericin B or Ambisome	3 mg/kg. Mucormycosis: 5–10 mg/kg	
Flucytosine	100–200 mg/kg/day in 4 divided doses	Frequency unknown: hepatotoxicity, bone marrow suppression
Terbinafine	250 mg once daily	Erythema, arthralgia, myalgia

BIBLIOGRAPHY

Dodds Ashley ES, Lewis R, Lewis JS, Martin C, Andes D. Pharmacology of systemic antifungal agents. *Clin Infect Dis.* August 2006;43(Issue Supplement 1).

Grayson ML. Kucers' the Use of Antibiotics: A Clinical Review of Antibacterial, Antifungal, Antiparasitic, and Antiviral Drugs. 2018.

Heffernan AJ, Sime FB, Taccone FS, Roberts JA. How to optimize antibiotic pharmacokinetic/ pharmacodynamics for Gram-negative infections in critically ill patients. *Curr Opin Infect Dis.* December 2018;31(6):555–565.

Joint Formulary Committee. *British National Formulary* (online). London: BMJ Group and Pharmaceutical Press <http://www.medicinescomplete.com> [Accessed on 19/11/2019]

Rhodes NJ, Liu J, O'Donnell JN, Dulhunty JM, Abdul-Aziz MH, Berko PY, Nadler B, Lipman J, Roberts JA. Prolonged infusion Piperacillin-Tazobactam decreases mortality and improves outcomes in severely Ill Patients: Results of a systematic review and meta-analysis. *Crit Care Med.* 2018 February;46(2):236–243.

Yu Z, Pang X, Wu X, Shan C, Jiang S. Clinical outcomes of prolonged infusion (extended infusion or continuous infusion) versus intermittent bolus of meropenem in severe infection: A meta-analysis. *PLOS ONE.* 30 July 2018;13(7):e0201667.

6.5 Pathogen-Specific Infection Control Precautions

Firza Alexander Gronthoud

Organism	Disease	Transmission	Incubation Period	Duration of Symptoms	Duration of Shedding	Isolation Precaution	Duration of Isolation
Adenovirus	Pneumonia/ gastroenteritis/ conjunctivitis	Droplets, fecal–oral	5 days (range 1–7 days)			Droplet or strict	Until symptoms resolved
Bordetella (para) pertussis	Whooping cough	Droplets	7–10 days (range 4–28 days)	6 weeks (adults)	After antibiotics, 5–7 days	Droplet	Until at least 5 days of antibiotics
Campylobacter jejuni	Gastroenteritis	Fecal–oral	3 days (range 1–7 days)	1–7 days, fever usually settles after 72 hours	2–7 weeks	Contact	Until symptoms resolved
Clostridioides difficile	Diarrhoea, pseudomembranous colitis, ileus, toxic megacolon	Fecal–oral	Variable	Variable	Intermittent or chronic, 28 days or longer after treatment	Strict	Until symptoms resolved
Novel coronaviruses	SARS-CoV-1 MERS-CoV SARS-CoV-2	Droplets, contact with bodily fluids	2–14 days	SARS-CoV-2: viable virus 7–8 days, RNA may be detectable for 3–4 weeks		Droplet and contact precautions. Airborne precautions during aerosol generating procedures	Until symptoms resolved
Diphtheria	Nasal/pharyngitis/ laryngeal/cutaneous	Droplets, contact	2–5 days (range 1–7 days)		2–4 weeks after infection, chronic carriers shed for >6 months	Cutaneous, contact; pharyngitis, droplet	Until antibiotics finished followed by two negative cultures collected 24 hours apart
E. coli O157:H7	Haemorrhagic gastroenteritis	Vegetables, fecal–oral	3–4 days (range 1–7 days), HUS may appear until 2 weeks after GI symptoms	4 days (range 2–9 days)	2–62 days	Strict	Until symptoms resolved

(Continued)

Organism	Disease	Transmission	Incubation Period	Duration of Symptoms	Duration of Shedding	Isolation Precaution	Duration of Isolation
Giardia lamblia	Gastroenteritis	Fecal oral	≥1 week	Acute giardiasis, 7–10 day but may be complicated by chronic infection with recurring symptoms	Intermittent	Standard precautions	
Hepatitis A	Hepatitis	Fecal oral	28 days (range 2–7 weeks)	Acute illness 1–2 weeks, full recovery 2 months, 10%–15% recovered by month 6	1 week before fever/icterus to 1 week after	Standard precautions	
Hepatitis B	Hepatitis	Bloodborne and sexually transmitted	3 months (range 2–5 months)	Acute HBV, 3 months	6 weeks before start symptoms until seroconversion to anti-Hbs	Standard precautions	
Hepatitis C	Hepatitis	Bloodborne	7 weeks (2–26 weeks)	85% or more do not clear infection; symptoms of HCV infection are non-specific	As long as HCV-RNA is detectable	Standard precautions	
Hepatitis E	Hepatitis	Fecal–oral, blood transfusion	40 days (range 2–8 weeks)	Acute/Chronic	One week prior to onset of symptoms until 30 days after jaundice	Standard precautions	
Herpes simplex 1	Vesicles	HSV 1, oral–oral, oral–genital, or genital–genital contact	2–12 days	12 days (range 7–18 days)	During primary infection, asymptomatic shedding occurs throughout life	Standard precautions	

(Continued)

Organism	Disease	Transmission	Incubation Period	Duration of Symptoms	Duration of Shedding	Isolation Precaution	Duration of Isolation
Herpes simplex 2	Vesicles, blisters	Sexual contact	4 days (range 2–12 days)	2–4 weeks	During primary infection, asymptomatic shedding occurs throughout life	Standard precautions	
Human immunodeficiency virus	Immunodeficiency with wide range of manifestations	Blood borne and sexual transmission	2–4 weeks; period until seroconversion, 2–6 weeks (range, 2 weeks to 6 months)	Acute HIV, 2–4 weeks	Lifelong	Standard precautions	
Influenza	Mild symptoms to respiratory failure	Droplets, contact	1–4 days (influenza B 1–2 days)	5–7 days	5–7 days	Droplet precautions. Airborne precautions during aerosol generating procedures	Until symptoms resolved
Legionella pneumophila	Pontiac fever and Legionnaire's disease/atypical pneumonia	inhalation of aerosols derived from water or soil	Pontiac fever, 4 hours to 3 days (median 32–36 hours); Legionnaire's disease, 1–14 days (median 4 days)	Pontiac fever, a week; Legionnaire's disease, longer than a week not uncommon	No human to human transmission 14 weeks or longer (urine antigen)	Standard precautions	
Listeria monocytogenes	Gastroenteritis, bacteraemia, meningoencephalitis	Fecal oral	8 days (range 1–67 days)	Gastroenteritis, 2 days	Until 7 days after giving birth detectable in urine and vaginal secretion	Gastroenteritis, strict precautions; if no gastroenteritis, standard precautions	If gastroenteritis, until resolution of symptoms
Measles	Measles	Aerosols	10–12 days, up to 21 days	10 days	4 days before the rash until 4 days after the rash	Airborne	4 days before the rash until 4 days after the rash

(Continued)

Organism	Disease	Transmission	Incubation Period	Duration of Symptoms	Duration of Shedding	Isolation Precaution	Duration of Isolation
MRSA	Cellulitis, pneumonia, bacteraemia, endocarditis, bone + joint	Contact	Variable	Depends on colonization site and symptoms	During period of colonization	Strict precautions	Until three negative MRSA screens whilst antibiotic free
Mycoplasma pneumoniae	Self-limiting resp. illness, atypical pneumonia, extrapulmonary manifestations	Droplets but requires prolonged contact	2–3 weeks	Few days to more than a month	After acute infection, asymptomatic carriage can persist weeks to months, median duration 7 weeks	Standard precautions	
Mycobacterium tuberculosis	Pulmonary tuberculosis, extrapulmonary tuberculosis, latent TB	Pulmonary TB Airborne Extrapulmonary TB only if in direct contact with infected body site Latent TB not transmissible	8 weeks to lifelong	Latent TB asymptomatic (Extra)Pulmonary TB chronic infections	Infectious only if pulmonary tuberculosis	Pulmonary TB, airborne Extrapulmonary TB, standard precautions	Until at least 2 weeks of treatment and 2 negative sputum samples
Neisseria meningitidis	Meningitis, invasive disease, pneumonia (uncommon)	Droplets through coughing, sneezing, talking, kissing, mouth-to-mouth resuscitation	3–4 days (range 2 to 10 days)	Rarely may initial infection lead to chronic meningococcaemia (lasting >1 week), without meningitis	7 days before onset symptoms until 24 hours after antibiotics, asymptomatic carriage few days to 2 years	Droplet	Until 24 hours after antibiotics

(Continued)

Organism	Disease	Transmission	Incubation Period	Duration of Symptoms	Duration of Shedding	Isolation Precaution	Duration of Isolation
Norovirus	Diarrhoea, vomiting	Fecal–oral. If projectile vomiting, then also aerosolized respiratory droplets	1–2 days	3 days	2–3 weeks, may be prolonged in immunocompromised	Contact	Until symptoms resolved
Parainfluenza	Croup, bronchiolitis, bronchitis, pneumonia. Parainfluenza type 3 potentially severe ARDS in immunocompromised	Droplets, contact	2–4 days (range 2–7 days)	Depends on respiratory illness, i.e. croup, bronchitis or pneumonia	4 days (but may be 2–3 weeks. Bone marrow Tx recipients can shed for months)	Droplet, contact	Until symptoms resolved
Rhinovirus	Common cold	Droplets, contact	2 days (range 1–7 days)	1–2 weeks	10–14 days, elderly and immunosuppressed may shed for >28 days	Standard precautions	
Rotavirus	Gastroenteritis, may be complicated by ARDS in immunocompromised	Fecal–oral	2–4 days	3–8 days	3 weeks or longer	Strict precautions	Until symptoms resolved
Respiratory syncytial virus	Mild illness to bronchiolitis to ARDS	Droplets, contact	5 days (range 2–7 days)		5–7 days; children <2 years, 3–4 weeks	Droplet, contact	Until symptoms resolved
Salmonella spp.	Gastroenteritis	Fecal–oral route	6–48 hours	2–7 days	3 weeks to more than 1 year	Strict precautions	Until symptoms resolved

(Continued)

Organism	Disease	Transmission	Incubation Period	Duration of Symptoms	Duration of Shedding	Isolation Precaution	Duration of Isolation
Salmonella Typhi or Paratyphi A	Enteric fever	Fecal–oral route	7–14 days (range, 3–60 days)	3 weeks to months	5 weeks, small proportion become a chronic carrier	Standard precautions strict precautions if diarrhoea/fecal incontinent/diapers/age <6 years	
Sarcoptes scabiei (*Scabies*)	Scabies, crusted scabies in immunocompromised	Direct and prolonged skin to skin contact	3–6 weeks (1–4 days if previous infection)	Until treatment	1–2 weeks after infection until 24 hours after effective treatment	Strict precautions	Until 24 hours of therapy
Shigella spp.	Gastroenteritis	Fecal–oral route	24–72 hours (range 1–7 days)	7 days	Up to 6 weeks after resolution of symptoms	Strict precautions	Until symptoms resolved
Simian B virus	Encephalomyelitis	Direct contact through saliva from macaques	2 days to 5 weeks, usually 5–21 days			Standard precautions	
Streptococcus pyogenes	Pharyngitis, pneumonia, invasive disease, open skin lesions/draining wounds/burns	Aerosolized respiratory droplets and contact	2–5 days	2–5 days	3–4 weeks	Droplet	Until 24 hours after antibiotics
Streptococcus pneumoniae	Pneumonia, invasive disease	Contact	24–72 hours			Standard precautions, contact precautions if penicillin resistant	
Varicella zoster	Chickenpox	Airborne, contact	10–21 days (usually 13–18 days)	Initial febrile illness, 2–3 days Vesicles, 5–7 days	Two days before symptoms until lesions dried in	Airborne + contact	Until lesions dried in

(Continued)

Organism	Disease	Transmission	Incubation Period	Duration of Symptoms	Duration of Shedding	Isolation Precaution	Duration of Isolation
Varicella zoster	Herpes zoster	Localized zoster, contact Disseminated or respiratory involvement, airborne + contact	Reactivation during periods of stress or lowered immune system	Vesicles following dermatomal distribution	Until lesions dried in	Localized, contact; if respiratory involvement or disseminated, airborne + contact	Until lesions dried in
Vibrio cholerae	Gastroenteritis	Fecal-oral route	2–3 days		Until several days after resolution of symptoms	Contact precautions	Until symptoms resolved
Vibrio parahaemolyticus	Gastroenteritis	Fecal-oral route	5–72 hours	3 days (range 8 hours to 12 days)		Contact precautions	Until symptoms resolved

Notes: Incubation period for *Listeria* depends on clinical manifestation: Overall incubation invasive listeriosis: 8 days (range: 1–67 days), pregnancy-associated cases (median: 27.5 days; range: 17–67 days), CNS cases (median: 9 days; range: 1–14 days), bacteraemia cases (median:2 days; range: 1–12 days). Gastroenteritis: The median incubation period was 24 hours with variation from 6 to 240 hours.

For enteropathogens normally isolated in standard precautions, consider strict precautions if in diapers or incontinent.

In general: Immunocompromised individuals may have a prolonged period of infectiousness and requiring extended duration of isolation.

Neisseria meningitis infection: Transmission: prolonged (>8 hours) contact while in close proximity (<3 feet) to the patient or who have been directly exposed to the patient's oral secretions during the 7 days before the onset of the patient's symptoms and until 24 hours after initiation of appropriate antibiotic therapy. Carriage: Infection leads in most cases to asymptomatic carriage. On the other hand, people can become asymptomatic carriers without preceding infection. Regardless of this, duration of asymptomatic carriage few days to 2 years but on average is 9 months.

BIBLIOGRAPHY

Drevets DA, Bronze MS. Listeria monocytogenes: Epidemiology, human disease, and mechanisms of brain invasion. *FEMS Immunol Med Microbiol.* July 2008;53(2):151–65.

Goulet V, King LA, Vaillant V, de Valk H. What is the incubation period for listeriosis?. *BMC Infect Dis.* 2013;13:11.

https://www.sahealth.sa.gov.au/wps/wcm/connect/Public+Content/SA+Health+Internet/Health+topics/Health+conditions+prevention+and+treatment/Infectious+diseases/

https://lci.rivm.nl/richtlijnen

https://www.canada.ca/en/public-health/services/infectious-diseases.html

https://www.cdc.gov/infectioncontrol/guidelines/index.html

https://www.cdc.gov/DiseasesConditions/

Kramer A, Schwebke I, Kampf G. How long do nosocomial pathogens persist on inanimate surfaces? A systematic review. *BMC Infect Dis.* 16 August 2006;6:130.

Lee RM, Lessler J, Lee RA, Rudolph KE, Reich NG, Perl TM, Cummings DA. Incubation periods of viral gastroenteritis: A systematic review. *BMC Infect Dis.* 25 September 2013;13:446.

Lessler J, Reich NG, Brookmeyer R, Perl TM, Nelson KE, Cummings DA. Incubation periods of acute respiratory viral infections: A systematic review. *Lancet Infect Dis.* May 2009;9(5):291–300.

Mukhopadhya I, Sarkar R, Menon VK et al. Rotavirus shedding in symptomatic and asymptomatic children using reverse transcription-quantitative PCR. *J Med Virol.* September 2013;85(9):1661–1668.

Olson ME, Goh J, Phillips M, Guselle N, McAllister TA. *Giardia* cyst and *Cryptosporidium* oocyst survival in water, soil, and cattle feces. *External J Environ Qual.* 1999;28(6):1991–1996.

Prabhu S, Harwell JI, Kumarasamy N. Advanced HIV: Diagnosis, treatment, and prevention. *Lancet HIV.* August 2019;6(8):e540–e551.

Sewnarine M, Kohn N, Tong S, Rubin L. Duration of parainfluenza virus detection in nasopharyngeal Swabs using a polymerase chain reaction-based detection. *Open Forum Infectious Diseases.* December 2015;2 (Issue suppl_1):516.

Zlateva KT, de Vries JJ, Coenjaerts FE, van Loon AM, Verheij T, Little P, Butler CC, Goossens H, Ieven M, Claas EC, GRACE Study Group. Prolonged shedding of rhinovirus and re-infection in adults with respiratory tract illness. *Eur Respir J.* July 2014;44(1):169–77.

6.6 Pillars of Infection Control

Firza Alexander Gronthoud

	PILLAR 1 Prevention of Transmission	PILLAR 2 Source Control	PILLAR 3 Decontamination	PILLAR 4 Antimicrobial Stewardship	PILLAR 5 Diagnostic Stewardship
Targets	Healthcare Workers + Patient	Patient	Environment	Patients + Healthcare Workers	Patients

Methods	Hand hygiene & PPE
	• Standard precautions
	• Transmission-based precautions
	  • Droplet
	  • Airborne
	  • Strict/Enhanced
		Isolation
		• Spacing between beds
		• Single rooms with en suite facilities
		• Cohorting
		• Transport
		Protective isolation
			Cleaning
			• Disinfecting & sterilization
			• Scopes
			• Sharps needles
			• Equipment
			• Waste/linen
			• Food handling
			• Environment
				Rational use of antibiotics
				Vaccination
				Prophylaxis pre- and post-exposure
				MRSA decolonization
					Targeted admission screens
					• Screening for MRSA, CPO, VRE, multidrug-resistant Gram-negative rods, SARS-CoV-2
					Rapid and accurate diagnosis of infections with early isolation or de-isolation

Pillar 2 Isolation is in normal pressure for contact or droplet precautions. Airborne transmission requires negative pressure with anteroom.

Pillar 5 Consider screening healthcare workers if, during their current employment, they have done a rotation in other healthcare settings with high prevalence of tuberculosis or multidrug-resistant organisms.

BIBLIOGRAPHY

Loveday HP, Wilson JA, Pratt RJ, Golsorkhi M, Tingle A, Bak A, Browne J, Prieto J, Wilcox M, UK Department of Health. epic3 national evidence-based guidelines for preventing healthcare-associated infections in NHS hospitals. *J Hosp Infect.* January 2014;86(Suppl 1):S1–S70.

Siegel JD, Rhinehart E, Jackson M, Chiarello L, and the Healthcare Infection Control Practices Advisory Committee. Guideline for Isolation Precautions: Preventing Transmission of Infectious Agents in Healthcare Settings, 2007.

6.7 Transmission-Based Precautions

Firza Alexander Gronthoud

Transmission-based precautions are in addition to standard precautions when use of standard precautions alone does not effectively prevent transmission of disease. There are three main categories of transmission-based precautions: (1) contact, (2) droplet and (3) airborne. Strict/enhanced precaution is a hybrid used for difficult-to-treat organisms such as CPOs. The category used depends on the mode of transmission of a specific disease. Some diseases require more than one type of transmission-based precaution. The proven most effective ways of infection control are hand hygiene and antimicrobial stewardship. Environmental decontamination is equally important to prevent spread. To illustrate this: for single room occupants, the risk of becoming a carrier with a drug-resistant organism is significantly increased if the previous occupant was colonized with a drug resistant organism.

Based on current data and guidelines, it is unclear how effective contact precaution and strict precaution/enhanced precaution are in preventing transmission and infection from ESB/de-repressed AmpC, VRE and MRSA. It is therefore recommended to adhere to local hospital guidance.

Precautions	Indication/Examples	Personal Protective Equipment	Single Room
Standard precautions	Standard precautions apply for all work practices to prevent the likelihood of transmission of infection.	Gloves, gowns/apron during procedures and/or patientcare where exposure to bodily fluids is likely to occur. Wear eye protection or face mask if splashes to the eye may occur.	No
Contact precautions	ESBL/de-repressed AmpC, multidrug-resistant Gram-negative rods, scabies.	In addition to standard precautions, wear gloves + gowns (or apron depending on own local hospital policy) for all patient contact. Surgical mask may be considered if in sputum.	No
Droplet precautions	*Neisseria meningitidis*, rubella, pertussis, respiratory viruses	In addition to standard precautions wear a surgical mask when within 2 metres distance + consider eye protection.	Normal pressure
Airborne precautions	*Mycobacterium tuberculosis*, measles, varicella zoster and during aerosol generating procedures in patients who potentially are infected with organisms that can spread through the respiratory route.	In addition to standard precautions, wear a N95 or FFP2/FFP3.	Negative Pressure with anteroom, 6–12 air changes per hour
Strict precautions/ Enhanced precautions	MRSA, carbapenemase-producing organisms, multidrug-resistant *Pseudomonas aeruginosa*, multidrug-resistant *Acinetobacter baumannii*, infective diarrhoea (i.e. *C. difficile*, norovirus).	Contact precautions in a single room. Surgical mask may be considered if in sputum or severe vomiting whereby aerosolized respiratory droplets are formed.	Normal pressure single room

BIBLIOGRAPHY

European Centre for Disease Prevention and Control. *Systematic Review of the Effectiveness of Infection Control Measures to Prevent the Transmission of Extended-Spectrum Beta-Lactamase-Producing Enterobacteriaceae Through Cross-Border Transfer of Patients.* Stockholm: ECDC, 2014.

Loveday HP, Wilson JA, Pratt RJ, Golsorkhi M, Tingle A, Bak A, Browne J, Prieto J, Wilcox M, UK Department of Health. epic3 national evidence-based guidelines for preventing healthcare-associated infections in NHS hospitals. *J Hosp Infect.* January 2014;86(Suppl 1):S1–S70.

Siegel JD, Rhinehart E, Jackson M, Chiarello L, and the Healthcare Infection Control Practices Advisory Committee. Guideline for Isolation Precautions: Preventing Transmission of Infectious Agents in Healthcare Settings, 2007.

Index

Printed in the United States
by Baker & Taylor Publisher Services

Printed in the United States
By Bookmasters